Third Edition

© by LEA & FEBIGER, 1957

Reprinted August, 1958
Reprinted August, 1960

First Edition, 1945

Reprinted March, 1946
Reprinted September, 1946
Reprinted January, 1947
Reprinted November, 1947
Reprinted June, 1949

Second Edition, 1952

Reprinted November, 1953
Reprinted September, 1955

Library of Congress Card Catalog Number: 57–12169

Printed in the United States of America

PHARMACEUTICA
CALCULATIONS

BY

WILLIS T. BRADLEY, A.B., A.M.
CARROLL B. GUSTAFSON, Ph.C., B.S., A.M.

AND

MITCHELL J. STOKLOSA, Ph.C., B.S., A.M.

OF THE FACULTY OF
THE MASSACHUSETTS COLLEGE OF PHARMACY
BOSTON, MASSACHUSETTS

Third Edition

LEA & FEBIGER
PHILADELPHIA

PREFACE TO THE THIRD EDITION

THE many satisfied teachers who have been using the Second Edition of this book will discover that the present revision introduces no radical changes.

The text has been carefully made to conform with the usage of the current revision of the *United States Pharmacopeia*.

An effort has been made here and there to clarify the exposition. Some problems have been revised, and many new ones, reflecting contemporary practice, have been added.

Almost every problem presented represents actual pharmaceutical experience, constantly suggesting the atmosphere of the laboratory or dispensing room. The student will calculate only with quantities that he will later deal with in his professional work, and stress is put upon the importance of his keeping track of significant figures and allowable percentage of error when he uses numbers representing measurement of weight or volume. Every drug and chemical referred to is familiar in present-day practice; and the only units of measure included are those that the pharmacist meets: the tables of measure have been pruned of all non-pharmaceutical denominations.

In short, this book is concerned exclusively with the arithmetic of today's *applied* pharmacy.

The material in Chapter I, some of it very elementary, is meant to be a check of certain arithmetic fundamentals with which the student should be thoroughly acquainted at the outset. The main body of the text thereafter shows a logical development; but the self-explanatory character of every section and the calculation of examples of every type of problem in full should permit any arrangement that suits the requirements of a particular course of study. The miscellaneous topics in the Appendix may be taken up in any order according to the discretion of the instructor or the needs of the individual. The problems at the end of the book are available for review and test purposes, and they may be used as a sort of "refresher" course.

Theoretical discussion, although cut to a minimum, is included whenever it seems to contribute to an understanding of a problem and its solution. However, the aim has been to teach by practice rather than by precept: sample problems set the pattern, and practice problems at the end of each chapter or section, half of them with answers for the purpose of checking, give the student an opportunity to master the form.

Most arithmetic problems can be solved in several ways. Occasionally alternate methods are suggested; but in general the methods recommended are those that have given the best results in the classroom. In the matter of theoretical discussion and choice of method, the authors will welcome correspondence with all teachers and students who have questions or suggestions.

W. T. B.

C. B. G.

M. J. S.

Boston, Massachusetts

CONTENTS

(5)

CHAPTER V

CHAPTER VI

CHAPTER VII

CHAPTER VIII

CHAPTER IX

CHAPTER X

CHAPTER XI

CHAPTER XII

CHAPTER XIII

8 CONTENTS

APPENDIX

CHAPTER I

SOME FUNDAMENTALS OF MEASUREMENT AND CALCULATION

NUMBERS AND NUMERALS

A *number* is a total quantity, or amount, of units. A *numeral* is a word or sign, or a group of words or signs, expressing a number.

For example, *3, 6,* and *48* are arabic numerals expressing numbers that are respectively *three times, six times,* and *forty-eight times* the unit *1.*

KINDS OF NUMBERS

In *arithmetic,* which is the science of calculating with positive, real numbers, a number will usually be (a) a natural or *whole* number, or *integer,* such as *549;* (b) a *fraction,* or subdivision of a whole number, such as $\frac{4}{7}$; or (c) a *mixed* number, consisting of a whole number plus a fraction, such as $3\frac{7}{8}$.

A number such as *4, 8,* or *12,* taken by itself, without application to anything concrete, is called an *abstract* or *pure* number. It merely designates how many times the unit *1* is contained in it, without implying that anything else is being counted or measured. An abstract number may be added to, subtracted from, multiplied by, or divided by any other abstract number. The result of any of these operations is always an abstract number designating a new total of units.

But a number that designates a quantity of objects or units of measure, such as *4 grams, 8 ounces, 12 grains,* is called a *concrete* or *denominate* number. It designates the total quantity of whatever has been measured. A denominate number may be added to or subtracted from any other number of the same denomination; but a denominate number may be multiplied or divided only by a pure number. The result of any of these operations is always a number of the same denomination.

Examples:

>   *10 grams + 5 grams = 15 grams*
>   *10 grams − 5 grams = 5 grams*
>   *300 grains × 2 = 600 grains*
>   *12 ounces ÷ 3 = 4 ounces*

If any one rule of arithmetic may take first place in importance, this is it: *Numbers of different denominations have no direct numerical connection with each other and cannot be used together in any arithmetical operation.* We shall see again and again that if quantities are to be added, or if one quantity is to be subtracted from another, they must be expressed in the same denomination. And when we apparently multiply or divide a denominate number by a number of different denomination, we are in fact using the multiplier or divisor as an abstract number. If, for example, *1 ounce* costs *5 cents* and we want to find the cost of *12 ounces*, we do not multiply *5 cents* by *12 ounces*, but by the abstract number *12*.

ARABIC NUMERALS

Our so-called "arabic" system of notation is properly called a *decimal* system. With only ten figures—a *zero* and nine *digits*—any number may be expressed by an ingenious system in which different values are assigned to the digits according to the *place* they occupy in a row. The central place in the row is usually identified by a sign placed to its right called the *decimal point.* Any digit occupying this place expresses its own value—in other words, a certain number of *ones;* but the former value of a digit is increased tenfold each time it moves one place to the left; and, conversely, its value is one-tenth of its preceding value each time it moves one place to the right.

Zero serves to mark a place not occupied by one of the digits.

Scheme of the decimal system:

Etc. ← millions, hundred thousands, ten thousands, thousands, hundreds, tens, ones . tenths, hundredths, thousandths, ten-thousandths, hundred-thousandths, millionths → Etc.

In this scheme, any digit occupying the central place expresses that number of *ones*, but in the first place to the left of center it expresses that number of *tens*, in the second place to the left, that number of *hundreds*, and so on. And in the first place to the right of center it expresses that number of *tenths*, and so on.

The total value of any number expressed in the arabic system, then, is the sum of the values of its digits as determined by their position.

Example:

3,085.673	means:	
3,000.000	or	3 thousands
+ 000.000		plus 0 hundreds
+ 80.000		plus 8 tens
+ 5.000		plus 5 ones
+ .600		plus 6 tenths
+ .070		plus 7 hundredths
+ .003		plus 3 thousandths

The universal use of this system has resulted from the ease—as compared with the difficulties encountered in the other ancient systems of notation—with which it may be adapted to the various purposes of arithmetical calculations.

ROMAN NUMERALS

Roman numerals can merely record quantities: they are of no use in computation. They customarily designate quantities on prescriptions when ingredients are measured by the common or apothecaries' systems.

To express quantities in the roman system, these eight letters of fixed values are used:[1]

ss = $\frac{1}{2}$	V or v = 5	L or l = 50	D or d = 500
I or i = 1	X or x = 10	C or c = 100	M or m = 1000

Other quantities are expressed by combining these letters by the general rule that when the second of two letters has a value equal to or smaller than that of the first, their values are to be added; but when the second has a value greater than that of the first, the smaller is to be subtracted from the larger. This rule may be illustrated as follows:

(1) Two or more letters express a quantity that is the *sum* of their values *if they are successively equal or smaller in value:*

ii = 2	xx = 20	ci = 101	dc = 600
iii = 3	xxii = 22	cv = 105	mi = 1001
vi = 6	xxxiii = 33	cx = 110	mv = 1005
vii = 7	li = 51	cl = 150	mx = 1010
viii = 8	lv = 55	cc = 200	ml = 1050
xi = 11	lx = 60	di = 501	mc = 1100
xii = 12	lxvi = 66	dv = 505	md = 1500
xiii = 13	lxxvii = 77	dx = 510	mdclxvi = 1666
xv = 15	lxxxviii = 88	dl = 550	mm = 2000

[1] Physicians tend to use capitals except for the letter *i*, which they dot for the sake of clarity; and many use *j* for a final *i*. Following the Latin custom, they put the symbol for the denomination first and the roman numeral second.

(2) Two or more letters express a quantity that is the *sum* of the values remaining *after the value of each smaller letter has been subtracted from that of a following greater:*

iv = 4	xxxix = 39	xcix = 99	cdxc = 490
ix = 9	xl = 40	cd = 400	cm = 900
xiv = 14	xli = 41	cdi = 401	cmxcix = 999
xix = 19	xliv = 44	cdxl = 440	mcdxcii = 1492
xxiv = 24	xc = 90	cdxliv = 444	mcmlvii = 1957

Practice Problems

1. Write the following in roman numerals:

   (*a*) 18.   (*d*) 126.
   (*b*) 64.   (*e*) 99.
   (*c*) 72.   (*f*) 37.

2. Interpret the *quantity* in each of these phrases taken from prescriptions:

   (*a*) Caps. no. xlv.
   (*b*) Gtts. M.
   (*c*) Tabs. no. xlviii.
   (*d*) Pil. no. lxiv.
   (*e*) Pulv. no. xvi.
   (*f*) Caps. no. lxxxiv.

3. Interpret the *quantities* in each of these prescriptions:

   (a) ℞ Zinc Oxide   part. v
          Wool Fat   part. xv
          Petrolatum   part. lxxx
          Disp. ℥ iv
          Sig. Apply.
   (b) ℞ Dilaudid   gr. iss
          Ammonium Chloride gr. xl
          Syrup ad   ℥ vi
          Sig. ℥ ss pro tuss.

SIGNIFICANT FIGURES

When we *count* objects accurately, *every* figure in the numeral expressing the total number of objects must be taken at its face value. Such figures may be said to be *absolute.*

But when we record a *measurement*, the last figure to the right must be taken to be an *approximation*, an admission that the limit of possible precision or of necessary accuracy has been reached, and that any further figures to the right would be non-significant—that is, either meaningless or, for a given purpose, needless.

Recognition of this truth is of fairly recent origin. You will find no discussion of significant figures in the old arithmetic texts— and in few recent ones. We are familiar, of course, with phrases like "roughly a yard" and "about a pint" and "a little over a pound"; but most of us find it difficult to grasp the fact that *every* measurement, no matter how precisely made, is only an approximation. Failure to grasp this fact has two unfortunate consequences: it encourages us (1) to retain too many figures in our calculations and thus waste time and run greater risk of careless error and (2) to record results that are invalid.

We should learn to interpret a denominate number like *325 grams* as follows: The *3* means *300 grams*, neither more nor less, and the *2* means *exactly 20 grams more;* but the final *5* means *approximately 5 grams more*—that is, *5 grams plus or minus some fraction of a gram.* Whether this fraction is, for a given purpose, negligible depends upon how precisely the quantity was (or is to be) weighed.

Significant figures, then, are consecutive figures that express the value of a denominate number accurately enough for a given purpose. The accuracy varies with the number of significant figures, which are all absolute in value except the last—and this is properly called *uncertain.*

Two-figure accuracy is liable to a deviation as high as 5% from the theoretic absolute measurement. For example, if a substance is reported to weigh *10 grams* to the nearest *gram*, its actual weight may be anything between *9.5 grams* and *10.5 grams.*

Three-figure accuracy is liable to a deviation as high as 0.5%; four-figure accuracy may deviate 0.05%; and five-figure accuracy, 0.005%.

In scientific work, three-figure or four-figure accuracy is a commonplace; but laymen are often surprised to hear that five-figure, six-figure, and higher degrees of accuracy are rare and are valid only if we have exercised the greatest skill in measuring with the finest instruments.

Any of the digits in a valid denominate number must be regarded as significant. Whether *zero* is significant, however, depends upon its position or upon known facts about a given number. The interpretation of *zero* may be summed up as follows:

Rule 1. Any zero between digits is significant.

Rule 2. Initial zeros to the left of the first digit are never significant: they are included merely to show the location of the decimal point and thus give place value to the digits that follow.

Rule 3. One or more final zeros to the right of the decimal point may be taken to be significant.

Rule 4. One or more final zeros in a whole number—that is, immediately to the left of the decimal point—sometimes merely serve to give place value to digits to the left, but they should be considered significant unless shown by the data to be non-significant.

Examples:

Assuming that the following numbers are all denominate—

(1) In *12.5* there are *three* significant figures; in *1.256, four* significant figures; and in *102.56, five* significant figures.

(2) In *0.5* there is *one* significant figure. The digit *5* tells us how many *tenths* we have. The non-significant *0* simply calls attention to the decimal point.

(3) In *0.05* there is still only *one* significant figure, and again in *0.005*.

(4) In *0.65* there are *two* significant figures, and likewise *two* in *0.065* and *0.0065*.

(5) In *0.0605* there are *three* significant figures. The first *0* calls attention to the decimal point; the second *0* shows the number of places to the right of the decimal point occupied by the remaining figures; and the third *0* significantly contributes to the value of the number. In *0.06050* there are *four* significant figures, since the final *0* also contributes to the value of the number.

(6) In *20000* there are *five* significant figures; but *20000* ± 50 (or, to express the same quantity another way, *20000 to the nearest 100*) contains only *three* significant figures.

It should go without saying that the ability to make proper and accurate measurements constitutes an essential qualification of a competent pharmacist; but his zeal for accuracy should not blind him to the truth that there is always bound to be a maximum degree beyond which he cannot go—and need not if he could. As already pointed out, one of the factors determining the degree of approximation to perfect measurement is the precision of the instrument used. It would be absurd for a pharmacist to pretend that he had measured *7.76 milliliters* in a graduate calibrated in units of *1 milliliter;* or that he had weighed *25.562 grains* on a balance sensitive to $\frac{1}{10}$ grain.

Other Examples:

(1) If a substance weighs *0.06 gram* according to a balance sensitive to *0.001 gram,* we may record the weight as *0.060 gram.* But if the balance is sensitive only to *0.01 gram,* the value should be recorded as *0.06 gram,* and a record of *0.060 gram* would be invalid.

(2) Again, when recording a length of *10 millimeters* found by use of an instrument accurate to *0.1 millimeter,* the value may be recorded as *10.0* millimeters.

(3) And again, if a volume of *5 milliliters* is measured with an instrument calibrated in *10ths of a milliliter,* the volume may be recorded as *5.0 milliliters.*

We must clearly distinguish *significant figures* from *decimal places.* When recording a measurement, the number of decimal places we include indicates *the degree of precision with which the measurement has been made,* whereas the number of significant figures retained indicates *the degree of accuracy* that is sufficient for a given purpose.

Sometimes we are asked to record a value "correct to (so-many) decimal places"; and we should never confuse this familiar expression with the expression "correct to (so-many) significant figures."

Examples:

(1) If the value of *27.625918* is rounded off to *five decimal places,* it is written *27.62592;* but when rounded off to *five significant figures* it is written *27.626.*

(2) The value *54.326,* when rounded off to *54.3,* is precise to *one decimal place* but accurate to *three significant figures.*

Now, when we *calculate* with denominate—that is, with approximate—numbers, it is very easy to get results that are invalid *because they pretend to a greater accuracy or precision than is supplied in the data.*

To emphasize and clarify this often-ignored point, every uncertain figure included in the following discussion is identified by a slanting line indicating that its value is not absolute.

Invalid results are commonly met with in division. Forgetting that the *last* figure in a denominate number is always *uncertain,* we add a succession of zeros to the dividend and drive our quotient into the meaningless darkness of *too many decimal places,* perhaps in the hope that it will "come out even." (By definition, a denominate quotient is *never* "even" in the absolute sense: if you divide approximately *8* fluidounces by 2, no matter how close the approximation is, you get approximately *4* fluidounces!)

Example:

> *Divide 3.9I grains by 8.*
>
>   8)3.9I000
>   ‾‾‾‾‾‾‾‾‾‾
>   0.48875 grain, *invalid answer.*

Since the I of 3.9I *grains* is uncertain, when we divide the next figure beyond it by 8 the quotient will be uncertain, and it is sheer waste of time to proceed any farther than one more place in order to get a rough approximation to guide us in rounding off the result to 0.489 *grain,* with only one uncertain figure.

It is equally tempting, and equally foolish, to retain meaningless figures in the product of multiplication.

Example:

> *Multiply 0.00563 grain by 7.*
>
>   0.00563
>   ×   7
>   ‾‾‾‾‾‾‾‾‾‾
>   2I
>   42
>   35
>   ‾‾‾‾‾‾‾‾‾‾
>   0.03941 grain, *invalid answer.*

Since the 3 of 0.00563 *grain* is uncertain, the product of 7 × 3 will be 2I. The final product should be rounded off to 0.0394 *grain,* again with only one uncertain figure.

The *principle* that *the result of any calculation involving an approximate number should be rounded off so as to contain only one uncertain figure* holds as well for sums and differences as for quotients and products.

With this principle in mind, we can get valid results, and save a good deal of time, by obeying the following rules for (a) recording measurements, (b) calculating with approximate numbers, and (c) recording the results of such calculations.

> *Rule 1. When recording a measurement, retain as many figures as will give only one uncertain figure.*

The uncertain figure will sometimes represent an estimate between graduations on a scale. Thus, if you use a ruler calibrated in centimeters, you might record a measurement as approximately 11.3 *centimeters,* but not as approximately 11.32 *centimeters.* Since the 3 is uncertain, no other figure should follow it.

> *Rule 2. When rejecting superfluous figures in the result of a calculation, add 1 to the last figure retained if the following figure is 5 or more.*

Thus, 2.4$\cancel{3}$ may be rounded off to 2.$\cancel{4}$, but 2.4$\cancel{6}$ should be rounded off to 2.$\cancel{5}$. Note that if a number like 2.5$\cancel{9}$7 is rounded off to three significant figures, the 1 added to the $\cancel{9}$ makes 1$\emptyset$, and the $\emptyset$ should be recorded for it is significant: 2.6$\emptyset$.

> *Rule 3.* Since you cannot increase the precision of the *least* precise number, therefore *before adding or subtracting approximate numbers, you may save time by rounding off each component so that it will contain one more decimal place than is contained in the component having the fewest decimal places. The result should always be rounded off to the same number of decimal places as are contained in that component.*

Example:
> *Add these approximate weights:* 162.$\cancel{5}$ *grams,* 0.56$\cancel{9}$ *gram,* 0.037$\cancel{3}$ *gram, and* 120.5$\cancel{8}$ *grams.*

If the last figure in each of the given numbers is uncertain, the *total* should be rounded off to one decimal place. Note that the shorter method (b) gives the same result as the longer method (a):

(a)	162.$\cancel{5}$	(b)	162.$\cancel{5}$
	0.56$\cancel{9}$		0.57
	0.037$\cancel{3}$		0.0$\cancel{4}$
	120.5$\cancel{8}$		120.5$\cancel{8}$
	283.$\cancel{6}$$\cancel{8}$$\cancel{6}$$\cancel{3}$ or		283.$\cancel{6}$9 or
	283.7 grams, *answer.*		283.7 grams, *answer.*

It is important to note that in filling a prescription, the pharmacist *must* assume that the physician means each quantity to be measured with *the same degree of precision.* Hence, if we add these quantities taken from a prescription:

$$5.5 \quad grams$$
$$0.01 \quad gram$$
$$0.005 \quad gram$$

we must *not* round off the total to one decimal place. Rather we must retain at least *three* decimal places in the total by interpreting the given quantities to mean 5.50$\emptyset$ *grams,* 0.01$\emptyset$ *gram,* and 0.00$\cancel{5}$ *gram.* Where greater precision is required, we may interpret the given quantities to mean 5.500$\emptyset$, 0.010$\emptyset$, and 0.005$\emptyset$, etc.

Rule 4. Since you cannot increase the accuracy of the *least* accurate number, therefore, *before multiplying or dividing one approximate number by another approximate number, you may save time by rounding off the component with the greater number of significant figures to one more than are contained in the component having fewer significant figures. The result should be rounded off to the same number of significant figures as are contained in the latter component.*

Example:

Multiply 1.65370 grams by 0.26.

If the last figure in each number is uncertain, each of these methods gives the same result:

	(a) 1.65370 grams		(b) 1.65 grams
	× 0.26		×0.26
	992220		990
	330740		330
	0.4299620 or		0.4290 or
	0.43 gram, *answer.*		0.43 gram, *answer.*

Here again, when calculating with denominate numbers taken from a prescription or official formula, since we must assume that each quantity is meant to be measured with the same degree of accuracy, we must interpret each quantity as having at least as many significant figures as appear in the quantity containing the greatest number of significant figures. So, if the quantities 0.25 *gram*, 0.5 *gram*, and 5 *grams* are included in a prescription, they should be interpreted as 0.25 *gram*, 0.50 *gram*, and 5.0 *grams* for purposes of multiplication or division (as when we enlarge or reduce a formula); and results should be rounded off to contain two significant figures. Where greater accuracy is required, we may interpret the given quantities to mean 0.2500, 0.5000, and 5.000, etc.[1]

---

[1] When converting from one system of measurement to another, we are expressly ordered by the *United States Pharmacopeia* as follows: "For converting specific quantities in a prescription which requires compounding, or in converting a pharmaceutical formula from one system of weights or measures to the other, 'exact' equivalents must be used." This order can mean only that we are required often to pretend that a denominate number in a prescription or formula contains a far greater number of significant figures than in practice it needs. Four-figure accuracy guarantees a margin of error no greater than about one per cent; five-figure accuracy, a margin of error no greater than about one-tenth per cent. But the *Pharmacopeia* requires us to interpret *1 gram* as the equivalent of *15.4324 grains*, which is a *six*-figure factor! Even more astonishing is the apparent inconsistency in the official Table of Equivalents: we may interpret *324 milligrams* as *5 grains* (a one-figure factor), *1 milligram* as $\frac{1}{64}$ *grain* (a two-figure factor), *10 grams* as *154.3 grains* (a four-figure factor), *100 grams* as *1543.2 grains* (a five-figure factor), and *1000 grams* as *15432.4 grains* (once more a six-figure factor).

Rule 5. After multiplying or dividing an approximate number by an absolute number, round off the result to the same number of significant figures as are contained in the approximate number.

This is consistent with Rule 4, for the denominate number contains fewer significant figures if the absolute number is interpreted as being followed by significant zeros to an infinite number of decimal places.

Example:

If a patient has taken 96 doses, each containing 2.54 milligrams of active ingredient, how much of the active ingredient has he taken in all?

2.54 milligrams
× 96
———
15 24
228 6
———
243.84 or
244 milligrams, *answer.*

Practice Problems

1. State the number of significant figures in each of the *italicized* quantities:

(a) One gram equals *15.4324* grains.
(b) One liter equalls *1000* milliliters.
(c) One inch equals *2.54* centimeters.
(d) The chemical costs *$1.05* a pound.
(e) One gram equals *1,000,000* micrograms.
(f) One microgram equals *0.001* milligram.

2. Assuming these numbers to be denominate, how many significant figures has each?

(a) 35.
(b) 609.
(c) 2.7.
(d) 9004.
(e) 506.03.
(f) 0.0047.
(g) 40.07.
(h) 350 (to the nearest 1).
(i) 350 (to the nearest 10).
(j) 5000 (to the nearest 100).

3. Round off each of the following to three significant figures:

   (a) 32.75.
   (b) 200.39.
   (c) 0.03629.
   (d) 21.635.
   (e) 0.00944.
   (f) 1.0751.
   (g) 27.052.
   (h) 0.86249.
   (i) 3.14159.

4. Round off each of the following to three decimal places:

   (a) 0.00083.
   (b) 34.79502.
   (c) 0.00494.
   (d) 6.12963.
   (e) 14.8997.

5. If a mixture of seven ingredients contains the following approximate weights, what can you validly record as the approximate total combined weight of the ingredients?

   26.8$\cancel{3}$ grains, 275.$\cancel{3}$ grains, 2.75$\cancel{6}$ grains, 4.0$\cancel{9}$ grains, 5.19$\cancel{7}$ grains, 16.$\cancel{6}$ grains, and 0.00$\cancel{1}$ grain.

6. You have 420.$\cancel{5}$ grams of a chemical weighed on a balance sensitive to 0.$\cancel{1}$ gram. After taking from this 0.01$\cancel{6}$ gram weighed on a balance sensitive to 0.00$\cancel{1}$ gram, what can you validly record to be the weight of what is left of the chemical?

7. If each of a batch of tablets contains 0.05$\cancel{0}$ grain of active ingredient, what approximate weight of active ingredient will be contained in 750 tablets?

8. If each tablet contains 0.0$\cancel{5}$ grain of active ingredient, what will be in the approximate weight of active ingredient in 750 tablets?

9. Perform the following operations and retain only significant figures in the results:

   (a) 6.3$\cancel{9}$ − 0.00$\cancel{8}$.
   (b) 7.0$\cancel{1}$ − 6.$\cancel{0}$.
   (c) 97.$\cancel{1}$ − 6.936$\cancel{8}$.
   (d) 5.$\cancel{0}$ × 48.$\cancel{3}$ grain.
   (e) 24 × 0.2$\cancel{5}$ gram.
   (f) 350 × 0.6015$\cancel{6}$ gram.
   (g) 0.72$\cancel{0}$ × 0.09$\cancel{5}$ grain.

 (h) 0.056 × 0.9626 gram.
 (i) 56.824 ÷ 0.090.
 (j) 250 ÷ 1.1.
 (k) 5.0001 ÷ 1.9.
 (l) 0.00729 ÷ 0.2735.
 (m) 71.425 ÷ 0.512.
 (n) 71.425 ÷ 3.

ESTIMATION

One of the best checks of the reasonableness of a numerical computation is an estimation of the answer. If we have arrived at a wrong answer by use of a wrong method, a thoughtless, mechanical final verification of our figuring may not show up the error. But an absurd result, such as occurs when the decimal point is put in the wrong place, will not likely slip past if we check it against a preliminary estimation of what the result should be.

Since it is imperative that the pharmacist insure the accuracy of his calculations by every means at his disposal, the student of pharmacy is urged to adopt estimation as one of those means; and since proficiency in estimating comes only from constant practice, he is urged to acquire the habit of estimating the answer to every problem he encounters before attempting to solve it. If so, he will discover, too, that his estimate not only will serve as a means for judging the reasonableness of the final result but also will very often serve as a guide in the solution of the problem.

Checking the accuracy of every calculation, of course, such as by adding a column first upwards and then downwards, is very important. Hence the student should follow this invariable procedure: (1) *estimate*, (2) *compute*, (3) *check*.

The estimating process is basically very simple. First the numbers given in a problem are mentally rounded off to slightly larger or smaller numbers containing fewer significant figures. So, the number *59* would be rounded off to *60*, and the number *732* to *700*. Then the required operations are performed, as far as possible mentally, and the result, although known to be somewhat greater or smaller than the exact answer, is close enough to serve as an estimate.

No set rules for estimating can be given to cover all the operations in arithmetic. But examples can illustrate some of the methods that can be used.

In *addition*, one way to obtain a reasonable estimate of the total is first to add the figures in the leftmost column. But the neglected remaining figures of each number are equally likely to express more or less than one-half the value of a unit of the order we have just added, and hence to the sum of the leftmost column should be added ½ for every number—or *1* for every two numbers—in the column.

Examples:

Add the following numbers: *7428, 3652, 1327, 4605, 2791, and 4490.*

Estimation:	*Calculation:*
The figures in the thou-	7428
sands column add up to	3652
21000, and with each	1327
number on the average	4605
contributing 500 more,	2791
or every pair 1000 more,	4490
we get 21000 + 3000 =	——
24000, *estimated answer.*	24293, *answer.*

Add the following numbers: *2556, 449, 337, 1572.*

Estimation:	*Calculation:*
The figures of the thousands	2556
column add up to 3000, and	449
with each pair of numbers	337
contributing approximately	1572
another 1000, we get 3000 +	——
2000 = 5000, *estimated answer.*	4914, *answer.*

In *multiplication*, the product of the two leftmost digits plus a sufficient number of *zeros* to give the right place value will serve as a fair estimate. The number of *zeros* supplied must equal the total number of all discarded figures to the left of the decimal point. A closer approximation to the correct answer will result if the discarded figures are used to round off the value of those retained.

Examples:

Multiply *612* by *413.*

Estimation:	*Calculation:*
	612
$4 \times 6 = 24$, and	$\times$ 413
since we have dis-	——
carded four fig-	1836
ures, four zeros	612
must be supplied,	2448
giving 240,000,	——
estimated answer.	252756, *answer.*

Multiply 2889 by 209.

Estimation:	*Calculation:*
	2889
The given numbers	$\times$ 209
round off to 3000	
and 200. $3 \times 2 = 6$,	26001
and supplying five	5778
zeros we get 600,000	
estimated answer.	603801, *answer.*

The correct place value is easier to keep track of if relatively insignificant decimal fractions are ignored. When the multiplier is a decimal fraction, the possibility of error is reduced if we first convert it to a common fraction of approximately the same value.

Examples:

Multiply 41.76 by 20.3.
Estimate: $42 \times 20 = 840$.

Multiply 730.5 by 321.
Estimate: $700 \times 300 = 210,000$.

Multiply 314.2 by 0.18.
Estimate: Since 0.18 or $\frac{18}{100}$ lies between $\frac{1}{6}$ and $\frac{1}{5}$, the answer will lie between 50 and 60.

Multiply 48.16 by 0.072.
Estimate: $\frac{7}{100}$ equals about $\frac{1}{15}$, and $\frac{1}{15}$ of 48 is about 3.

In *division*, the given numbers may be rounded off to convenient approximations, but here again care must be exercised to preserve correct place values.

Example:
Divide 2456 by 5.91.

Estimate: The numbers may be rounded off to 2400 and 6. We may divide 24 by 6 mentally; but we must not forget the two zeros substituted for the given 56 in 2456, and our estimated answer will be 400.

The use of short cuts and variations in arithmetical operations contributes to both speed and accuracy in mental calculation. Facility in the use of short cuts can be developed only if we select or devise variations that appeal to us and practice them constantly. Here are some short cuts that may suggest other possibilities:

(1) To multiply by 10, 100, 1000, etc., move the decimal place one, two, three places to the right, etc. To divide by 10, 100, 1000, etc., move the decimal place one, two, three places to the left, etc.

(2) To multiply by 200, 300, 500, etc., multiply by 2, 3, 5, etc., and then multiply by 100. To divide by the same numbers, divide by 2, 3, 5, etc., and divide by 100.

(3) To multiply by 2000, 4000, 6000, etc., multiply by 2, 4, 6, etc., and then multiply by 1000. To divide by these numbers, divide by 2, 4, 6, etc., and divide by 1000.

(4) To multiply by $87\frac{1}{2}$, which is $\frac{7}{8}$ of a hundred, multiply by 700 and divide by 8. To divide by $87\frac{1}{2}$, multiply by 8 and divide by 700.

(5) To multiply by $83\frac{1}{3}$, which is $\frac{5}{6}$ of a hundred, multiply by 500 and divide by 6. To divide by $83\frac{1}{3}$, multiply by 6 and divide by 500.

(6) To multiply by 75, which is $\frac{3}{4}$ of a hundred, multiply by 300 and divide by 4. To divide by 75, multiply by 4 and divide by 300.

(7) To multiply by $66\frac{2}{3}$, which is $\frac{2}{3}$ of a hundred, multiply by 200 and divide by 3. To divide by $66\frac{2}{3}$, multiply by 3 and divide by 200.

(8) To multiply by $62\frac{1}{2}$, which is $\frac{5}{8}$ of a hundred, multiply by 500 and divide by 8. To divide by $62\frac{1}{2}$, multiply by 8 and divide by 500.

(9) To multiply by 50, which is $\frac{1}{2}$ of a hundred, multiply by 100 and divide by 2. To divide by 50, multiply by 2 and divide by 100.

(10) To multiply by $37\frac{1}{2}$, which is $\frac{3}{8}$ of a hundred, multiply by 300 and divide by 8. To divide by $37\frac{1}{2}$, multiply by 8 and divide by 300.

(11) To multiply by $33\frac{1}{3}$, which is $\frac{1}{3}$ of a hundred, multiply by 100 and divide by 3. To divide by $33\frac{1}{3}$, multiply by 3 and divide by 100.

(12) To multiply by 25, which is $\frac{1}{4}$ of a hundred, multiply by 100 and divide by 4. To divide by 25, multiply by 4 and divide by 100.

(13) To multiply by $16\frac{2}{3}$, which is $\frac{1}{6}$ of a hundred, multiply by 100 and divide by 6. To divide by $16\frac{2}{3}$, multiply by 6 and divide by 100.

(14) To multiply by 15, multiply by 10 and add half the product. To divide by 15, divide $\frac{2}{3}$ of the dividend by 10 (or divide by 10 and multiply by $\frac{2}{3}$).

(15) To multiply by $12\frac{1}{2}$, which is $\frac{1}{8}$ of a hundred, multiply by 100 and divide by 8. To divide by $12\frac{1}{2}$, multiply by 8 and divide by 100.

(16) To multiply any two-digit number by 11, first add the two digits. If the sum is less than ten, place it between the digits; if the sum is ten or more, place the unit figure between the digits and add 1 to the left digit.

$$11 \times 43: \ 4 + 3 = 7, \text{ hence } 473$$
$$11 \times 83: \ 8 + 3 = 11, \text{ hence } 913$$

To multiply any number by eleven, multiply by 10 and add the multiplicand.

(17) To multiply by 0.25 and 0.50, divide by 4 and 2. To divide by 0.25 and 0.50, multiply by 4 and 2.

$$6947 \times 0.25 = 6947 \div 4$$
$$6947 \div 0.50 = 6947 \times 2$$

(18) Reduce inconvenient multipliers to their more convenient factors.

$$16 \times 55 = 8 \times 2 \times 55 = 8 \times 110 = 880$$

Practice Problems

1. In estimating the result of multiplying 8,329 by 7,242, how many zeros will follow 56?

2. In estimating the result of dividing 811500 by 16.23, how many zeros will follow 5?

3. How many terminal zeros are there in the product obtained by multiplying 5.100 by 90,000?

4. How many terminal zeros are there in the quotient obtained by dividing 8.100 by 0.009?

Estimate the sums:

5.	5641	7.	3298	9.	953
	2177		368		1020
	294		5192		171
	8266		627		580
	3503		4835		856
6.	9874	8.	7466	10.	5544
	6018		5288		9636
	459		9013		4824
	1297		8462		670
	3361		716		7846
	396		4369		465

Estimate the products:

11. $17 \times 22 =$
12. $28 \times 31 =$
13. $8 \times 48 =$
14. $19 \times 38 =$
15. $28 \times 62 =$
16. $39 \times 77 =$
17. $42 \times 39 =$
18. $125 \times 92 =$
19. $365 \times 98 =$
20. $473 \times 102 =$
21. $596 \times 204 =$
22. $604 \times 122 =$
23. $675 \times 19 =$
24. $998 \times 13 =$
25. $6549 \times 830 =$
26. $1073 \times 972 =$

27. $8431 \times 9760 =$
28. $7183 \times 19 =$
29. $5106 \times 963 =$
30. $2349 \times 5907 =$
31. $2\frac{1}{2} \times 14\frac{1}{2} =$
32. $\frac{2}{3} \times 400 =$
33. $21\frac{1}{3} \times 6\frac{2}{3} =$
34. $\frac{3}{4} \times 816 =$
35. $\frac{2}{3} \times 425.65 =$
36. $5.8 \times 7165 =$
37. $2.04 \times 705.3 =$
38. $0.016 \times 589.4 =$
39. $0.0726 \times 6951 =$
40. $98 \times 0.0031 =$
41. $6.1 \times 67.39 =$
42. $7569 \times 0.0963 =$

Estimate the quotients:

43. $171 \div 19 =$
44. $165 \div 15 =$
45. $184 \div 2300 =$
46. $3080 \div 144 =$
47. $160 \div 3200 =$
48. $36900 \div 41 =$
49. $86450 \div 72 =$
50. $1078 \div 98 =$

51. $98000 \div 49 =$
52. $17015 \div 57 =$
53. $1.0745 \div 500 =$
54. $18.954 \div 0.39 =$
55. $1.9214 \div 0.026 =$
56. $19.223 \div 47 =$
57. $458.4 \div 8 =$
58. $448.32 \div 0.048 =$

Estimate the final results:

59. $\dfrac{272103 \times 300}{901}$

60. $\dfrac{750 \times 300 \times 380.5}{760 \times 375}$

61. $\dfrac{270\ (15 - 10)}{91 \times 5}$

62. $\frac{1}{120} \times \frac{1}{10} \times 11.95$

63. $\dfrac{437.5}{8.05} \times \frac{1}{16}$

64. $\dfrac{809 \times (35 - 25)}{4.01 \times 20}$

65. $\dfrac{\frac{1}{100}}{\frac{1}{2}} \times 5123$

66. $\dfrac{627 \times (25 - 10)}{30 \times 15}$

67. $\dfrac{750 \times 380 \times 319.53}{760 \times 750}$

68. What should be the approximate total cost of 625,250 tablets at $\frac{1}{5}$ cent each?

69. Estimate the approximate cost of 32,560 capsules at \$12.50 per M.

70. Estimate the approximate cost of 30,125 capsules at 75 cents per hundred.

71. What should be the approximate cost of 120,050 tablets at $33\frac{1}{3}$ cents per C?

72. A formula for 1,250 capsules contains 3.635 grams of a medicament. Estimate the amount of medicament that should be used in preparing 325 capsules.

73. Approximately how many teaspoonful- (5 milliliter-) doses can be obtained from 1 gallon (3,784 milliliters) of a liquid?

74. The cost of 1000 capsules is \$15.00. If they are sold at the rate of \$1.50 for 48 capsules, estimate the profit that can be realized from the sale of 1000 capsules.

75. The cost of 5000 capsules is \$50.00. If they are sold at the rate of 75 cents for 24 capsules, estimate the profit that can be realized from the sale of 500 capsules.

PERCENTAGE OF ERROR

Since measurements are never absolutely accurate, it is important for the pharmacist to recognize the limitations of his measuring instruments and to know the magnitude of the errors that may be incurred when he uses them.

When he weighs a substance, for instance, he may record the weight as a single quantity, such as *50 milligrams;* but he should be aware that a truer record of the weight should include two quantities, expressing (1) the apparent weight and (2) the possible excess or deficiency calculated from the known sensitivity of the balance.[1] The second quantity is called the *maximum potential error.* So, if the pharmacist weighs *"50 milligrams"* on a balance sensitive to *2 milligrams,* he has actually weighed something between *48* and *52 milligrams,* for the maximum potential error is ± *2 milligrams.* This potential error may be used to calculate the percentage of possible error in order to determine whether an error of this magnitude may be allowed.

Percentage of error may be defined as *the maximum potential error multiplied by 100 and divided by the quantity desired.* The calculation may be formulated as follows:

$$\frac{\text{Error} \times 100\%}{\text{Quantity desired}} = \text{Percentage of error}$$

This formula is valid only if the error and the quantity desired are expressed in the same denomination.

Example:

> *When the maximum potential error is* ± *2 milligrams in a total of 50 milligrams, what is the percentage of error?*

$$\frac{2 \times 100\%}{50} = 4\%, \text{ answer.}$$

Now, if the sensitivity of an instrument of dubious accuracy is not known, its performance may be checked with that of an instru-

---

[1] The sensitivity of a balance may be defined as the smallest weight that will disturb its equilibrium.

It may be determined by the following procedure:

1. Place the balance in a level position.
2. Adjust the balance to equilibrium.
3. Determine the smallest weight that will disturb the equilibrium.

ment of known high accuracy. If the two instruments are used to measure the same thing, the difference between the two results will not be a potential error but a close approximation of an actual error; and given this, we may calculate the percentage of error actually committed by the less accurate instrument.

Example:

A prescription calls for 800 milligrams of a substance. After weighing this amount on a balance, the pharmacist decides to check by weighing it again on a much more sensitive balance. Now he finds that he has only 750 milligrams. Since the first weighing was 50 milligrams short of the desired amount, what was the percentage of error?

$$\frac{50 \times 100\%}{800} = 6.25\%, \text{ answer.}$$

Finally, if a certain percentage of error is not to be exceeded, and the maximum potential error of an instrument is known, it is possible to calculate the smallest quantity that can be measured within the desired accuracy. Here is a convenient formula:

$$\frac{100 \times \text{maximum potential error}}{\text{Permissible percentage of error}} = \text{Smallest quantity}$$

Example:

What is the smallest quantity that can be weighed with a potential error of not more than 4% on a balance sensitive to 2 milligrams?

$$\frac{100 \times 2 \text{ milligrams}}{4} = 50 \text{ milligrams, } answer.$$

Practice Problems

1. A pharmacist attempts to weigh 75 milligrams of arsenic trioxide on a balance having a sensitivity of 5 milligrams. Calculate the maximum potential error in terms of percentage.

2. In compounding a prescription, a pharmacist weighed 0.050 gram of a substance on a balance insensitive to quantities smaller than 0.004 gram. What was the maximum potential error in terms of percentage?

3. A pharmacist wants to weigh 5 grains of a substance on a balance having a sensitivity of $\frac{1}{4}$ grain. Calculate the maximum potential error in terms of percentage.

4. A pharmacist weighed 825 milligrams of a substance. When checked on another balance, the weight was found to be 805 milligrams. Calculate the deviation from the original weighing in terms of percentage.

5. A pharmacist weighed 475 milligrams of a substance on a balance of dubious accuracy. When checked on a balance of high accuracy, the weight was found to be 445 milligrams. Calculate the percentage of error in the first weighing.

6. A 10-milliliter graduate weighs 42.745 grams. When 5 milliliters of distilled water are measured in it, the combined weight of graduate and water is 47.675 grams. By definition, 5 milliliters of water should weigh 5 grams. Calculate the weight of the measured water and express any deviation from 5 grams as percentage of error.

7. A graduate weighs 35.825 grams. When 10 milliliters of water are measured in it, the weight of the graduate and water is 45.835 grams. Calculate the weight of the water and express any deviation from 10 grams as percentage of error.

8. In compounding a certain prescription, a pharmacist used 45.5 grains instead of the 48 grains called for. Calculate the percentage of error on the basis of the desired quantity.

9. A pharmacist attempts to weigh 0.375 gram of carmine on a balance of dubious accuracy. When checked on a highly accurate balance, the weight is found to be 0.400 gram. Calculate the percentage of error in the first weighing.

10. On a balance having a sensitivity of 0.012 gram, what is the smallest amount that can be weighed with a maximum potential error of not more than 5%?

11. On a balance having an accuracy of $\frac{1}{30}$ grain, what is the smallest amount that can be weighed with a potential error of not more than 2%?

12. If an accuracy of 2% is desired, what is the minimum amount that should be weighed on a balance having a sensitivity of 0.004 gram?

13. A pharmacist measured 60 milliliters of glycerin by difference, starting with 100 milliliters. After completing the measurement, he noted that the graduate which he used contained 45 milliliters of glycerin. Calculate the percentage of error that was incurred in the measurement.

14. A pharmacist failed to place the balance in equilibrium before weighing three grains of a medicament. Later, he discovered that the balance was out of equilibrium and that a 20% error was incurred. If the balance pan on which he placed the medicament was heavy, how many grains of the medicament did he actually weigh?

ALIQUOT METHOD OF MEASURING

When a degree of precision in measurement is required that is beyond the capacity of the instrument at hand, the pharmacist may achieve the desired precision by measuring and calculating in terms of aliquot parts.

An *aliquot part* may be defined as any part that is contained a whole number of times in a quantity. Thus, *2* is an aliquot part of *10;* and since *10 ÷ 2 = 5, 2* is called the *fifth aliquot* of *10.* Again, *4* is an aliquot part of *16;* and since *16 ÷ 4 = 4, 4* is the *fourth aliquot* of *16.*

To Weigh by the Aliquot Method:

The aliquot method of weighing is a method by which small quantities of a substance may be obtained within the degree of accuracy desired. The procedure may be summed up as follows:

Step 1. Select some multiple of the desired quantity that can be weighed with the required precision. Weigh this multiple.

Step 2. Using an inert substance that is compatible with the given preparation, dilute the multiple quantity.

Step 3. Weigh the aliquot part of the dilution that contains the desired quantity.

To select the multiple quantity in Step 1, first calculate the smallest quantity of the substance that can be weighed with the required precision (see Percentage of Error, p. 28). To insure an error no greater than *5%*, for instance, a quantity at least twenty times the sensitivity of the balance (the sensitivity being the smallest amount that will upset the equilibrium of the balance) must be weighed; and hence, if the sensitivity of a balance is *4 milligrams, 20 × 4 milligrams,* or *80 milligrams*, is the smallest amount that can be weighed. If *50 milligrams* were weighed on such a balance, the maximum potential error would be *8%* (see p. 28). Convenience in multiplying, availability of weights, and the cost of the substance are other factors that help determine the choice of the multiple quantity.

The amount of inert diluent used in Step 2 is determined by the fact that the aliquot part of the dilution to be weighed in *Step 3* must be a quantity large enough to be weighed within the desired degree of accuracy. In *Step 1* we have already calculated the minimum quantity that satisfies this condition. The aliquot must weigh at least as much as the multiple quantity weighed in *Step 1;* and to reduce the potential error its weight should usually be somewhat greater. So, if the multiple quantity weighs *80 milligrams*, the aliquot must weigh at least *80 milligrams*, but preferably *100 milligrams* or more. When we multiply the chosen aliquot by the multiple selected in *Step 1*, we get the quantity of the dilution, and have only to add sufficient diluent to the multiple quantity to equal this weight of dilution.

The aliquot weighed in Step 3 will contain the quantity originally desired, for if, say, *20* times the original quantity is diluted, $\frac{1}{20}$ of the dilution will contain the original quantity. And by arbitrarily selecting a sufficiently large multiple quantity and a sufficiently large dilution, we can be sure that we have measured within the required degree of precision.

Example:

> *Assuming a balance sensitivity of 4 milligrams, explain how you would weigh 5 milligrams of atropine sulfate with an accuracy of ± 5 %, using lactose as the diluent.*

> Since 4 milligrams (mg.) is the potential balance error, 80 milligrams is the smallest amount that should be weighed to achieve the required precision.

> If 100 milligrams, or 20 times the desired amount of atropine sulfate, is chosen as the multiple quantity to be weighed in Step 1, and if 150 milligrams is set as the aliquot to be weighed in Step 3, then —

> (1) Weigh 20 × 5 mg., or   100 mg. of atropine sulfate
> (2) Dilute with   2900 mg. of lactose
>   to get $\overline{3000}$ mg. of dilution
> (3) Weigh $\frac{1}{20}$ of dilution, or 150 mg. of dilution,
>   which contain 5 milligrams of atropine sulfate, *answer.*

In this example the weight of the aliquot was arbitrarily set as *150 milligrams*, which exceeds the weight of the multiple quantity, as it preferably should. If *100 milligrams* had been set as the aliquot, the multiple quantity should have been diluted with *1900 milligrams* of lactose to get *2000 milligrams* of dilution, and its twentieth aliquot, or *100 milligrams*, would have contained *5 milligrams* of atropine sulfate. On the other hand, if *200 milligrams* had been set as the aliquot, the multiple quantity of atropine sulfate should have been diluted with *3900 milligrams* of lactose to get *4000 milligrams* of dilution.

Another example:

> *Assuming a balance sensitivity of $\frac{1}{10}$ grain, explain how you would weigh $\frac{1}{4}$ grain of strychnine sulfate with an accuracy of ± 5%, using lactose as the diluent.*

Since $\frac{1}{10}$ grain (gr.) is the potential balance error, 2 grains is the smallest amount that should be weighed to achieve the required precision.

If 12 is chosen as the multiple, and if 3 grains is set as the weight of the aliquot, then—

(1) Weigh 12 × $\frac{1}{4}$ gr., or   3 gr. of strychnine sulfate
(2) Dilute with $\underline{33}$ gr. of lactose
       to get $\overline{36}$ gr. of dilution
(3) Weigh $\frac{1}{12}$ of dilution, or 3 gr. of dilution, which contain $\frac{1}{4}$ grain of strychnine sulfate, *answer*.

To Measure Volume by the Aliquot Method:

The aliquot method of measuring volume, which is identical in principle to the aliquot method of weighing, may be used when relatively small volumes must be measured with great precision:

Step 1. Select a multiple of the desired quantity that can be measured with the required precision.

Step 2. Dilute the multiple quantity with a compatible diluent (usually a solvent for the liquid to be measured) to an amount evenly divisible by the multiple selected.

Step 3. Measure the aliquot of the dilution that contains the quantity originally desired.

Examples:

> *A prescription calls for 0.25 milliliter of hydrochloric acid. Using a 10-milliliter graduate calibrated in units of 1 milliliter, explain how you would obtain the desired quantity of hydrochloric acid by the aliquot method.*

If 4 is chosen as the multiple, and if 2 milliliters is set as the volume of the aliquot, then—

(1) Measure 4 × 0.25 ml., or 1 ml. of the acid
(2) Dilute with $\underline{7}$ ml. of water
       to get $\overline{8}$ ml. of dilution

3

(3)   Measure $\frac{1}{4}$ of dilution, or 2 ml. of dilution, which contain 0.25 milliliter of hydrochloric acid, *answer.*

A prescription calls for $\frac{1}{2}$ minim of clove oil. Using a 60-minim graduate calibrated in units of 5 minims, explain how you would obtain the clove oil by the aliquot method. Use alcohol as the diluent.

If 10 is chosen as the multiple, and if 5 minims is set as the volume of the aliquot, then—

(1)   Measure $10 \times \frac{1}{2}$ minim, or 5 minims of clove oil

(2)   Dilute with   45 minims of alcohol

to get $\overline{50}$ minims of dilution

(3)   Measure $\frac{1}{10}$ of dilution, or 5 minims of dilution, which contain $\frac{1}{2}$ minim of clove oil, *answer.*

Practice Problems

1. If 1000 milliliters of a certain solution contain 30 milligrams of a dye, (a) what is the volume of the tenth aliquot? and (b) how many milligrams of the dye will the tenth aliquot contain?

2. A balance has a sensitivity of 0.005 gram. Explain how you would weigh 0.012 gram of atropine sulfate with an error not greater than 5%, using lactose as a diluent.

3. A balance has a sensitivity of 4 milligrams. Explain how you would weigh 5 milligrams of strychnine sulfate with an error not greater than 5%. Use lactose as the diluent.

4. The sensitivity of a balance is $\frac{1}{20}$ grain. Explain how you would weigh $\frac{1}{10}$ grain of atropine sulphate with an error not greater than 5%. Use milk sugar as the diluent.

5. A balance has a sensitivity of 6 milligrams. Explain how you would weigh 20 milligrams of a substance with an error not greater than 2%.

6. A balance has a sensitivity of $\frac{1}{6}$ grain. Explain how you would weigh 1 grain of a substance with an error not greater than 5%.

7. A balance has a sensitivity of 0.003 gram. Explain how you would weigh 0.008 gram of a substance with an error not greater than 5%.

8. A balance has a sensitivity of $\frac{1}{8}$ grain. Explain how you would weigh $\frac{3}{4}$ grain of a substance with an error not greater than 5%.

9. A formula calls for 0.6 milliliter of a coloring solution. Using a 10-milliliter graduate calibrated in units of 1 milliliter, how could you obtain the desired quantity of the coloring solution by the aliquot method? Use water as the diluent.

10. In preparing 100 milliliters of a dilute solution of hydrochloric acid, 0.75 milliliter of hydrochloric acid is required. Using the graduate described in Problem 9, how could you obtain the desired 0.75 milliliter of the acid with satisfactory accuracy? Use water as the diluent.

11. A prescription calls for 0.2 milliliter of a stock solution of a chemical. Using the graduate described in Problem 9, how could you obtain the desired 0.2 milliliter of stock solution with satisfactory accuracy? Use water as the diluent.

12. Using a 10-milliliter graduate calibrated in units of 1 milliliter, explain how you would measure 0.125 milliliter of a dye solution by the aliquot method. Use water as the diluent.

13. A prescription calls for 2 minims of rose oil. Using a 60-minim graduate calibrated in units of 5 minims, explain how you would obtain the rose oil by the aliquot method. Use alcohol as the diluent.

14. Using a balance having a sensitivity of $\frac{1}{10}$ grain, explain how you would obtain $\frac{8}{50}$ grain of menthol. Menthol is soluble in alcohol.

15. ℞ Sodium Citrate   5.0   Gm.
    Tartar Emetic   0.015 Gm.
    Cherry Syrup q.s. ad 120.0   ml.
    Sig. Use for cough.
Assuming a balance sensitivity of 0.004 gram (Gm.), state how you would obtain the correct quantity of tartar emetic. Use water as the solvent for tartar emetic.

COMMON AND DECIMAL FRACTIONS

Much of the arithmetic of pharmacy requires facility in the handling of common fractions and decimal fractions. Even if the student already has a good working knowledge of their use, the following brief review of certain principles and rules governing them should be helpful, and the practice problems should provide him with the means of gaining accuracy and speed in their manipulation.

COMMON FRACTIONS

A number in the form $\frac{1}{8}$, $\frac{3}{16}$, and so on, is called a *common fraction*, or very often simply a *fraction*. Its *denominator*, or second or lower figure, always indicates the number of aliquot parts into which *1* is divided; and its *numerator*, or first or upper figure, specifies the number of those parts with which we are concerned.

The *value* of a fraction is the quotient when its numerator is divided by its denominator. If the numerator is smaller than the denominator, the fraction is called *proper*, and its value is less than *1*. If the numerator and denominator are alike, its value is *1*. If the numerator is larger than the denominator, the fraction is called *improper*, and its value is greater than *1*.

Now, two principles must be understood by anyone attempting to calculate with common fractions.

First Principle. Multiplying the numerator increases the value of a fraction, and multiplying the denominator decreases the value; but *when both numerator and denominator are multiplied by the same number, the value does not change.*

$$\frac{2}{7} = \frac{3 \times 2}{3 \times 7} = \frac{6}{21}$$

This principle allows us to reduce two or more fractions to a common denomination when necessary. We usually want the *lowest common denominator*, which is the smallest number divisible by all the given denominators. It is most easily found by testing successive multiples of the largest given denominator until we reach a number divisible by all the other given denominators. Then we multiply both numerator and denominator of each fraction by the number of times its denominator is contained in the common denominator.

Example:

Reduce the fractions $\frac{3}{4}$, $\frac{4}{5}$, and $\frac{1}{3}$ to a common denomination.

By testing successive multiples of 5, we discover that 60 is the smallest number divisible by 4, 5, and 3.

4 is contained 15 times in 60; 5, 12 times; and 3, 20 times.

$$\frac{3}{4} = \frac{15 \times 3}{15 \times 4} = \frac{45}{60},$$

$$\frac{4}{5} = \frac{12 \times 4}{12 \times 5} = \frac{48}{60}, \quad answers.$$

$$\frac{1}{3} = \frac{20 \times 1}{20 \times 3} = \frac{20}{60},$$

Second Principle. Dividing the numerator decreases the value of a fraction, and dividing the denominator increases the value; but *when both numerator and denominator are divided by the same number, the value does not change.*

$$\frac{6}{21} = \frac{6 \div 3}{21 \div 3} = \frac{2}{7}$$

This principle allows us to reduce an unwieldy fraction to more convenient lower terms, either at any time during a series of calculations or when recording a final result. To reduce a fraction to its *lowest terms,* divide both the numerator and the denominator by the largest common divisor.

Example:

Reduce $\frac{36}{2880}$ to its lowest terms.

The largest common divisor is 36.

$$\frac{36}{2880} = \frac{36 \div 36}{2880 \div 36} = \frac{1}{80}, \text{ } answer.$$

These principles often suggest direct solutions to practical problems.

Examples:

A prescription calls for $\frac{3}{50}$ grain of atropine sulfate. How many $\frac{1}{200}$-grain tablets will supply the required amount?

50 is contained 4 times in 200.

$$\frac{3}{50} \text{ gr. } = \frac{4 \times 3}{4 \times 50} \text{ gr. } = \frac{12}{200} \text{ gr.}$$

Twelve $\frac{1}{200}$-grain tablets would supply $\frac{12}{200}$ gr. which equals the $\frac{3}{50}$ gr. required, *answer.*

Justify the assertion that nine $\frac{1}{150}$-grain tablets would supply the $\frac{3}{50}$ grain of atropine sulfate called for.

Nine $\frac{1}{150}$-grain tablets would supply $\frac{9}{150}$ gr.

50 is contained 3 times in 150.

$$\frac{9}{150} \text{ gr. } = \frac{9 \div 3}{150 \div 3} \text{ gr. } = \frac{3}{50} \text{ gr. required, } answer.$$

Besides developing a firm grasp of these two principles, the student should follow two rules before indulging in any short cuts.

Rule 1. Before performing any arithmetical operation involving fractions, *reduce every mixed number to an improper fraction.* To do so, multiply the integer, or whole number, by the denominator of the fractional remainder, add the numerator, and write the result over the denominator.

For example, before attempting to multiply $\frac{3}{4}$ by $1\frac{1}{5}$, first reduce the $1\frac{1}{5}$ to an improper fraction:

$$1\frac{1}{5} = \frac{(1 \times 5) + 1}{5} = \frac{6}{5}$$

If the final result of a calculation is an improper fraction, you may, if you like, reduce it to a mixed number. To do so, simply divide the numerator by the denominator and express the remainder as a common, not a decimal, fraction:

$$\frac{6}{5} = 6 \div 5 = 1\frac{1}{5}$$

Rule 2. When performing an operation involving a fraction and a whole number, *express (or at least visualize) the whole number as a fraction having 1 for its denominator.*
Think of *3* as $\frac{3}{1}$, *42* as $\frac{42}{1}$, and so on.
As will be seen, this visualization is desirable when a fraction is subtracted from a whole number, and it is necessary when a fraction is divided by a whole number.

To add fractions:

To add common fractions, reduce them to a common denomination, add the numerators, and write the sum over the common denominator. If whole and mixed numbers are involved, the safest (though not the quickest) procedure is first to apply *Rules 1* and *2.* If the sum is an improper fraction, you may want to reduce it to a mixed number.

Examples:

A prescription for a capsule contains $\frac{3}{80}$ grain of ingredient A, $\frac{1}{200}$ grain of ingredient B, $\frac{1}{50}$ grain of ingredient C, and $\frac{3}{16}$ grain of ingredient D. What is the total weight of these four ingredients?

The lowest common denominator of the four fractions is 400.

Reducing to a common denomination:

$\frac{3}{80} = \frac{15}{400}$, $\frac{1}{200} = \frac{2}{400}$, $\frac{1}{50} = \frac{8}{400}$, and $\frac{3}{16} = \frac{75}{400}$

Adding the numerators:

$$\frac{15 + 2 + 8 + 75}{400} \text{ gr.} = \frac{100}{400} \text{ gr.}$$

Reducing the sum to its simplest terms:

$\frac{100}{400}$ gr. $= \frac{1}{4}$ gr., *answer.*

A patient receives the following doses of a certain drug: $\frac{1}{4}$ grain, $\frac{1}{12}$ grain, $\frac{1}{8}$ grain, and $\frac{1}{6}$ grain. Calculate the total amount of the drug received by the patient.

The lowest common denominator of the fractions is 24.

$\frac{1}{4} = \frac{6}{24}$, $\frac{1}{12} = \frac{2}{24}$, $\frac{1}{8} = \frac{3}{24}$, and $\frac{1}{6} = \frac{4}{24}$

$$\frac{6 + 2 + 3 + 4}{24} \text{ gr.} = \frac{15}{24} \text{ gr.}$$

$\frac{15}{24}$ gr. $= \frac{5}{8}$ gr., *answer.*

To subtract fractions:

To subtract one fraction from another, reduce them to a common denomination, subtract, and write the difference over the common denominator. If a whole or mixed number is involved, first apply *Rule 1* or *2*. If the difference is an improper fraction, you may want to reduce it to a mixed number.

Examples:

A patient's medication chart shows that he has received a total of $\frac{7}{12}$ grain of morphine sulfate. If he had not been given the last dose of $\frac{1}{8}$ grain, what quantity would he have received?

The lowest common denominator is 24.

$\frac{7}{12} = \frac{14}{24}$ and $\frac{1}{8} = \frac{3}{24}$.

$$\frac{14 - 3}{24} \text{ gr.} = \frac{11}{24} \text{ gr.}, \text{ *answer.*}$$

A capsule is to weigh 3 grains. If it contains $\frac{1}{24}$ grain of ingredient A, $\frac{1}{4}$ grain of ingredient B, and $\frac{1}{3}$ grain of ingredient C, how much diluent should be added?

The lowest common denominator of the fractions is 24.

$\frac{1}{24} = \frac{1}{24}$, $\frac{1}{4} = \frac{6}{24}$, and $\frac{1}{3} = \frac{8}{24}$.

$$\frac{1 + 6 + 8}{24} \text{ gr.} = \frac{15}{24} \text{ gr.} = \frac{5}{8} \text{ gr.}$$

Interpreting the given 3 grains as $\frac{3}{1}$ grains, and reducing it to a fraction with 8 for a denominator:

$\frac{3}{1}$ gr. $= \frac{24}{8}$ gr.

Subtracting:

$$\frac{24 - 5}{8} \text{ gr.} = \frac{19}{8} \text{ gr.}$$

Changing the difference to a mixed number:

$\frac{19}{8}$ gr. $= (19 \div 8)$ gr. $= 2\frac{3}{8}$ gr., *answer.*

To multiply fractions:

To multiply fractions, multiply the numerators and write the product over the product of the denominators. If either or both is a mixed number, first apply *Rule 1*. If the multiplier is a whole number, simply multiply the numerator of the fraction and write the product over the denominator.

Examples:

How much active ingredient is represented in 24 tablets each containing $\frac{1}{320}$ grain of the ingredient?

$$24 \times \frac{1}{320} \text{ gr.} = \frac{24 \times 1}{320} \text{ gr.} = \frac{24}{320} \text{ gr.} = \frac{3}{40} \text{ gr., } answer.$$

The adult dose of a drug is $\frac{3}{20}$ grain. Calculate the dose for a child if it is $\frac{1}{12}$ of the adult dose.

$$\frac{1}{12} \times \frac{3}{20} \text{ gr.} = \frac{1 \times 3}{12 \times 20} \text{ gr.} = \frac{3}{240} \text{ gr.} = \frac{1}{80} \text{ gr., } answer.$$

To divide fractions:

To divide by a fraction, invert its terms and multiply. When a fraction is to be divided by a whole number, *Rule 2* must be first applied, and when the number is inverted it will have *1* for its numerator.

Examples:

If $\frac{1}{2}$ ounce is divided into 4 equal parts, how much will each part contain?

Interpreting 4 as $\frac{4}{1}$:

$$\frac{1}{2} \text{ oz.} \div \frac{4}{1} = \frac{1}{2} \text{ oz.} \times \frac{1}{4} = \frac{1 \times 1}{2 \times 4} \text{ oz.} = \frac{1}{8} \text{ oz., } answer.$$

The dose of a drug is $\frac{1}{60}$ grain. How many doses can be made from $\frac{1}{5}$ grain?

$$\frac{1}{5} \div \frac{1}{60} = \frac{1}{5} \times \frac{60}{1} = \frac{1 \times 60}{5 \times 1} = 12 \text{ doses, } answer.$$

A child is given $\frac{5}{8}$ grain of a drug. If this represents $\frac{1}{16}$ of the adult dose, what is the adult dose?

If $\frac{1}{16}$ of (that is, *times*) the adult dose is $\frac{5}{8}$ grain, then $\frac{5}{8}$ grain divided by $\frac{1}{16}$ must equal the adult dose.

$$\frac{5}{8} \text{ gr.} \div \frac{1}{16} = \frac{5}{8} \text{ gr.} \times \frac{16}{1} = \frac{5 \times 16}{8 \times 1} \text{ gr.} = 10 \text{ gr., } answer.$$

DECIMAL FRACTIONS

A fraction whose denominator is 10 or any power of ten is called a *decimal fraction*, or simply a *decimal*. The denominator of a decimal fraction is never written, since the decimal point serves to indicate the place value of the numerals. The numerator and the decimal point are sufficient to express the fraction. So, $\frac{1}{10}$ is written 0.1, $\frac{45}{100}$ is written 0.45, and $\frac{65}{1000}$ is written 0.065.

All operations with decimal fractions are carried out in the same manner as with whole numbers, but care must be exercised in putting the decimal point in its proper place in the results.

Three familiar operations are worth recalling.

(1) As a direct consequence of the place value in the decimal notation, moving the decimal point one place to the right multiplies a number by 10, two places to the right multiplies it by 100, and so on. Likewise, moving the point one place to the left divides a number by 10, two places to the left divides it by 100, and so on.

(2) A decimal fraction may be changed to a common fraction by writing the numerator over the denominator and (if desired) reducing to lowest terms:

$$0.125 = \tfrac{125}{1000} = \tfrac{1}{8}$$

(3) A common fraction may be changed to a decimal by dividing the numerator by the denominator (note that the result may be a repeating or endless decimal fraction):

$$\tfrac{3}{8} = 3 \div 8 = 0.375$$
$$\tfrac{1}{3} = 1 \div 3 = 0.3333 \ldots .$$

Practice Problems

1. Add each of the following:
   (a) $\frac{5}{8}$ gr. $+ \frac{9}{32}$ gr. $+ \frac{1}{4}$ gr.
   (b) $\frac{1}{150}$ gr. $+ \frac{1}{200}$ gr. $+ \frac{1}{100}$ gr.
   (c) $\frac{1}{60}$ gr. $+ \frac{1}{20}$ gr. $+ \frac{1}{16}$ gr. $+ \frac{1}{32}$ gr.

2. Find the difference:
   (a) $3\frac{1}{2}$ gr. $- \frac{15}{64}$ gr.
   (b) $\frac{1}{30}$ gr. $- \frac{1}{40}$ gr.
   (c) $2\frac{1}{3}$ gr. $- 1\frac{1}{2}$ gr.

3. Find the product:
   (a) $\frac{30}{75} \times \frac{15}{32} \times 25$.
   (b) $2\frac{1}{2} \times 12 \times \frac{7}{8}$.
   (c) $\frac{1}{125} \times \frac{9}{20}$.

4. Find the quotient:
   (a) $\frac{2}{3} \div \frac{1}{24}$.
   (b) $\frac{1}{5000} \div 12$.
   (c) $6\frac{1}{4} \div \frac{1}{2}$.

5. A prescription contains $\frac{5}{8}$ grain of ingredient A, $\frac{1}{4}$ grain of ingredient B, $\frac{1}{100}$ grain of ingredient C, and $\frac{3}{50}$ grain of ingredient D. Calculate the weight of the four ingredients in the prescription.

6. How many $\frac{1}{2000}$-grain doses can be obtained from $\frac{3}{80}$ grain of a certain drug?

7. A patient received the following doses of a drug:

   3 doses each containing $\frac{1}{20}$ grain
   3 doses each containing $\frac{1}{24}$ grain
   2 doses each containing $\frac{1}{32}$ grain
   2 doses each containing $\frac{1}{64}$ grain

Calculate the total amount of the drug received by the patient.

8. A capsule contains $\frac{1}{40}$ grain of ingredient A, $\frac{1}{4}$ grain of ingredient B, $\frac{1}{120}$ grain of ingredient C, and enough of ingredient D to make 4 grains. How many grains of ingredient D are in the capsule?

9. The adult dose of a certain drug is $\frac{1}{120}$ grain. If the child dose is $\frac{1}{6}$ of an adult dose, what fraction of a grain will be given if 8 doses are administered to a child?

10. Calculate the fractional difference between a $\frac{1}{100}$-grain tablet and a $\frac{1}{150}$-grain tablet of atropine sulfate.

11. The dose of a drug is $\frac{1}{120}$ grain. How many doses can be made from $\frac{2}{3}$ grain?

12. Write the following as decimals and add:

$$\frac{3}{1000}, \frac{75}{100}, \frac{3}{20}, \frac{5}{8}, \frac{13}{25}$$

13. Write the following as decimals and add:

$\frac{3}{5}$, $\frac{1}{20}$, $\frac{65}{1000}$, $\frac{19}{40}$, $\frac{3}{8}$

14. How many 0.000065-gram doses can be made from 0.130 gram of a drug?

15. Calculate the fractional difference between a $\frac{1}{30}$-grain and a $\frac{1}{120}$-grain tablet of strychnine sulfate.

16. Calculate the fractional difference between a $\frac{1}{24}$-grain and $\frac{1}{32}$-grain tablet of dihydromorphinone hydrochloride.

17. A patient received the following doses of a drug:

4 doses each containing $\frac{1}{120}$ grain
4 doses each containing $\frac{1}{100}$ grain
2 doses each containing $\frac{1}{150}$ grain
4 doses each containing $\frac{1}{200}$ grain

Calculate the total amount of the drug received by the patient.

18. A pharmacist had three grains of dihydromorphinone hydrochloride. He used it in preparing the following:

8 capsules each containing $\frac{1}{32}$ grain
8 capsules each containing $\frac{1}{24}$ grain
20 capsules each containing $\frac{1}{48}$ grain

How many grains of dihydromorphinone hydrochloride were left after he prepared the capsules?

CHAPTER II

RATIO AND PROPORTION

THE relative magnitude of two like quantities is called their *ratio.* Ratio is sometimes defined as *the quotient of two like numbers.* But in order not to lose sight of the fact that *two* quantities are being *compared,* this quotient is always expressed as an *operation,* not as a *result:* in other words, it is expressed as a *fraction,* and the fraction is interpreted as indicating the operation of dividing the numerator by the denominator.

The ratio of *20* and *10*, for example, is not expressed as *2* (that is, the quotient of *20* divided by *10*), but as the fraction $\frac{20}{10}$. And when this fraction is to be interpreted as a ratio, it is traditionally written *20:10* and always read *twenty to ten.* Similarly, when the fraction $\frac{1}{2}$ is to be interpreted as a ratio, it is traditionally written *1:2*, and it is read not as *one-half* but as *one to two.*

All the rules governing common fractions equally apply to a ratio. Of particular importance is the principle that *if the two terms of a ratio are multiplied or are divided by the same number, the value is unchanged*—the *value,* of course, being the quotient of the first term divided by the second.

For example, the ratio *20:4* has a value of *5*. Now, if both terms are multiplied by *2*, the ratio becomes *40:8*, still with a value of *5;* and if both terms are divided by *2*, the ratio becomes *10:2*, again with a value of *5*.

The terms of a ratio must be of the same kind: they may be two abstract numbers, or else they may be concrete numbers of the same denomination. Thus, we can have a ratio of *20* to *4*, or of *20 grains* to *4 grains.* The value of a ratio is always an abstract number expressing how many *times* greater or smaller the first term is than the second.

An expression that two ratios are equal in value is called a *proportion. Three* 5-grain tablets, for example, should contain *15* grains of active ingredient, and *twelve* 5-grain tablets should contain *60* grains. The ratio of *3* tablets to *12* tablets equals the ratio of *15* grains to *60* grains, for each ratio has the value of $\frac{1}{4}$. We may say, then, that the number of grains is *in proportion to* the number of tablets. And just as with equal fractions we may express the equation $\frac{3}{12} = \frac{15}{60}$, so with equal ratios we may express the proportion $3:12 = 15:60$, which is read *as three is to twelve, so fifteen is to sixty* or *three is to twelve as fifteen to sixty.*

The first and fourth terms of a proportion are called its *extremes,* and the second and third terms its *means:*

$$\textit{Means}$$

$$\overbrace{3:12}^{} = 15:60$$

Extremes

In any proportion *the product of the extremes is equal to the product of the means.* It follows, too, that *either extreme of a proportion is equal to the product of the means divided by the other extreme;* and *either mean is equal to the product of the extremes divided by the other mean.* This important rule is often called the *Rule of Three,* and it allows us to find the missing term of any proportion when the other three terms are known.

Most experienced calculators are indifferent to the order of terms in the proportions they devise. But both for the sake of clarity in exposition and for the greater mechanical accuracy gained if one gets into the habit of using a familiar routine when performing similar operations, the pattern used throughout this book follows the old custom of always putting the unknown term (represented by x) in the *fourth* place.

In setting up a proportion, we must remember that a proportion is an assertion that two ratios are *equal.* Hence, if the given facts indicate that the unknown fourth term must be greater than the third, then the second must be greater than the first. Otherwise the two ratios could not have the same value. And conversely, if the unknown fourth is to be smaller than the third, the second must be smaller than the first.

The following steps minimize the possibility of error in setting up a proportion:

Step 1. Write x *in the fourth position and indicate its denomination.* (In problems in applied arithmetic, every number in a proportion is a denominate number.)

Step 2. From the data, select or calculate a number of the same denomination as x *and write it in the third position.*

Step 3. Examine the condition of the problem. *If* x *is to be greater than the third term, write the greater of the remaining given numbers in the second position and the other in the first position; but if* x *is to be smaller, write the smaller of the remaining numbers in the second position and the greater in the first position.*

Having set up your proportion in this way, *and having checked to make sure that the terms of the first ratio are of a common denomination,* you may "solve for x" by the Rule of Three.

Examples:

If 3 tablets contain 15 grains of active ingredient, how many grains should be contained in 12 tablets?

Let x stand for the unknown number of grains, which inspection indicates will be greater in *12* tablets than the *15* grains contained in *3* tablets.

3 (tablets):12 (tablets) = 15 (grains):x (grains)

Or: 3:12 = 15:x (grains)

$$x = \frac{12 \times 15}{3} \text{ grains} = 60 \text{ grains, } \textit{answer.}$$

If 3 tablets contain 15 grains of active ingredient, how many tablets should contain 60 grains?

15 (grains):60 (grains) = 3 (tablets):x (tablets)

Or: 15:60 = 3:x (tablets)

$$x = \frac{60 \times 3}{15} \text{ tablets} = 12 \text{ tablets, } \textit{answer.}$$

If 12 tablets contain 60 grains of active ingredient, how many grains should 3 tablets contain?

12 (tablets):3 (tablets) = 60 (grains):x (grains)

Or: 12:3 = 60:x (grains)

$$x = \frac{3 \times 60}{12} \text{ grains} = 15 \text{ grains, } \textit{answer.}$$

If 12 tablets contain 60 grains of active ingredient, how many tablets should contain 15 grains?

60 (grains):15 (grains) = 12 (tablets):x (tablets)

Or: 60:15 = 12:x (tablets)

$$x = \frac{15 \times 12}{60} \text{ tablets} = 3 \text{ tablets, } \textit{answer.}$$

Note that in each of these problems you are given (*a*) a quantity of grains or of tablets and (*b*) another quantity of the same kind, with which you can set up your first ratio, using the pattern a:b or b:a according to what your common sense tells you must be the relationship between the third term and the unknown *x*. Obviously you cannot even make a start unless you can foresee whether *x* must be greater or smaller than the third term.

Proportions need not contain whole numbers. If common or decimal fractions are supplied in the data, they may be included in the proportion without changing the method.

Example:

> *If 35 pounds of a chemical cost $78.75, how much will 47 pounds cost?*
>
> 35 (pounds):47 (pounds) = ($)78.75:x (dollars)
>
> Or: 35:47 = 78.75:x (dollars)
>
> $x = \dfrac{47 \times 78.75}{35}$ dollars = $105.75, *answer.*

But, since calculating with common fractions is more complicated than with whole numbers or decimal fractions, it is useful to know— and wherever possible to apply—these two facts:

(1) *Two fractions having a common denominator are directly proportional to their numerators.*

$$\frac{\frac{60}{100}}{\frac{50}{100}} = \frac{60}{50}$$

Proof: $\dfrac{60}{100} \div \dfrac{50}{100} = \dfrac{60}{100} \times \dfrac{100}{50} = \dfrac{60}{50}$

(2) *Two fractions having a common numerator are inversely proportional to their denominators.*

$$\frac{\frac{2}{3}}{\frac{2}{7}} = \frac{7}{3}$$

Proof: $\frac{2}{3} \div \frac{2}{7} = \frac{2}{3} \times \frac{7}{2} = \frac{7}{3}$

Examples:

If 1½ grains of a drug represent 18 doses, how many doses are represented in ¼ grain?

1½ grains = $\frac{3}{2}$ grains = $\frac{6}{4}$ grains

$\frac{6}{4}$ (grains):$\frac{1}{4}$ (grain) = 18 (doses):x (doses)

Or: 6:1 = 18:x (doses)

$$x = \frac{1 \times 18}{6} \text{ doses} = 3 \text{ doses, } answer.$$

If 30 milliliters represent $\frac{1}{6}$ of the volume of a prescription, how many milliliters will represent $\frac{1}{4}$ of the volume?

$\frac{1}{6}$ (volume):$\frac{1}{4}$ (volume) = 30 (ml.):x (ml.)

Or: 4:6 = 30:x (ml.)

$$x = \frac{6 \times 30}{4} \text{ ml.} = 45 \text{ ml., } answer.$$

The use of proportion in pharmaceutical problems is abundantly illustrated in the text. The following miscellany reveals a variety of applications of the method.

Practice Problems

Solve by proportion:

1. If 250 pounds of a chemical cost $60.00, what will be the cost of 135 pounds?

2. If 75 pounds of a chemical cost $250, what will be the cost of 95 pounds?

3. A formula for 1,250 capsules contains 3.25 grams of arsenic trioxide. How much arsenic trioxide should be used in preparing 350 capsules?

4. If 100 capsules contain $\frac{3}{8}$ grain of an active ingredient, how much of the ingredient will 48 capsules contain?

5. If 450 pounds of Medicinal Soft Soap cost $103.50, what will be the cost of 33 pounds?

6. If 50 tablets contain 0.625 gram of an active ingredient, how many tablets can be prepared from 31.25 grams of the ingredient?

7. If 24 pounds of a chemical cost $15.60, how many pounds can be bought for $26.00?

8. If 15 gallons of a certain liquid cost $7.25, how much will 4 gallons cost?

9. If 125 gallons of a mouth rinse contain 20 grams of a coloring agent, how many grams will 160 gallons contain?

10. If 50 tablets contain 1.5 grams of active ingredient, how much of the ingredient will 1,375 tablets contain?

11. If 3 doses of a liquid preparation contain 7.5 grains of a substance, how many grains will 32 doses contain?

12. If 1.625 grams of a coloring agent are used to color 250 liters of a certain solution, how many liters could be colored by using 0.750 gram?

13. How many grains of a substance are needed for 350 tablets if 75 tablets contain 3 grains of the substance?

14. If 48 pints of a preparation contain $2\frac{1}{2}$ grains of a certain substance, how much will 5 pints contain?

15. If 12 pounds of a drug cost $9.60, how many pounds can be bought for $58.00?

16. If 1000 grams of an ointment contain 0.875 gram of a certain ingredient, how much of the ingredient will 625 grams contain?

CHAPTER III

THE METRIC SYSTEM

THE *measure* of a quantity is the number of times that it contains a standard quantity taken as a *unit*. A 5-pound weight, for instance, contains five times the weight of a standard 1-pound unit. Some kinds of quantities measured are temperature, length, area, volume, and time—respectively measured in such familiar units as degrees, feet, square miles, gallons, and hours.

The standard subdivisions and multiples of the unit in any system of measurement are called *denominations*, and we have seen that figures specifying their number are called *denominate numbers*. So, in the expression "ten cents" the term "cents" designates a denomination in our monetary system, and "ten" is a denominate number. We find it convenient, as a rule, to express large quantities in terms of large denominations, and small quantities in small—as great distances are measured by the common system in miles, short intervals in inches. Denominations are understood to stand in a fixed ratio with the unit upon which the system is based—as a cent has a fixed value of $\frac{1}{100}$ of a dollar—and therefore they have a fixed ratio with each other. A statement of the mutual relationships of denominations of the same kind is called a *table of measure*.

The *metric* or *decimal system* of measure, formulated by the revolutionary French government in the late eighteenth century, has been the legal standard in the United States since 1893, and all other systems are referred to it for official comparison.

Its acceptance by scientists the world over has resulted from these two merits: (1) its tables are simple, for they are based upon the decimal system of notation, and the greater of two consecutive denominations of the same kind is always ten times the less; (2) its tables of length, volume, and weight are conveniently correlated, for the meter is the fundamental unit of the system.

Each table of the metric system contains a definitive unit. The *meter* is the unit of length, the *liter* of volume, and the *gram* of weight.

Subdivisions and multiples of these principal units are indicated respectively by Latin and Greek prefixes:

Latin:
  milli-   to denote one-thousandth of the unit,
  centi-   to denote one-hundredth of the unit,
  deci-   to denote one-tenth of the unit;

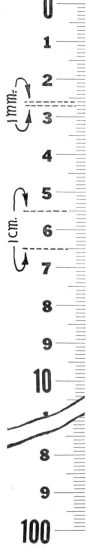

Section of Meter Stick (actual scale).

Greek:

deka-   to denote ten times the unit,
hekto-   to denote one hundred times the unit,
kilo-   to denote one thousand times the unit,
myria-   to denote ten thousand times the unit.

Anyone who wishes to become quickly used to the system should note that our money is "metrically" or decimally computed. The names of the chief fractions of the dollar unit are a clue to their value: a *mill* (for which we have no coin) is one-thousandth, a *cent* one-hundredth, and a *dime* one-tenth of the unit.

MEASURE OF LENGTH

The meter is the fundamental unit of this system. It has been determined as approximately one-ten-millionth part of the distance from the earth's equator to the north pole.

Table of metric length:

$$
\begin{aligned}
10 \text{ millimeters (mm.)} &= 1 \text{ centimeter (cm.)} \\
10 \text{ centimeters} &= 1 \text{ decimeter (dm.)} \\
10 \text{ decimeters} &= 1 \text{ meter (M.)} \\
10 \text{ meters} &= 1 \text{ dekameter (Dm.)} \\
10 \text{ dekameters} &= 1 \text{ hektometer (Hm.)} \\
10 \text{ hektometers} &= 1 \text{ kilometer (Km.)} \\
10 \text{ kilometers} &= 1 \text{ myriameter (Mm.)}
\end{aligned}
$$

Further subdivisions of the unit are occasionally used. A millionth of a meter (a thousandth of a millimeter) is the *micron* (μ) used to express such small things as the diameter of a red blood corpuscle. A thousandth of a micron is the *millimicron* (mμ).

As indicated in the table, pharmaceutical custom requires small letters for abbreviations of subdivisions, and initial capital letters for abbreviations of the unit and multiples of the unit.

The table may also be written:

$$
\begin{aligned}
1 \text{ meter} &= 1000 \text{ millimeters} \\
&= 100 \text{ centimeters} \\
&= 10 \text{ decimeters} \\
&= 0.1 \text{ dekameter} \\
&= 0.01 \text{ hektometer} \\
&= 0.001 \text{ kilometer} \\
&= 0.0001 \text{ myriameter}
\end{aligned}
$$

The most commonly used denominations are the millimeter, centimeter, and meter, as if the table were:

1000 mm. or 100 cm. = 1 M.

MEASURE OF VOLUME

The *liter* is the metric unit of volume. It represents the volume of the cube of one-tenth of a meter—that is, of one cubic decimeter.

Table of metric volume:

10 milliliters (ml. or mils)	= 1 centiliter (cl.)
10 centiliters	= 1 deciliter (dl.)
10 deciliters	= 1 liter (L.)
10 liters	= 1 dekaliter (Dl.)
10 dekaliters	= 1 hektoliter (Hl.)
10 hektoliters	= 1 kiloliter (Kl.)

This table may also be written:

1 liter	= 1000 milliliters
	= 100 centiliters
	= 10 deciliters
	= 0.1 dekaliter
	= 0.01 hektoliter
	= 0.001 kiloliter

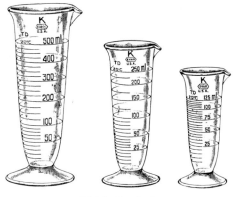

Metric Graduates.

Although in theory the liter was meant to have the volume of one cubic decimeter, or a thousand cubic centimeters, precise modern measurement has discovered that the standard liter contains slightly less than this volume. But the discrepancy is insignificant for most practical purposes; and since the milliliter has so very nearly the volume of a cubic centimeter, the *United States Pharmacopeia* states: "One milliliter (ml.) is used herein as the equivalent of 1 cubic centimeter (cc.)."

The most commonly used denominations are the milliliter and liter, as if the table were simply:

$$1000 \text{ ml.} = 1 \text{ L.}$$

MEASURE OF WEIGHT

The unit of weight in the metric system is the *gram*, which is the weight of 1 cubic centimeter of water at 4 degrees Centigrade, its temperature of greatest density.

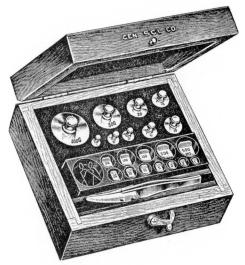

A set of Metric Weights.

Table of metric weight:

10 milligrams (mg.) = 1 centigram (cg.)
10 centigrams = 1 decigram (dg.)
10 decigrams = 1 gram (Gm.)
10 grams = 1 dekagram (Dg.)
10 dekagrams = 1 hektogram (Hg.)
10 hektograms = 1 kilogram (Kg. or *kilo*)

This table may also be written:

$$1 \text{ gram } = 1000 \text{ milligrams}$$
$$= 100 \text{ centigrams}$$
$$= 10 \text{ decigrams}$$
$$= 0.1 \text{ dekagram}$$
$$= 0.01 \text{ hektogram}$$
$$= 0.001 \text{ kilogram}$$

The denominations most commonly used are the milligram, gram, and kilogram, as if the table were:

$$1000 \text{ milligrams } = 1 \text{ gram}$$
$$1000 \text{ grams } = 1 \text{ kilogram}$$

Metric weight also includes the *microgram*, which is one-thousandth of a milligram:

$$1 \text{ microgram (mcg.) } = 0.001 \text{ mg.}$$
$$1000 \text{ (mcg.) } = 1 \text{ mg.}$$

According to the *United States Pharmacopeia*, "The abbreviation 'mcg.' has come into general use in pharmaceutical literature and labeling. The term 'gamma,' symbolized by γ, is customarily used for microgram in biochemical literature, while 'μg' is generally accepted as the abbreviation in the literature of physics and physical chemistry. As yet, there is no international convention on the abbreviation and symbol."

When prescriptions are written in the metric system, arabic numerals are always used and are written *before* the abbreviations for the denominations, if such abbreviations are used. Quantities of weight are written as grams and *decimals* of a gram and volumes are written as milliliters and *decimals* thereof.

Example:

℞	Codeine Phosphate	0.26 Gm.
	Ammonium Chloride	6.0 Gm.
	Cherry Syrup ad	120.0 ml.
	Sig. 4 ml. as directed.	

FUNDAMENTAL OPERATIONS

To reduce to lower or higher denominations:

The restatement of a given quantity in terms of a higher or lower denomination is called *reduction*. "Thirty minutes" may equally be expressed as a "half hour" or, if occasion requires, as

"1800 seconds." The process of changing from higher to lower denominations is known as *reduction descending;* from lower to higher, *reduction ascending.*

A length, a volume, or a weight expressed in one denomination of the metric system may be expressed in another denomination by simply moving the decimal point. In doing this, it is generally best to reduce the given quantity first to the *unit* and then to the required denomination.

To change a metric denomination to the next smaller denomination, move the decimal point one place to the right. To change to the next larger denomination, move the decimal point one place to the left.

Examples:

   Reduce 0.25 kilogram to milligrams.

     0.25 Kg. = 250 Gm. = 250000 mg., *answer.*

   Reduce 250 micrograms to grams.

     250 mcg. = 0.250 mg. = 0.000250 Gm., *answer.*

   Reduce 85 microns to centimeters.

     85 μ = 0.085 mm. = 0.0085 cm., *answer.*

   Reduce 2.525 liters to milliliters

     2.525 L. = 2525 ml., *answer.*

To add or subtract:

To add or subtract quantities in the metric system, we must reduce them to a *common denomination*—preferably the unit of the table—and arrange their denominate numbers for addition or subtraction as ordinary decimals.

Examples:

   Add 1 Kg., 250 mg., and 7.5 Gm. Express the total in grams.

$$
\begin{array}{rcl}
1 \text{ Kg.} & = & 1000. \quad \text{Gm.} \\
250 \text{ mg.} & = & 0.250 \text{ Gm.} \\
7.5 \text{ Gm.} & = & 7.5 \quad \text{Gm.} \\
\hline
\end{array}
$$

     1007.750 Gm. or 1008 Gm., *answer.*

Add 4 L., 375 ml., and 0.75 L. Express the total in milliliters.

4 L. = 4000 ml.
375 ml. =   375 ml.
0.75 L. =   750 ml.
———————
5125 ml , *answer.*

*A capsule contains the following amounts of medicinal substances:
0.075 Gm., 20 mg., 0.0005 Gm., 4 mg., and 500 mcg.   What is
the total weight of the substances in the capsule?*

0.075 Gm. = 0.075 Gm.
20 mg. = 0.020 Gm.
0.0005 Gm. = 0.0005 Gm.
4 mg. = 0.004 Gm.
500 mcg. = 0.0005 Gm.
———————
0.1000 Gm. or 100 mg., *answer.*

Subtract 2.5 mg. from 4.850 Gm.

4.850 Gm. = 4.850 Gm.
2.5 mg. = 0.0025 Gm.
———————
4.8475 Gm. or 4.848 Gm., *answer.*

*A prescription calls for 0.060 Gm. of one ingredient, 2.5 mg. of
another, and enough of a third to make 0.5 Gm.   How many milligrams of the third ingredient should be used?*

Interpreting all quantities as accurate to the nearest tenth of
a milligram—

1st ingredient: 0.0600 Gm. = 0.0600 Gm.
2nd ingredient: 2.5 mg. = 0.0025 Gm.
———————
0.0625 Gm.

Total weight: 0.5000 Gm.
Weight of 1st and 2nd: 0.0625 Gm.
———————
Weight of 3rd: 0.4375 Gm. or 437.5 mg., *answer.*

To multiply or divide:

Since all measurements in the metric system are expressed in
single denominations, problems involving multiplication and division are solved by the methods used for any decimal numbers.

Examples:

> *Multiply 820 ml. by 12.5 and express the result in liters.*
>
> 820 ml. $\times$ 12.5 = 10250 ml. = 10.25 L., *answer.*
>
> *Divide 0.465 Gm. by 15 and express the result in milligrams.*
>
> 0.465 Gm. $\div$ 15 = 0.031 Gm. = 31 mg., *answer.*

Practice Problems

1. Add 0.5 Kg., 50 mg., and 2.5 Gm.   Reduce the result to grams.

2. Add 7.25 L. and 875 ml. Reduce the result to milliliters.

3. Reduce 25 mcg. to grams.

4. Divide 0.875 Gm. by 15 and reduce the result to milligrams.

5. Reduce 0.5 mg. to grams.

6. Multiply 30 mg. by 24 and reduce the result to grams.

7. How many 4-ml. doses may be obtained from 2 L. of a liquid?

8. Multiply 875 ml. by 12.5 and reduce the result to liters.

9. Multiply 0.00025 Gm. by $\frac{9}{20}$ and reduce the result to milligrams.

10. Multiply 0.4 mg. by 630 and reduce the result to grams.

11. Add 1 Kg., 150 mg., and 6.5 Gm.

12. Reduce the tenth aliquot of 0.2 Gm. to milligrams.

13. Reduce the eighth aliquot of 2 L. to milliliters.

14. What fraction of 0.002 Gm. is 0.5 mg.?

15. A capsule contains the following amounts of medicinal substances: 0.075 Gm., 20 mg., 0.0005 Gm., and 3 mg. What is the total amount of material in the capsule?

16. Add 0.040 Gm. and 0.5 mg., multiply the result by $\frac{2}{15}$, and reduce the result to milligrams.

17. A 1000-ml. solution contains 0.065 Gm. of active ingredient. What is the volume of the twelfth aliquot? How many milligrams of active ingredient will it contain?

18. Reduce the sixth aliquot of 4.55 Gm. to milligrams.

19. Reduce 1.256 Gm. to micrograms, to milligrams, and to kilograms.

20. How many 0.1-ml. doses may be obtained from 1 L. of a liquid?

21. Multiply 16.99 mg. by 75 and subtract the result from 3.968 Gm.

22. Divide 10.79 mg. by 100, multiply the result by 675, and reduce the result to grams.

23. Multiply 255 mg. by 380, divide the result by 0.85, and reduce the result to grams.

24. Divide 0.03 Gm. by 8000 and reduce the result to milligrams.

25. Multiply 0.003 Gm. by 500 and reduce the fiftieth aliquot of the result to milligrams.

26. Divide 8 Gm. by 3000 and reduce the result to milligrams.

27. Divide 4 Gm. by 8000, subtract the result from 4 Gm., and reduce the result to milligrams.

28. Divide 2 L. by 150 and reduce the result to milliliters.

29. Add 19 mg., 0.016 Gm., and 2.0 Gm.; multiply the result by 75; and express the result in grams.

30. Multiply 0.05 mg. by the quotient of 120 ÷ 0.5 and reduce the result to grams.

31. Subtract 250 mg. from 4.85 Gm.

32. What is the twelfth aliquot of 72 × 0.0006 mg.?

33. Multiply 50.32 mg. by 35, subtract the result from 2 Gm., divide the result by 10, and express the result in milligrams.

34. Multiply 0.45 Gm. by 0.33 and reduce the result to milligrams.

35. Adhesive Plaster has a tensile strength of not less than 20.41 Kg. per 2.54 cm. of width. Reduce these quantities to grams and millimeters.

36. Reduce 85 μ to millimeters.

37. Reduce 125 mcg. to milligrams.

38. Reduce 9520 μ to millimeters.

39. Subtract 245 mg. from 135.004 Gm.

40. Subtract 125 mg. from 10 Gm.

41. Divide 0.04 Gm. by 64 and express the result in milligrams.

42. A liquid contains 0.25 mg. of a substance per milliliter. How many milligrams of the substance will 3.5 L. contain?

43. Add 280 Gm. and 700 mg., divide by 8, and express the result in grams.

44. A prescription calls for 0.060 Gm. of one ingredient, 2.5 mg. of another, and enough of a third to make 2 Gm. How many milligrams of the third ingredient are required?

45. A pill contains 45 mg. of one ingredient, 65 mg. of a second, and 1.3 mg. of a third. Express in grams the amount of each ingredient needed for 200 pills.

46. Multiply 0.004603 Gm. by 48 and subtract the product from 1 Gm.

47. Multiply 0.005585 Gm. by 65 and reduce the product to milligrams.

48. If 2 mcg. of riboflavin is the indicated minimum daily adult requirement, how many milligrams of riboflavin are in a vitamin capsule containing ⅛ the minimum requirement?

49. A vitamin capsule contains 1.5 mg. of Ingredient A, 0.130 Gm. of Ingredient B, 250 mcg. of Ingredient C, and enough of Ingredient D to make 0.500 Gm. How many milligrams of Ingredient D are in the capsule?

50. If 480 ml. of a certain solution contain 0.24 Gm. of a chemical, (a) what is the volume of the thirtieth aliquot? (b) how many milligrams of the chemical will the thirtieth aliquot contain? (c) how many micrograms of the chemical are in this aliquot?

51. One tablet of thyroid extract represents 125 mcg. of thyroxin. How many tablets should be taken by a person requiring 0.0005 Gm. of thyroxin?

52. How many grams of thiamine hydrochloride should be used to prepare 500 tablets each containing 200 mcg. of thiamine hydrochloride?

53. A prescription for a capsule specifies 0.05 mg. of Ingredient A, 50 mg. of Ingredient B, and 0.5 mg. of Ingredient C. How many grams of each ingredient are needed to make 250 capsules?

54. A certain formula specifies 0.625 Gm. of a substance in 2.5 L. How many milligrams of the substance are in each milliliter?

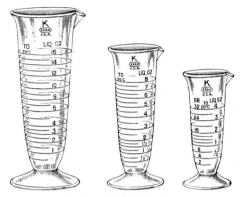

Apothecaries' Graduates.

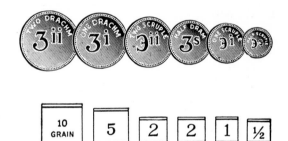

A set of Apothecaries' Weights.

Table of avoirdupois measure of weight:

$437\frac{1}{2}$ or 437.5 grains (gr.) = 1 ounce (oz.)

16 ounces (7000 grains) = 1 pound (lb.)

This table may also be written:

lb.	oz.	gr.
1	16	7000
	1	437.5

Only one denomination has a value common to the apothecaries' and avoirdupois systems of measuring weight, namely, the *grain*. The other denominations bearing the same name have quite different values. It is to prevent possible confusion with *gr.*, the abbreviation of *grain*, that the abbreviation for *gram*, in the metric system, is capitalized: *Gm.*

The pharmacist buys by the avoirdupois system, for manufacturers and wholesalers customarily supply drugs and chemicals, when they are sold by weight, in avoirdupois units only. The pharmacist likewise sells in bulk "over the counter" by the avoirdupois system.

In contrast with the invariable use of *simple* quantities in the metric system, in the common systems measurements are recorded whenever possible in *compound quantities*—that is, quantities expressed in two or more denominations. So, *20 f℥* may be used during the process of calculating, but as a final result it should be recorded as *1 pt. 4 f℥*. The process of reducing a quantity to a compound quantity beginning with the highest possible denomination is called *simplification*. Decimal fractions may be used in calculation, but the subdivision of a minim or grain in a final result is recorded as a *common fraction*.

When prescriptions are written in the common system, the numbers are written in roman numerals and *follow* the abbreviations or symbols for the denominations.

Example:

℞	Codeine Phosphate	gr. iv
	Ammonium Chloride	ℨ iss
	Cherry Syrup ad	f℥ iv
	Sig. ℥i as directed.	

FUNDAMENTAL OPERATIONS

To reduce a compound quantity to a simple quantity:

Before a compound quantity can be used in a calculation it must usually be expressed in terms of a single denomination. To do so, reduce each of the denominations in the compound quantity to the required denomination and add the results.

Examples:

Reduce ℥ss ℨii ℈i to grains.

$$℥ss = \tfrac{1}{2} \times 480 \text{ gr.} = 240 \text{ gr.}$$
$$ℨii = 2 \times 60 \text{ gr.} = 120 \text{ gr.}$$
$$℈i = 1 \times 20 \text{ gr.} = 20 \text{ gr.}$$

                    380 gr., *answer.*

Reduce f℥ iv f℈ iiss to fluidrachms.

$$f℥iv = 4 \times 8 \text{ f℈} = 32 \text{ f℈}$$
$$f℈iiss = 2\tfrac{1}{2} \text{ f℈}$$

                    $34\tfrac{1}{2}$ f℈, *answer.*

To reduce simple quantities to weighable or measurable denominations:

Before being weighed, a given quantity should be expressed in denominations equal to the actual weights on hand; and before a volume is measured, a given quantity should be expressed in denominations represented by the calibrations on the graduate.

Examples:

Change 165 grains to weighable apothecaries' units.

By selecting larger weight units to account for as many of the required grains as possible, beginning with the largest, we find that we may use the following weights:

ʒii, ʒss, ℈ss, 5 gr., *answer.*

Check: ʒii = 120 gr.
      ʒss = 30 gr.
      ℈ss = 10 gr.
    5 gr. =   5 gr.
           165 gr., *total.*

In enlarging a formula, we find that we are to measure 90 fʒ of a liquid. Using two graduates, if necessary, in what denominations may we measure this quantity?

11 f℥ and 2 fʒ, *answer.*

Check: 11 f℥ = 88 fʒ
     2 fʒ = 2 fʒ
          90 fʒ, *total.*

To add or subtract:

To add or subtract quantities in the common systems, reduce to a common denomination, add or subtract, and reduce the result (unless it is to be used in further calculation) to a compound quantity.

Examples:

A formula contains ℈ii of Ingredient A, ʒi of Ingredient B, ℥iv of Ingredient C, and gr. viiss of Ingredient D. Calculate the total weight of the ingredients.

    ℈ii = 2 × 20 gr. =   40 gr.
    ʒi = 1 × 60 gr. =   60 gr.
    ℥iv = 4 × 60 gr. = 240 gr.
        gr. viiss =   7½ gr.

       347½ gr. = 5 ʒ 2 ℈ 7½ gr., *answer.*

A pharmacist had 1 gallon of alcohol. At different times he dispensed f℥iv, Oii, f℥viii, and f℈iv. What volume of alcohol was left?

$$
\begin{aligned}
\text{f℥ iv} &= 4 \ \ \text{f℥} \\
\text{Oii} = 2 \times 16 \ \text{f℥} &= 32 \ \ \text{f℥} \\
\text{f℥ viii} &= 8 \ \ \text{f℥} \\
\text{f℈ iv} &= \tfrac{1}{2} \ \text{f℥}
\end{aligned}
$$

$44\frac{1}{2}$ f℥, *total dispensed.*

$$
\begin{aligned}
1 \text{ gal.} &= 128 \ \ \text{f℥} \\
&-44\tfrac{1}{2} \ \text{f℥}
\end{aligned}
$$

$83\frac{1}{2}$ f℥ $= 5$ pt. 3 f℥ 4 f℈, *answer.*

To multiply or divide:

A *simple* quantity may be multiplied or divided by any *pure* number—as *12 × 10 oz. = 120 oz.* or *7 lb. 8 oz.*

But if *both* terms in division are derived from denominate numbers (as when we express one quantity as a fraction of another) they must be reduced to a *common* denomination before division can be performed.

A *compound* quantity is most easily multiplied or divided, and with least chance of careless error, if it is first reduced to a *simple* quantity: *2 × 8 f℥ 6 f℈ = 2 × 70 f℈ = 140 f℈ or 17 f℥ 4 f℈.*

The *result* of multiplication should be (1) left as it is, if it is to be used in further calculations, (2) simplified, or (3) reduced to weighable or measureable denominations.

Examples:

A prescription for 24 powders calls for gr. ¼ of Ingredient A, ℈ss of Ingredient B, and gr. v of Ingredient C in each powder. How much of each ingredient should be used in compounding the prescription?

24 × gr.¼ = 6 gr. of Ingredient A,
24 × ½ ℈ = 12 ℈, or 4 ʒ of Ingredient B,
24 × gr.v = 120 gr., or 2 ʒ of Ingredient C, *answers.*

A formula for 24 capsules contains ℈ss of one ingredient, ʒi of another, and ʒiiss of a third. How many grains of each ingredient will be contained in each capsule?

℈ss = 10 gr., and $\frac{10}{24}$ gr. = $\frac{5}{12}$ gr.,
ʒi = 60 gr., and $\frac{60}{24}$ gr. = $2\frac{1}{2}$ gr.,
ʒiiss = 150 gr., and $\frac{150}{24}$ gr. = $6\frac{1}{4}$ gr., *answers.*

How many 15-minim doses can be obtained from a mixture containing fℨ iii of one ingredient and fʒ ii of another?

fℨ iii = 3 × 480 ℳ = 1440 ℳ
fʒ ii = 2 × 60 ℳ = 120 ℳ
_____

1560 ℳ, *total.*

$\frac{1560}{15}$ doses = 104 doses, *answer.*

RELATIONSHIP OF AVOIRDUPOIS AND APOTHECARIES' WEIGHTS

As noted above, the *grain* is the same in both the avoirdupois and apothecaries' systems of weight, but other denominations with the same names are not equal.

To convert from either system to the other, first reduce the given quantity to grains in the one system, and then reduce the result to any desired denomination in the other system.

The custom of buying drugs by avoirdupois weight and dispensing them by apothecaries' weight leads to problems many of which can be most conveniently solved by proportion.

Examples:

Convert ℨ ii ʒ ii to avoirdupois weight.

ℨ ii = 2 × 480 gr. = 960 gr.
ʒ ii = 2 × 60 gr. = 120 gr.
_____

Total: 1080 gr.

1 oz. = 437.5 gr.
$\frac{1080}{437.5}$ oz. = 2 oz. 205 gr., *answer.*

How many grains of a chemical are left in a 1-oz. bottle after ʒ vii are dispensed from it?

1 oz. = 1 × 437.5 gr. = 437.5 gr.
ʒ vii = 7 × 60 gr. = 420.0 gr.
_____

Difference: 17.5 gr., *answer.*

If a drug costs $1.75 per oz., what is the cost of 2 ʒ?

1 oz. = 437.5 gr., and 2 ʒ = 120 gr.

437.5 (gr.): 120 (gr.) = 1.75 ($): x ($)

x = $0.48, *answer.*

Practice Problems

1. Reduce each of the following quantities to grains:
   - (a) ʒii ℈ss.
   - (b) ℥ii ʒss.
   - (c) ℥i ʒss ℈i.
   - (d) ʒi ℈i gr.x.

2. Reduce 0i ℥ii to fluidrachms.

3. Reduce each of the following quantities to weighable apothecaries' denominations:
   - (a) 158 gr.
   - (b) 175 gr.
   - (c) 210 gr.
   - (d) 75 gr.
   - (e) 96 gr.

4. What is the weight, in grains, of a mixture containing ℥ii of one ingredient, ʒii of another, and ℈i of a third?

5. A pharmacist had ½ gallon of alcohol. At different times he dispensed f℥iss, 0i, f℥iv, and f℥iv. What volume of alcohol was left?

6. How many f℥ii doses can be obtained from f℥xii of a liquid preparation?

7. How many 15-grain doses can be obtained from ℥ss of a powder?

8. How many f℥iv bottles of iodine tincture can be obtained from 2 pt. of iodine tincture?

9. How many f℥ii bottles of cough syrup can be obtained from 5 gal. of the cough syrup?

10. How many grains of a chemical are left in a 1-oz. package after ʒii and ℈i have been dispensed?

11. How many 5-grain capsules of aspirin can be made from a 4-oz. package of aspirin?

12. How many 10-grain capsules of reduced iron can be made from ½ lb. of reduced iron?

13. How many ¼-gr. tablets of morphine sulfate can be made from ⅛ oz. of morphine sulfate?

14. What is the volume, in fluidounces, of a mixture containing ½ gal. of one liquid, 2 pt. of another, and 96 f℥ of a third?

15. What volume should a physician prescribe if he wishes to write a prescription for 32 f℥ii doses?

16. A prescription contains gr.x of one ingredient, ℥i of a secon and Ɔii of a third. How many 5-grain doses can be made fr the mixture?

17. A formula for 40 powders contains Ɔi of one ingredient, ℥i of another, and ℥iv of a third. Express the amount, in grains, of each ingredient in each powder.

18. How many grains of a chemical are left in a 1-oz. bottle after enough of it has been used to make 2000 tablets each containing $\frac{1}{200}$ gr. of the chemical?

19. If a chemical costs $1.75 per oz., what is the cost of ℥iii?

20. A pharmacist compounded a prescription for 100 capsules each containing $\frac{1}{4}$ gr. of codeine phosphate. If 1 oz. of codeine phosphate costs $17.50, calculate the cost of the amount used in compounding the prescription.

21. How many $\frac{1}{120}$-gr. doses of atropine sulfate can be obtained from $\frac{1}{8}$-oz. bottle of atropine sulfate?

22. A cough syrup contains Ɔss of ammonium chloride in f℥iv. How many grains should be used in preparing 1 gallon of the syrup?

23. How many $\frac{1}{32}$-gr. tablets can be made from $\frac{1}{8}$ oz. of Dilaudid?

24. If a chemical costs $2.50 per oz., what is the cost of ℥iv?

25. How many grains of a chemical are left in a $\frac{1}{4}$-oz. bottle after enough of it is used to make 5000 tablets each containing $\frac{1}{200}$ gr. of the chemical?

26. A pharmacist bought 2 oz. of a chemical from a wholesaler. At different times he dispensed ℥i, ℥ii, 15 gr., and ℥iv. How many grains of the chemical were left?

27. In checking a narcotic file, a pharmacist found that the following quantities of codeine phosphate had been used from an originally 1-oz. bottle:

$$\text{℞ # 1—gr.v}$$
$$\text{℞ # 2—Ɔi}$$
$$\text{℞ # 3—℥ss}$$
$$\text{℞ # 4—Ɔss}$$
$$\text{℞ # 5—gr.iiss}$$

How many grains of codeine phosphate were left in the bottle?

CHAPTER V

CONVERSION

WHEN we want to measure something, we are theoretically privileged to select any system of measure we please. But when we are required to measure a given quantity, in a formula, say, or in a prescription, the instrument at hand—the graduate or set of weights—may not happen to measure in the system specified. Consequently, a quantity called for in one system may have to be translated to its equivalent in the system of our available instrument. This translation is called *conversion*.

Conversion is frequently required in pharmacy, for the metric and common systems are sometimes jumbled together in everyday experience. Pounds may not be added to grams, nor may scruples be subtracted from avoirdupois ounces, nor may a ratio be made between liters and fluidounces; and we must convert to a single system (as well as reduce to a common denomination) all miscellaneous quantities that are to be in any way compared.

Denominations in the metric system are incommensurate with those of the common systems. Hence there can be no *exact* equivalence. But the International Bureau of Standards has measured the meter in terms of inches and the kilogram in terms of pounds so precisely as to be able to express the linear equivalence with 7-figure accuracy and the weight equivalence with 9-figure accuracy. Such precision, of course, is not intended to have any ordinary practical application. From these figures the relationships of other denominations can be calculated as accurately as necessary for a given purpose.

The measurement of a denomination of one system in terms of another system is properly called a *conversion factor*. Any one conversion factor is sufficient to serve as a bridge between two systems; but in practice it is convenient to have a choice of several. We may use the equation *1 Gm.* = *15.432 gr.*, for example, in converting a number of grams to grains; but in converting grains to grams, a more useful equation is *1 gr.* = *0.065 Gm.* Again, it is convenient to have one equation for converting a large denomination directly to a large denomination, and another for converting a small denomination to a small denomination.

The question just how accurate our conversion factors should be has not been satisfactorily established. The *United States Pharmacopeia* allows very rough approximations when our calculations concern dosage (see Chapter VI), but insists that we use "exact" equivalents when we convert quantities in a prescription or official formula. Yet, as previously pointed out (footnote, p. 18), the tables of "exact" equivalents in the *Pharmacopeia* itself admit of a range from 1- or 2-figure up to 6-figure accuracy.

Ordinary pharmaceutical procedure actually seeks something between 2- and 3-figure accuracy in final results, and the following convenient figures, although not wholly consistent, are in widespread use and are more than sufficient for all practical purposes. *These should be memorized.*

SOME PRACTICAL EQUIVALENTS

1 M. = 39. 37 in.
1 in. = 2.54 cm.

1 ml. = 16.23 ℳ
1 f℥ = 29.57 ml.
1 pt. = 473 ml.

know this cold

1 Gm. = 15.432 gr.
1 Kg. = 2.2 lb.[1]
1 gr. = 0.065 Gm. or 65 mg.
1 oz. = 28.35 Gm.
1 ℥ = 31.1 Gm.
1 lb. = 454 Gm.
1 oz. = 437.5 gr.
1 ℥ = 480 gr.

[1] Since this conversion factor is an abbreviation of 2.20, it is really accurate to 3 figures.

Note that such equivalents may be used in two ways. For example, to convert a number of fluidounces to milliliters, *multiply* by *29.57;* and to convert a number of milliliters to fluidounces, *divide* by *29.57.*

Note likewise that to the question: *Must we round off results so as to contain no more significant figures than are contained in the conversion factor?*—the answer is *Yes.* If we desire greater accuracy, we should use a more accurate conversion factor. But to the question:

*If a formula includes the 1-figure quantity 5 Gm., and we convert it
to grains, must we round off the result to 1 significant figure?*—the
answer is decidedly *No.* We should interpret the quantity given
in a formula as expressing the precision we are expected to achieve
in compounding—usually not less than 3-figure accuracy. Hence,
5 Gm. in a formula or prescription should be interpreted as meaning
at least *5.00 Gm.*

CONVERSION OF LINEAR QUANTITIES

To convert metric lengths to common equivalents:

We may reduce any given metric length to meters—by moving
the decimal point—and then multiply this quantity by *39.37* (the
number of inches equivalent to each meter) to get inches. But if
the metric quantity is small, it may be more convenient to reduce
it to centimeters and divide by *2.54* to get inches.

Example:

> *The fiber length of a sample of purified cotton is 6.35 mm.
> Express the length in inches.*

> 6.35 mm. = 0.635 cm.

> $\frac{0.635}{2.54}$ in. = 0.250 in., or $\frac{1}{4}$ in., *answer.*

To convert common lengths to metric equivalents:

If given a length of a yard or more, reduce it to inches and divide
by *39.37* to get meters. If given a shorter length, reduce it to
inches and multiply by *2.54* to get centimeters.

Example:

> *A medicinal plaster measures 4½ in. by 6½ in. What are its
> dimensions in centimeters?*

> Assuming 3-figure precision in the measurement,

> 4½ or 4.50 × 2.54 cm. = 11.4 cm. wide,

> 6½ or 6.50 × 2.54 cm. = 16.5 cm. long, *answers.*

CONVERSION OF LIQUID QUANTITIES

To convert metric volumes to apothecaries' fluid equivalents:

For small volumes, multiply the number of milliliters by *16.23* to
get minims—and reduce the result to measurable units if necessary.

For larger volumes, reduce the given volume to milliliters and divide by *29.57* to get fluidounces or by *473* to get pints.

Examples:

Convert 0.4 ml. to minims.

To achieve 2-figure precision,

0.40 × 16.23 ℳ = 6.492 or 6.5 ℳ, *answer.*

Convert 2.5 L. to fluidounces.

2.5 L. = 2500 ml.

Assuming 3-figure precision,

$\frac{2500}{29.57}$ = 84.5 f℥, *answer.*

To convert apothecaries' fluid volumes to metric equivalents:

For small volumes, reduce to minims and divide by *16.23* to get milliliters.

For larger volumes, reduce to fluidounces and multiply by *29.57* to get milliliters.

Examples:

Convert f℥ iiss to milliliters.

f℥ iiss = $2\frac{1}{2}$ × 60 ℳ = 150 ℳ

$\frac{150}{16.23}$ ml. = 9.24 ml., *answer.*

Convert Oiiss to milliliters.

Oiiss = $2\frac{1}{2}$ × 16 f℥ = 40 f℥

40 × 29.57 ml. = 1182.8 or 1180 ml., *answer.*

CONVERSION OF WEIGHTS

To convert metric weights to common weights:

Reduce a given small quantity to grams and multiply by *15.432* or divide by *0.065* (whichever gives the answer more readily) to get grains, and reduce the quantity to any desired denominations.

For a larger quantity, divide the number of grams by *31.1* to get apothecaries' ounces, or by *28.35* to get ounces avoirdupois.

For a still larger quantity, divide the number of grams by *454* to get pounds avoirdupois.

Examples:

Convert 12.5 Gm. to grains.

12.5 × 15.432 gr. = 192.9 or 193 gr., *answer.*

Alternate solution (about 0.5% less accurate):

$\frac{12.5}{0.065}$ gr. = 192.3 or 192 gr., *answer.*

Convert 5 mg. to grains.

5 mg. = 0.005 Gm.

$\frac{0.005}{0.065}$ gr. = $\frac{1}{13}$ gr., *answer.*

Alternate solution, using a more convenient conversion factor:

Since 1 grain = 65 milligrams,

$\frac{5}{65}$ gr. = $\frac{1}{13}$ gr., *answer.*

Convert 15 Kg. to pounds avoirdupois.

15 Kg. = 15000 Gm.

$\frac{15000}{454}$ lb. = 33.0 lb., *answer.*

To convert common weights to metric equivalents:

Reduce a given small quantity to grains and multiply by *65* to get milligrams; or reduce the quantity to grains and multiply by *0.065* or divide by *15.432* (whichever gives the answer more readily) to get grams. Reduce the result to any required denomination.

For larger quantities, reduce to apothecaries' ounces and multiply by *31.1*, or to ounces avoirdupois and multiply by *28.35*, to get grams.

For still larger quantities, reduce to pounds avoirdupois and multiply by *454* to get grams, and then reduce, if required, to kilograms; or, more directly, reduce the given quantity to pounds avoirdupois and divide by 2.2 to get kilograms.

Examples:

Convert 6.2 gr. to milligrams.

6.2 × 65 mg. = 403 or 400 mg., *answer.*

How many grams are represented by 850 grains?

850 × 0.065 Gm. = 55.25 or 55 Gm., *answer.*

Convert 176 pounds avoirdupois to kilograms.

$\frac{176}{2.2}$ Kg. = 80.0 Kg., *answer.*

Practice Problems

1. Convert 8 cm. and 12 cm. to inches.

2. Convert 1.35 M. to inches.

3. How many inches are equivalent to 800 mm.?

4. Convert 250 ml. to fluidounces.

5. Convert f℥i ℳxx to milliliters.

6. Convert 4.5 L. to fluidounces.

7. Convert 2 gal. 20 f℥ to liters.

8. A medicinal plaster measures 12 cm. by 16 cm. What is its size in inches?

9. Express a micron as a fraction of an inch.

10. The average diameter of the oil globules in an emulsion is 2.5 microns. What is the average diameter in inches?

11. A pharmacist orders a 100-mm. funnel. What is its size in inches?

12. A mercury barometer reads 760 mm. Express this pressure reading in inches.

13. Convert 3 gal. 1 pt. 10 f℥ to milliliters.

14. A mercury barometer reads 29.2 in. Express this pressure in mm.

15. The U.S.P. states that urethral suppositories weighing about 2 Gm. should be 7 cm. in length. Express the weight in grains and the length in inches.

16. If a mixture weighing 30 Gm. is divided into 100 dosage forms, how many grains will each dose weigh?

17. How many ½-gr. tablets can be made from 10 Gm. of a chemical?

18. Convert $\frac{1}{1000}$ gr. to milligrams, $2\frac{1}{2}$ gr. to grams, 5ℳ to milliliters, and 2.4 ml. to minims.

19. Convert each of the following to the metric system:

        (a) $\frac{1}{60}$ gr.
        (b) f℥ii.
        (c) $\frac{3}{8}$ gr.
        (d) 30 ℳ.
        (e) $\frac{1}{200}$ gr.

20. Convert each of the following to apothecaries' units:

    (a) 150 ml.
    (b) 0.3 ml.
    (c) 0.001 Gm.
    (d) 0.65 mg.

21. A plaster has a tensile strength of 40.82 Kg. per 76.5 mm. in width. Convert this strength to pounds per inches.

22. A certain drug is available in 15-, 25-, and 30-mg. tablets. Express these amounts in the apothecaries' system.

23. Convert 50 micrograms to a fraction of a grain.

24. If 2 f$\mathfrak{Z}$ of a solution contain $7\frac{1}{2}$ gr. of a chemical, how many grams would be contained in 125 ml. of the solution?

25. If a chemical costs $3.50 a pound, what is the cost of 15 Gm.?

26. If the cost of 10 Gm. of merbromin is $1.25, what is the cost of $4\frac{1}{2}$ gr.?

27. How many 6.5-mg. tablets can be obtained from $\mathfrak{Z}$ ss of a chemical?

28. If f$\mathfrak{Z}$ i of a cough syrup contains 10 gr. of sodium citrate, how many grams are contained in 2500 ml.?

29. Convert $\frac{1}{1000}$ gr. to micrograms.

30. The dose of a drug is $\frac{1}{10}$ gr. per kilogram of body weight. How many milligrams should be given to a person weighing 70 kilograms?

31. A prescription calls for $\frac{4}{5}$ gr. of atropine sulfate to be divided into 80 doses. How many milligrams will each dose weigh?

32. A prescription calls for 2 grains of epinephrine bitartrate. If 1 Gm. of epinephrine bitartrate costs $2.00, what is the cost of the amount needed in the prescription?

33. In the compounding of a prescription, a pharmacist used a $\frac{1}{4}$-grain dispensing tablet of atropine sulfate. How many 0.000325-Gm. doses were prescribed on the prescription?

34. A certain elixir contains 0.325 Gm. of potassium thiocyanate per f$\mathfrak{Z}$ i. At $1.75 per lb., what is the cost of the potassium thiocyanate required to make 1 gallon of the elixir?

35. A formula for a cough syrup calls for $\frac{1}{8}$ gr. of codeine phosphate per f$\mathfrak{Z}$ i. How many Gm. of codeine phosphate should be used in preparing one pint of the cough syrup?

CHAPTER VI

CALCULATION OF DOSES

ONE of the prime responsibilities of the pharmacist is the checking of doses specified in prescriptions against his knowledge of the average and maximum dispensing doses of the medicines prescribed. If he should note an unusual dose, he would be ethically bound, if possible, to consult the physician, to make sure that the dosage as he reads it is correct.

For the patient, dosage is almost invariably measured in "household" terms—the teaspoonful, the tablespoonful, and sometimes even the wineglassful. In *calculating* doses, pharmacists and physicians refer to a table of approximate metric and common equivalents of these denominations, although any given "household" container is likely to hold a somewhat larger or smaller quantity than its "equivalent" in the table.

According to the *United States Pharmacopeia*, "Agreement has not been reached with respect to a standard pharmacopeial teaspoon, in spite of the need for such a standard measure in connection with compounding and labeling liquid medicines. For household purposes, an American Standard Teaspoon has been established by the American Standards Association as containing 4.93 ± 0.24 ml. In view of the almost universal practice of employing teaspoons ordinarily available in the household for the administration of medicines, the teaspoon may be regarded as representing 5 ml."

For calculation of dosage problems, the following commonly used Table is suggested.

TABLE OF APPROXIMATE EQUIVALENTS

"Household" measure:		*Metric measure:*		*Apothecaries' measure:*
1 teaspoonful	=	4 ml.	=	f℥i
1 dessertspoonful	=	8 ml.	=	f℥ii
1 tablespoonful	=	15 ml.	=	f℥iv
1 wineglassful	=	60 ml.	=	f℥ii
1 teacupful	=	120 ml.	=	f℥iv
1 tumblerful	=	240 ml.	=	f℥viii

In *judging the safety* of doses of potent substances that are prescribed in liquid form where the liquid is to be administered in teaspoonful doses, it should be emphasized that it may make a significant difference whether the pharmacist checks the dosage on the basis of 8 or 6 doses per fluidounce. Since it is quite likely that fewer than 8 and, in some instances, only 6 teaspoonful doses can be obtained from a fluidounce of liquid medication, it is advisable to use 6 as the basis for checking questionable doses.

Frequently, the "drop" is used as a measure for medicines. It does not represent a definite quantity, since drops of different liquids vary greatly. The "drop" should not, therefore, be used as a measure until the volume that it represents has been determined for each specific liquid. This is done by *calibrating* the dispensing dropper. The calibrated dropper is the only one that should be used for the measurement of medicine.

CALIBRATION OF DROPPERS

A dropper may be calibrated by counting the drops of a liquid as they fall into a graduate until a measurable volume is obtained. The volume of the drop is then calculated in terms of a definite unit (ml. or ♏).

It is common practice for pharmacists to employ calibrated droppers for measuring small volumes.

All doses in the *United States Pharmacopeia* and *National Formulary* are given in the metric system. "Approximate" equivalents in the apothecary system may be calculated by reference to the "Table of Metric Doses with Approximate Apothecary Equivalents" in the *Pharmacopeia*. The *"approximate"* dose equivalents represent the quantities usually prescribed, under identical conditions, by physicians trained, respectively, in the metric or in the apothecary systems of weights and measures.

"When prepared dosage forms such as tablets, capsules, pills, etc., are prescribed in the metric system, the pharmacist may dispense the corresponding *approximate* equivalent in the apothecary system, and vice versa."

But, warns the *Pharmacopeia*, these *approximate* dose equivalents cannot be used for the conversion of specific quantities in a prescription *which requires compounding*, nor in converting a pharmaceutical formula from one system of weights or measures to the other system. For such purposes *exact* equivalents must be used.

MISCELLANEOUS DOSAGE PROBLEMS

To calculate the number of doses in a specified amount of medicine, given the size of each dose:

$$\text{Number of doses} = \frac{\text{Total amount}}{\text{Size of dose}}$$

The *total amount* and the *dose* must be measured in a common denomination.

Examples:

If the dose of a drug is 200 milligrams, how many doses are contained in 10 grams?

10 Gm. = 10000 mg.

$$\text{Number of doses} = \frac{10000 \ (\text{mg.})}{200 \ (\text{mg.})} = 50 \text{ doses, } answer.$$

How many 20-minim doses are contained in 40 ml. of a liquid?

40 ml. = 40 × 16.23 ℳ = 649.2 ℳ

$$\text{Number of doses} = \frac{649.2 \ (\text{ℳ})}{20 \ (\text{ℳ})} = 32 \text{ doses, } answer.$$

If the dose of a medicine is ⅕ grain, how many doses are contained in ½ drachm?

½ ℨ = ½ × 60 gr. = 30 gr.

$$\text{Number of doses} = \frac{30}{\frac{1}{5}} = 30 \times \frac{5}{1} = 150 \text{ doses, } answer.$$

If 1 tablespoonful is prescribed as the dose of a medicine, approximately how many doses will be contained in 12 fluidounces?

1 tablespoonful = 4 fℨ
12 f℥ = 96 fℨ

$$\text{Number of doses} = \frac{96}{4} = 24 \text{ doses, } answer.$$

If the dose of a drug is 50 micrograms, how many doses are contained in 0.020 Gm.?

0.020 Gm. = 20 mg.

50 mcg. = 0.05 mg.

$$\text{Number of doses} = \frac{20}{0.05} = 400 \text{ doses, } answer.$$

To calculate the size of each dose, given a specified amount of medicine and the number of doses it contains:

$$\text{Size of dose} = \frac{\text{Total amount}}{\text{Number of doses}}$$

The *size of the dose* will be expressed in whatever denomination is chosen for measuring the given total amount.

Examples:

How many teaspoonfuls would be prescribed in each dose of a medicine if f℥ iv contained 16 doses?

f℥ iv = 32 f℥ = 32 teaspoonfuls

$$\text{Size of dose} = \frac{32 \text{ (tsp.)}}{16} = 2 \text{ teaspoonfuls, } answer.$$

How many drops would be prescribed in each dose of a medicine if 15 ml. contained 60 doses? The dispensing dropper calibrates 32 drops per ml.

15 ml. = 15 × 32 = 480 drops

$$\text{Size of dose} = \frac{480 \text{ (drops)}}{60} = 8 \text{ drops, } answer.$$

To calculate the amount of a medicine, given the number of doses it contains and the size of each dose:

Total amount = number of doses × size of dose

It is convenient first to convert the given dose to the denomination in which the total amount is to be expressed.

Examples:

How many ml. of a medicine would provide a customer with 2 tablespoonfuls twice a day for 8 days?

Number of doses = 16

Size of dose = 2 tablespoonfuls or 30 ml.

Total amount = 16 × 30 ml. = 480 ml., *answer.*

How many fluidounces of a mixture would provide a customer with a half-teaspoonful dose to be taken 3 times a day for 16 days?

Number of doses = 16 × 3 = 48

Size of dose = $\frac{1}{2}$ teaspoonful = $\frac{1}{2}$ f℥

Total amount = 48 × $\frac{1}{2}$ f℥ = 24 f℥ = 3 f℥, *answer.*

How many milligrams of a drug will be needed to prepare 72 dosage forms if each is to contain $\frac{1}{12}$ grain?

Number of doses = 72

Size of dose $= \frac{1}{12}$ grain $= 5.4$ mg.

Total amount $= 72 \times 5.4$ mg. $= 390$ mg., *answer.*

To calculate the quantity of an ingredient in each specified dose of a medicine, given the quantity in a total amount:

When the number of doses in the total amount is given or can be quickly calculated, this is a convenient equation:

$$\text{Quantity in each dose} = \frac{\text{Quantity in total amount}}{\text{Number of doses}}$$

The quantity of the ingredient in the total amount should first be reduced or converted to the denomination desired in the answer.

But when the number of doses is not given, it is sometimes more convenient to use this proportion:

Total amount : Size of dose $=$ Quantity of ingredient in total : x

x $=$ Quantity in each dose

Examples:

If 0.050 Gm. of a substance is used in preparing 125 tablets, how many micrograms are represented in each tablet?

0.050 Gm. $= 50$ mg. $= 50000$ mcg.

$$\frac{50000 \text{ (mcg.)}}{125} = 400 \text{ mcg.}, \text{ *answer.*}$$

If a preparation contains 5 Gm. of a drug in 500 ml., how many Gm. are contained in each tablespoonful dose?

1 tablespoonful $= 15$ ml.

By the proportion:

500 (ml.) : 15 (ml.) $= 5$ (Gm.) : x

x $= 0.15$ Gm., *answer.*

A cough mixture contains $\frac{3}{4}$ gr. of dihydromorphinone hydrochloride in f℥ viii. How much dihydromorphinone hydrochloride is there in each dessertspoonful dose?

1 dessertspoonful $= 2$ f℥

f℥ viii $= 64$ f℥

$64 \div 2 = 32$ doses

$\frac{3}{4} \div 32 = \frac{3}{128}$ gr., *answer.*

Or,

By the proportion:

$$64 \ (f\text{℥}):2 \ (f\text{℥}) = \tfrac{3}{4} \ (\text{gr.}):x$$
$$x = \tfrac{3}{128} \ \text{gr., } answer.$$

How much codeine sulfate and how much ammonium chloride will be contained in each dose of the following prescription?

R̨ Codeine Sulfate   gr.iv
    Ammonium Chloride   ℥i
    Cherry Syrup ad   f℥iv
    Sig. Dessertspoonful for cough.

$$f\text{℥}iv = 32 \ f\text{℥}$$
$$1 \ \text{dessertspoonful} = 2 \ f\text{℥}$$

$$32 \div 2 = 16 \ \text{doses}$$

$$4 \ \text{gr.} \div 16 = \tfrac{1}{4} \ \text{gr. of codeine sulfate, } and$$

$$\text{℥i or } 60 \ \text{gr.} \div 16 = 3\tfrac{3}{4} \ \text{gr. of ammonium chloride, } answers.$$

Or,

By the proportions:

$$32 \ (f\text{℥}):2 \ (f\text{℥}) = 4 \ (\text{gr.}):x$$
$$x = \tfrac{1}{4} \ \text{gr. of codeine sulfate, } and$$

$$32 \ (f\text{℥}):2 \ (f\text{℥}) = 60 \ (\text{gr.}):y$$
$$y = 3\tfrac{3}{4} \ \text{gr. of ammonium chloride, } answers.$$

To Calculate the quantity of an ingredient in a specified total amount of medicine, given the quantity of the ingredient in each specified dose:

As always, we can make a sound ratio of two amounts only by measuring them in a common denomination.

Here again, when the number of doses is known or can be quickly calculated, this equation is convenient:

Quantity in total = Quantity in dose × Number of doses

Otherwise this proportion may be used:

Size of dose:Total amount=Quantity of ingredient in each dose:x

x = Quantity in total amount

Examples:

How many grains of a chemical are required to make f℥iv of a solution each teaspoonful of which will contain $\tfrac{1}{20}$ grain of the chemical?

1 teaspoonful = 1 f℥

4 f℥ = 32 f℥

By the proportion:

1 (f℥):32 (f℥) = $\frac{1}{20}$ (gr.):x

x = 1$\frac{3}{8}$ gr., *answer*.

A f℥iv cough mixture is to contain, in each f℥ii, $\frac{1}{8}$ gr. of codeine phosphate, $\frac{1}{2}$ minim of chloroform, and 2$\frac{1}{2}$ grains of sodium citrate. Calculate the quantity of each ingredient to be used in compounding the prescription.

4 f℥ = 32 f℥

Number of doses = 32 ÷ 2 = 16

16 × $\frac{1}{8}$ gr. = 2 gr. of codeine phosphate,

16 × $\frac{1}{2}$ ♏ = 8 ♏ of chloroform,

16 × 2$\frac{1}{2}$ gr. = 40 gr. or ℈ii of sodium citrate, *answers*.

To calculate the dose of a drug, given the amount per kilo of body weight:

Example:

The dose of a drug is $\frac{1}{10}$ grain per kilo of body weight. How many milligrams should be given to a person weighing 154 lb.?

$\frac{1}{10}$ gr. = 6.5 mg.

1 kilo (kilogram) = 2.2 lb.

By the proportion:

2.2 (lb.):154 (lb.) = 6.5 (mg.):x

x = 455 mg., *answer*.

CALCULATION OF DOSES FOR CHILDREN

To calculate approximate doses for children, given adult doses:

The method most commonly used for calculating doses for children is based on Young's Rule: *Divide the age of the child by the age plus 12 and multiply by the adult dose.* The rule may better be expressed as a mathematical formula:

$$\text{Dose for child} = \frac{\text{Age}}{\text{Age} + 12} \times \text{Adult dose}$$

Examples:

If the adult dose of a drug is 5 mg., what is the dose for a child 8 years old?

$$\frac{8}{8 + 12} \times 5 \text{ mg.} = \frac{2}{5} \times 5 \text{ mg.} = 2 \text{ mg., } answer.$$

If the adult dose of a drug is 3 grains, what is the dose for a child 6 years old?

$$\frac{6}{6 + 12} \times 3 \text{ gr.} = \frac{1}{3} \times 3 \text{ gr.} = 1 \text{ gr., } answer.$$

If the adult dose of a drug is 0.1 ml., what is the dose for a child 12 years old?

$$\frac{12}{12 + 12} \times 0.1 \text{ ml.} = \frac{1}{2} \times 0.1 \text{ ml.} = 0.05 \text{ ml., } answer.$$

Other methods:

Cowling's Rule: $\dfrac{\text{Age at next birthday (in years)} \times \text{Adult dose}}{24}$

Fried's Rule for Infants: $\dfrac{\text{Age (in months)} \times \text{Adult dose}}{150}$

✶ Clark's Rule for Infants: $\dfrac{\text{Weight (in pounds)} \times \text{Adult dose}}{150}$

Practice Problems

1. If the dose of a drug is 150 micrograms, how many doses are contained in 0.120 Gm.?

2. How many 15-minim doses are contained in 60 ml. of a tincture?

3. How many 6-grain doses are contained in 12 Gm. of a powder?

4. If the dose of a drug is $\frac{1}{16}$ gr., how many doses are contained in ℥i?

5. A medicine is to be taken in 5-minim doses. How many doses are contained in 15 ml. of the medicine?

6. If a medicine is to be taken three times daily, and if 180 ml. are to be taken in four days, how many tablespoonfuls should be prescribed for each dose?

7. What is the dosage in teaspoonfuls if 400 ml. of a medicine contain 50 doses?

8. How many teaspoonfuls per day must be taken if f℥ viii of a medicine are to be taken four times a day for eight days?

9. If a medicine is to be taken three times daily, and if 180 ml. are to be taken in four days, how many teaspoonfuls should be prescribed for each dose?

10. What is the dosage in teaspoonfuls if 480 ml. of a medicine contain 60 doses?

11. How many fluidounces of a mixture contain 24 dessertspoonful doses?

12. If a prescription contains 0.2 Gm. of codeine phosphate in 120 ml., how much is contained in each teaspoonful dose?

13. If a prescription contains 0.03 Gm. of atropine sulfate in 240 ml., what fraction of a grain is contained in 1 teaspoonful?

14. How many grains of a chemical are contained in each capsule if a mixture containing $1\frac{1}{4}$ grains of the chemical is divided into 30 capsules?

15. A powder contains $\frac{1}{20}$ gr. of atropine sulfate. If the powder is divided into 12 dosage forms, how much atropine sulfate will each dose contain?

16. If f℥ vi of a cough mixture contain $\frac{3}{4}$ gr. of Dilaudid, how much is contained in 1 dessertspoonful of the mixture?

17. If f℥ iv of a mixture contain 8 gr. of phenobarbital, how much is contained in each teaspoonful dose?

18. If a solution of atropine sulfate contains 1 grain in each fluidounce, what volume will contain $\frac{1}{120}$ gr.?

19. If 240 ml. of a liquid contain 0.150 Gm. of a chemical and 2 teaspoonfuls are taken at a dose, what fraction of a grain will each dose contain?

20. A prescription for 480 ml. of a liquid contains 0.030 Gm. of atropine sulfate and specifies a dose of 8 ml. Calculate the fraction of a grain of atropine sulfate contained in each dose.

21. If 500 ml. of a liquid contain 12.5 Gm. of a chemical, and 4 ml. are taken at a dose, how many grains will each dose contain?

22. ℞ Sodium Bromide   ℥ i
        Nux Vomica Tincture   ℥ ss
        Lactated Pepsin Elixir ad   Oi
        Sig. Tablespoonful t.i.d.

How much sodium bromide and how much nux vomica tincture will be contained in each dose?

23. ℞ Phenobarbital Sodium   1.0
        Belladonna Tincture   10.0
        Peppermint Water ad   120.0
        Sig. 4 ml. t.i.d.

How much phenobarbital sodium and how much belladonna tincture will be contained in each dose?

24. Potassium Bromide Elixir contains 175 Gm. of potassium bromide in each 1000 ml. How many grains of potassium bromide will be contained in a half-teaspoonful dose of the elixir?

25. One liter of Compound Squill Syrup contains 2 Gm. of tartar emetic. The official average dose of the syrup is 2 ml. Calculate the quantity, in grains, of tartar emetic in each average dose.

26. ℞   Codeine Phosphate   0.26 Gm.
       Sodium Citrate   4.0   Gm.
       Chloroform   0.5   ml.
       Tolu Syrup ad   120.0   ml.
       Sig. ℥ss ut dict.

How many grains of codeine phosphate and how many minims of chloroform are contained in each dose?

27. ℞   Belladonna Tincture   ℥iii
       Codeine Sulfate   gr.iv
       Phenobarbital Elixir ad   ℥iv
       Sig. Teaspoonful ex aq.

How much belladonna tincture and how much codeine sulfate will be contained in each dose?

28. A powder is divided into 36 capsules. If each capsule contains 0.5 mg. of one ingredient, 15 mg. of a second, and enough of a third to make 0.300 Gm., how much of each was there in the original powder?

29. How many grains of a chemical are required to make 3 fluidounces of a solution 1 fluidrachm of which is to contain $\frac{1}{80}$ gr.?

30. How many grams of a chemical are required to make 2 fluidounces of a mixture each teaspoonful of which is to contain $\frac{1}{25}$ gr.?

31. A f℥vi mixture is to contain, in each tablespoonful, 15 gr. of bismuth subcarbonate and f℥ss of paregoric. Calculate the quantity of each that should be used in preparing the mixture.

32. A prescription for 240 ml. of a mixture calls for 4 mg. of one ingredient and 200 mg. of another in each teaspoonful dose. How much of each ingredient should be used in compounding the prescription?

33. A solution contains gr. xvi of phenobarbital in each pint. What fraction of a grain of phenobarbital is contained in each dessertspoonful dose?

34. A solution contains 30 mg. of a chemical per 120 ml. and has a dose of 10 drops. If the dispensing dropper calibrates 25 drops per ml., how many mcg. of the chemical are contained in each dose?

35. How many minims of a solution containing 2 grains of hyoscine per fluidounce should be used in a four-fluidounce prescription, each teaspoonful dose of which is to contain 0.5 mg. of hyoscine?

36. ℞ Codeine Phosphate   8.5   mg.
       Chloroform   0.016 ml.
       Ammonium Chloride   0.1   Gm.
       Tolu Syrup ad   4.0   ml.
       Disp. 240 ml.
       Sig. 4 ml. as directed.

How many grains of codeine phosphate and how many minims of chloroform should be used in compounding the prescription?

37. ℞ Potassium Thiocyanate
       Spearmint Water aa q.s.
       Make a solution to contain gr. iii per f℥ii
       Dispense f℥viii
       Sig. ℥ii in water daily.

How many grains of potassium thiocyanate should be used in compounding the prescription?

38. ℞ Sodium Bromide   gr. x per ℥ii
       Compound Pepsin Elixir
       Aromatic Elixir aa ad   ℥vi
       Sig. 4 ml. t.i.d.

How many grains of sodium bromide should be used in compounding the prescription?

39. ℞ Codeine Phosphate   gr. ¼ per ℥i
       Hydriodic Acid Syrup
       Cherry Syrup aa   ℥iii
       Sig. ℥i every two hours for cough.

How many grains of codeine phosphate should be used in compounding the prescription?

40. The dose of a drug is 5 mg. per kilogram of body weight. How many grams should be given to a child weighing 55 lb.?

41. The dose of a drug is 0.2 mg. per kilo of body weight. How many grains should be given to a person weighing 209 lb.?

42. The rectal dose of tribromoethanol is 0.06 ml. for each kilogram of body weight. How many milliliters should be given to a person weighing 150 lb.?

43. The dose of iodophthalein sodium is 0.3 Gm. per 10 Kg. of body weight. What is the dose for a person weighing 135 lb.?

44. If the adult dose of a drug is 324 mg., what is the dose for a child 6 years old?

45. If the adult dose of a drug is 0.10 Gm., what is the dose for a child 4 years old?

46. If the adult dose of a drug is 0.25 Gm., what is the dose for a child 9 years old?

47. If the adult dose of a drug is 8 grains, what is the dose for a child 4 years old?

48. If the average adult dose of paregoric is 60 minims, what is the dose for a child 4 years old?

49. If the adult dose of atropine sulfate is $\frac{1}{120}$ gr., what is the dose for a child 6 years old?

50. If the adult dose of a prescription is a teaspoonful, how many minims should be prescribed for a child 8 years old?

51. The adult dose of a drug is 15 mg. Calculate the dose, in grains, for a child 6 years old.

52. The average dose of Dilaudid is 2 mg. How much Dilaudid should be used in 120 ml. of a cough syrup so that each 4 ml. will contain the dose for a child 6 years old?

53. The adult dose of a drug is 0.0004 Gm. What is the dose, expressed in grains, for a child of five years?

54. The adult dose of tetracycline hydrochloride is 250 mg. What would be the dose for a child of twelve months?

55. The adult dose of atropine sulfate is $\frac{1}{120}$ gr. Using Fried's Rule, calculate the dose for an infant of six months.

56. The adult dose of a drug is $\frac{1}{60}$ gr. Calculate (a) the dose for a 25-lb. child, (b) the dose for an infant of 7 months, and (c) the dose for a child of six years.

57. The average adult dose of a certain solution is 0.5 ml. (a) What is the dose for a child 4 years old? (b) If the solution is to be dispensed in a dropper bottle, the dropper of which calibrates 24 drops per ml., how many drops should be given to obtain the correct dose for the child?

58. ℞ Atropine Sulfate   q.s.
       Distilled Water ad   ℥ viii
       Sig. ℨi in each feeding.

How much atropine sulfate should be used to provide the proper dose for an infant of nine months?

CHAPTER VII

REDUCING AND ENLARGING FORMULAS

In dispensing, the pharmacist must frequently reduce official formulas, and in manufacturing, he is often called upon to enlarge them to quantity production. Official formulas may be for quantities of 1000 ml. or 1000 Gm., whereas prescriptions may call for relatively small amounts such as 30 ml. or 30 Gm., and formulas for quantity manufacturing may call for relatively large amounts such as 5 gallons or 25 pounds.

When a formula specifies a *total amount*, we may determine how much of each ingredient is needed to obtain a desired total amount by this proportion:

$$\begin{pmatrix} \text{Total amount} \\ \text{specified in} \\ \text{formula} \end{pmatrix} : \begin{pmatrix} \text{Total amount} \\ \text{desired} \end{pmatrix} = \begin{pmatrix} \text{Quantity of each} \\ \text{ingredient in} \\ \text{formula} \end{pmatrix} : x$$

x = Quantity of each ingredient in amount desired

Although all problems specifying a total amount may be solved by this proportion, it is usually more convenient—particularly if the quantities are given in the metric system—to solve them by the use of short cuts. Thus, given a formula for 1000 ml. or 1000 Gm., we may divide or multiply the quantity of each ingredient by a power of 10 simply by moving the decimal point to the left or right the required number of places. Or, given a formula for the same amounts, we may reduce or enlarge it by using factors. For example, if we wish to prepare 1 gallon (3785 ml.) of a formula whose specified total amount is 1000 ml., we would multiply the quantity of each ingredient by the factor 3.785. And, if we were to prepare 50 Gm. of a formula whose specified total amount is 1000 Gm., we would multiply the quantity of each ingredient by $\frac{1}{20}$ (since 50 Gm. is $\frac{1}{20}$ of 1000 Gm.).

Some formulas, however, do not specify a total amount, instead indicating relative quantities of ingredients or *proportional parts* to be used in obtaining any desired total amount. Such problems may be solved by this proportion:

$$\begin{pmatrix} \text{Total number} \\ \text{of parts in} \\ \text{formula} \end{pmatrix} : \begin{pmatrix} \text{Number of} \\ \text{parts of each} \\ \text{ingredient} \end{pmatrix} = \begin{pmatrix} \text{Total amount} \\ \text{desired} \end{pmatrix} : x$$

x = Quantity of each ingredient in amount desired

(89)

In solving problems that involve reducing and enlarging formulas, these facts should be noted:

(1) To make a valid ratio, the total amounts compared must be expressed in a common denomination, whether in grams, fluidounces, pounds, or anything else. Consequently, if they are unlike to start with, one or the other must be reduced or converted. If, for example, the formula is given in the metric system and the required quantity is in the common system, it is generally best to convert the required quantity into the metric system. The answers may then be converted into weighable or measurable denominations in the common system or, if this is not indicated, the results may be left in the metric system.

(2) Since the quantity of each ingredient is calculated separately, it does not matter if the formula includes an assortment of terms (pounds and fluidounces, grams and milliliters, and so on.)

FORMULAS THAT SPECIFY AMOUNTS OF INGREDIENTS

To calculate the quantities of ingredients to be used when reducing or enlarging a formula for a specified total amount:

Examples:

> *From the following formula, calculate the quantities of each ingredient required to make 240 ml. of Chalk Mixture.*

Prepared Chalk	60	Gm.
Saccharin Sodium	0.3	Gm.
Bentonite Magma	500	ml.
Cinnamon Water	400	ml.
Distilled Water ad	1000	ml.

Using the factor 0.24 (since 240 ml. is 0.24 × 1000 ml.), the quantity of each ingredient is calculated as follows:

Prepared Chalk	=	60	×	0.24	=	14.4	Gm.
Saccharin Sodium	=	0.3	×	0.24	=	0.072	Gm.
Bentonite Magma	=	500	×	0.24	=	120	ml.
Cinnamon Water	=	400	×	0.24	=	96	ml.

Distilled Water, a sufficient quantity to make 240 ml.,

answers.

If, in this problem, the required amount were *60 ml.*, we should *move the decimal point one place to the left and multiply by 0.6.* Or, if the required amount were *50 ml.*, we could either *divide by 20* or *move the decimal point one place to the left and divide by 2.* And, if the required amount were *125 ml.*, we should *multiply by the fraction* $\frac{1}{8}$ (since 125 ml. is $\frac{1}{8}$ of 1000 ml.).

From the following formula, calculate the quantity of each ingredient required to make 1 gallon of Compound Benzoin Tincture.

Benzoin	100 Gm.
Aloe	20 Gm.
Storax	80 Gm.
Tolu Balsam	40 Gm.
Alcohol ad	1000 ml.

1 gallon = 3785 ml.

Using the factor 3.785, the quantity of each ingredient is calculated as follows:

Benzoin	=	100	×	3.785	=	378.5 Gm.
Aloe	=	20	×	3.785	=	75.7 Gm.
Storax	=	80	×	3.785	=	302.8 Gm.
Tolu Balsam	=	40	×	3.785	=	151.4 Gm.

Alcohol, a sufficient quantity, to make   3785   ml.

or 1 gal. *answers.*

From the following formula, calculate the quantity of each ingredient required to make 1 lb. of the ointment.

Coal Tar	50 Gm.
Starch	250 Gm.
Zinc Oxide	150 Gm.
Petrolatum	550 Gm.

1 lb. = 454 Gm.

Since the formula is for 1000 Gm., and using the factor 0.454, the quantity of each ingredient is calculated as follows:

Coal Tar	=	50	×	0.454	=	22.7 Gm.
Starch	=	250	×	0.454	=	113.5 Gm.
Zinc Oxide	=	150	×	0.454	=	68.1 Gm.
Petrolatum	=	550	×	0.454	=	249.7 Gm.

454.0 Gm.

or 1 lb., *answers.*

From the following formula for 100 capsules, calculate the quantities of each ingredient required to make 24 capsules.

Belladonna Extract	1.0 Gm.
Ephedrine Sulfate	1.6 Gm.
Phenobarbital	2.0 Gm.
Phenacetin	32.0 Gm.

Using the factor 0.24 (since 24 capsules are represented by 0.24 × 100), the quantity of each ingredient is calculated as follows:

Belladonna Extract	=	1.0	×	0.24	=	0.24 Gm.
Ephedrine Sulfate	=	1.6	×	0.24	=	0.384 Gm.
Phenobarbital	=	2.0	×	0.24	=	0.48 Gm.
Phenacetin	=	32.0	×	0.24	=	7.68 Gm.,

answers.

FORMULAS THAT SPECIFY PROPORTIONAL PARTS

To calculate the quantities of ingredients required to prepare a desired amount of a formula when it specifies proportional parts:

If a formula gives us quantities in terms of *proportional parts,* these facts should be noted:

(1) When parts by weight are specified, we can convert only to weights and not to volumes, whereas when parts by volume are specified, we can convert only to volumes.

(2) Just as the formula measures all quantities in a common denomination (namely, in terms of parts), so will our calculations result in a single denomination, and this will be the denomination we select at the outset for measuring the desired total amount.

Examples:

From the following formula, calculate the quantity of each ingredient required to make 1000 Gm. of the ointment.

Cade Oil	5 parts
Zinc Oxide	10 parts
Hydrophilic Ointment	50 parts

Total number of parts (by weight) = 65
1000 Gm. will contain 65 parts

By the proportions:

$65: 5 = 1000$ (Gm.)$:x$	$x = 76.92$ Gm. of Cade Oil,
$65:10 = 1000$ (Gm.)$:y$	$y = 153.85$ Gm. of Zinc Oxide,
$65:50 = 1000$ (Gm.)$:z$	$z = 769.23$ Gm. of Hydrophilic
	Ointment, *answers.*

(Check total: 1000.00 Gm.)

From the same formula, calculate the quantities of each ingredient required to make ℥i of the ointment.

Total number of parts (by weight) = 65
℥i or 480 grains will contain 65 parts

By the proportions:

65: 5 = 480 (gr.):x   x = 36.9 gr. of Cade Oil,

65:10 = 480 (gr.):y   y = 73.9 gr. of Zinc Oxide,

65:50 = 480 (gr.):z   z = 369.2 gr. of Hydrophilic

Ointment, *answers.*

(Check total: $\overline{480}$ gr. or ℥i)

From the following formula, calculate the quantity of each ingredient required to make 5 lb. of the powder.

Bismuth Subcarbonate	8 parts
Kaolin	15 parts
Magnesium Oxide	2 parts
Total number of parts =	$\overline{25}$ parts

5 lb. (454 Gm. × 5) or 2270 Gm. will contain 25 parts

By the proportions:

25: 8 = 2270 (Gm.):x   x = 726.4 Gm. of Bismuth

Subcarbonate,

25:15 = 2270 (Gm.):y   y = 1362. Gm. of Kaolin,

25: 2 = 2270 (Gm.):z   z = 181.6 Gm. of Magnesium

Oxide, *answers.*

(Check total: $\overline{2270.}$ Gm.)

To calculate the quantities of ingredients in a desired amount when proportional parts may be reckoned from the formula:

If the ingredients are all measured by weight, or all by volume, we may consider the sum of the weights (or volumes) when expressed in a common denomination as specifying a total number of parts.

Example:

From the following formula, calculate the quantity of each ingredient required to make 500 Gm. of the powder.

Boric Acid	5 Gm.
Starch	20 Gm.
Talc	50 Gm.

Total number of parts (by weight) = 75

500 Gm. will contain 75 parts

By the proportions:

75: 5 = 500 (Gm.):x   x = 33.3 Gm. of Boric Acid,

75:20 = 500 (Gm.):y   y = 133.3 Gm. of Starch,

75:50 = 500 (Gm.):z   z = 333.3 Gm. of Talc, *answers.*

(Check total: 500.0 Gm.)

Practice Problems

1. From the following formula, calculate the quantities required to make 180 ml. of Benzyl Benzoate Lotion.

Benzyl Benzoate	250 ml.
Triethanolamine	5 Gm.
Oleic Acid	20 Gm.
Water ad	1000 ml.

2. From the following formula, calculate the quantities required to make 5 gallons of Ferrous Sulfate Syrup.

Ferrous Sulfate	40	Gm.
Citric Acid	2.1	Gm.
Peppermint Spirit	2	ml.
Sucrose	825	Gm.
Distilled Water ad	1000	ml.

3. From the following formula, calculate the quantities required to make 5 lb. of Hydrophilic Ointment.

Methylparaben		0.25 Gm.
Propylparaben		0.15 Gm.
Stearyl Alcohol	250	Gm.
White Petrolatum	250	Gm.
Propylene Glycol	120	Gm.
Polyoxyl 40 Stearate	50	Gm.
Purified Water ad	1000	Gm.

4. From the following formula, calculate the quantities of each ingredient required to prepare ½ gallon of Orange Syrup.

Sweet Orange Peel Tincture	50 ml.
Citric Acid	5 Gm.
Talc	15 Gm.
Sucrose	820 Gm.
Water ad	1000 ml.

5. From the following formula, calculate the quantities of each ingredient required to prepare 10 lb. of Medicinal Soft Soap.

Vegetable Oil	380	Gm.
Oleic Acid	20	Gm.
Potassium Hydroxide	91.7	Gm.
Glycerin	50	ml.
Distilled Water ad	1000	Gm.

6. From the following formula for 100 capsules, calculate the quantities of each ingredient required to prepare 36 capsules.

Codeine Phosphate	1.6	Gm.
Acetophenetidin	4.0	Gm.
Acetylsalicylic Acid	16.0	Gm.
Atropine Sulfate	0.025	Gm.

7. From the following formula, calculate the quantities of each ingredient required to prepare one pint of a compound ephedrine solution.

Ephedrine Sulfate	0.30 Gm.
Chlorobutanol	0.15 Gm.
Menthol	0.15 Gm.
Alcohol	0.60 ml.
Sodium Chloride	0.15 Gm.
Dextrose	0.90 Gm.
Amaranth Solution	0.03 ml.
Water ad	30.00 ml.

8. From the following formula, calculate the quantities of each ingredient required to make 1500 Gm. of the powder.

Calcium Carbonate	5 parts
Magnesium Oxide	1 part
Sodium Bicarbonate	4 parts
Bismuth Subcarbonate	3 parts

9. From the following formula, calculate the number of grams of each ingredient required to make 1 lb. of Zinc Oxide Paste.

Zinc Oxide	1 part
Starch	1 part
White Petrolatum	2 parts

10. From the following formula, calculate the quantities of each ingredient required to make ℥ii of the ointment.

Zinc Oxide	2 parts
Coal Tar	2 parts
Starch	15 parts
Petrolatum	25 parts

11. From the following formula, calculate the quantities of each ingredient required to make one liter of the lotion.

Witch Hazel	4 parts (by volume)
Glycerin	1 part
Boric Acid Solution	15 parts

12. From the following formula, calculate the number of grams of each ingredient required to make 5 lb. of the powder.

Camphor	6 Gm.
Starch	16 Gm.
Zinc Oxide	32 Gm.

13. From the following formula, calculate the quantities of each ingredient required to prepare 5 pints of the liniment.

Arnica Tincture	10 parts
Methyl Salicylate	20 parts
Isopropyl Alcohol	25 parts

14. From the following formula, calculate the quantities of each ingredient required to prepare 1 gallon of Tolu Balsam Syrup.

Tolu Balsam Tincture	50 ml.
Magnesium Carbonate	10 Gm.
Sucrose	820 Gm.
Distilled Water ad	1000 ml.

15. From the following formula, calculate the quantities of each ingredient required to prepare 5 pints of the solution.

Resorcinol Monoacetate	50 ml.
Castor Oil	25 ml.
Chloral Hydrate	75 Gm.
Isopropyl Alcohol ad	1000 ml.

16. Calculate the quantities of each ingredient that should be used in preparing 2000 Gm. of the following ointment.

Salicylic Acid	2 parts
Precipitated Sulfur	3 parts
Petrolatum	30 parts

17. How much of each ingredient should be used to prepare 5 lb. of the following ointment base?

Stearic Acid	14.0 Gm.
Triethanolamine	1.0 Gm.
Cetyl Alcohol	4.0 Gm.
Glycerin	8.0 Gm.
Water	63.0 Gm.

18. From the following formula, calculate the quantities of each ingredient that should be used in preparing 2500 Gm. of the ointment.

Resorcinol	0.6 Gm.
Zinc Oxide	3.0 Gm.
Starch	4.0 Gm.
White Petrolatum ad	30.0 Gm.

19. Calculate the quantities of each ingredient required to make ℥iv of aluminum paste.

Aluminum	1 part
Boric Acid Ointment	2 parts

20. From the following formula, calculate the quantities of each ingredient that should be used in preparing ℥ii of the ointment.

Crude Coal Tar	5.0 Gm.
Diglycol Stearate	10.0 Gm.
Petrolatum ad	100.0 Gm.

21. A formula for 500 capsules contains 2.5 Gm. of amphetamine, 32.5 Gm. of thyroid, 0.5 Gm. of thiamine hydrochloride, 4.0 Gm. of phenobarbital, and enough lactose to make 50 Gm. How much of each ingredient should be used in preparing 36 capsules?

22. From the following formula, calculate the quantities of each ingredient required to prepare 1 gallon of the mixture.

Belladonna Tincture	10 ml.
Nux Vomica Tincture	15 ml.
Iso-Alcoholic Elixir	95 ml.

23. How much of each ingredient is required to prepare 5 gallons of Hydriodic Acid Syrup?

Diluted Hydriodic Acid	140 ml.
Sucrose	450 Gm.
Distilled Water ad	1000 ml.

24. How much of each ingredient is required to prepare one hundred 5-grain capsules of Compound Acetanilid Powder?

Acetanilid	70 Gm.
Caffeine	10 Gm.
Sodium Bicarbonate	20 Gm.

7

25. From the following formula, calculate the quantities of each ingredient required to prepare 25 lb. of the cream.

Stearic Acid	220 Gm.
Wool Fat	40 Gm.
Triethanolamine	15 Gm.
Carbitol	75 Gm.
Distilled Water ad	1000 Gm.

26. From the following formula, calculate the quantities of each ingredient required to prepare 10 pints of the lotion.

Coal Tar Solution	10.0 ml.
Salicylic Acid	7.5 Gm.
Isopropyl Alcohol ad	120.0 ml.

27. How much of each ingredient is required to prepare 240 ml. of preserved water?

Methylparaben	0.26 Gm.
Propylparaben	0.14 Gm.
Distilled Water ad	1000 ml.

28. From the following formula, calculate the quantities of each ingredient required to prepare 5 gallons of mouth wash.

Zinc Chloride	2.4 Gm.
Menthol	0.8 Gm.
Soluble Saccharin	0.4 Gm.
Formalin	0.4 ml.
Clove Oil	0.4 ml.
Cinnamon Oil	1.6 ml.
Alcohol	100.0 ml.
Distilled Water ad	1000 ml.

29. A formula for 30 suppositories contains the following:

Bismuth Subgallate	6.0 Gm.
Peruvian Balsam	2.5 Gm.
Zinc Oxide	4.5 Gm.
Cocoa Butter	50.0 Gm.

How much of each ingredient should be used to prepare 8 suppositories?

30. Calculate the quantities of each ingredient required to prepare 1 lb. of the following ointment base.

Cetyl Alcohol	22.5 Gm.
White Wax	1.5 Gm.
Glycerin	15.0 Gm.
Sodium Lauryl Sulfate	3.0 Gm.
Water	108.0 Gm.

31. From the following formula, calculate the quantities of each ingredient required to prepare 60 ml. of the buffer solution.

Boric Acid	12.4	Gm.
Potassium Chloride	7.4	Gm.
Distilled Water ad	1000	ml.

32. From the following formula, calculate the quantities of each ingredient required to prepare 1 pint of thiamine elixir.

Thiamine Hydrochloride	0.1	Gm.
Simple Syrup	50.0	ml.
Sherry Wine ad	100	ml.

33. Calculate the quantities of each ingredient required to prepare 1 gallon of Salicylic Acid Lotion.

Salicylic Acid	1.0 Gm.
Polysorbate 80	1.5 Gm.
2-propyl Palmitate	3.0 Gm.
Isopropyl Alcohol	70.0 ml.
Distilled Water ad	100.0 ml.

34. From the following formula, calculate the quantities, in Gm., of each ingredient required to prepare 5 lb. of Hydrated Petrolatum (MGH).

Sorbitan Sesquioleate	5%
Petrolatum	45%
Distilled Water	50%

35. Calculate the quantities of each ingredient required to prepare 1 pint of Scott's Solution.

Merbromin	2 Gm.
Water	35 ml.
Acetone	10 ml.
Neutralized Alcohol ad	100 ml.

CHAPTER VIII

DENSITY, SPECIFIC GRAVITY, AND SPECIFIC VOLUME

THE relative weights of equal volumes of substances are shown by their densities and their specific gravities.

DENSITY

Density is mass per unit volume of a substance, *e.g.*, the number of grams per cubic centimeter or milliliter, or the number of grains per fluidounce, or the number of pounds per gallon, and so on. It is *usually* expressed as *Gm. per cc.* Since the *gram* is defined as the mass of 1 cc. of water at $4°$ C., the density of water is *1 Gm. per cc.* Since the *Pharmacopeia* states that 1 ml. may be used as the equivalent of 1 cc., for our purposes the density of water may be expressed as *1 Gm. per ml.* One (1) ml. of mercury, on the other hand, weighs 13.6 Gm., hence its density is *13.6 Gm. per ml.*

Density may be calculated by dividing mass by volume. Thus, if 10 ml. of sulfuric acid weigh 18 Gm., its density =

$$\frac{18 \text{ (Gm.)}}{10 \text{ (ml.)}} = 1.8 \text{ Gm. per ml.}$$

SPECIFIC GRAVITY

Specific gravity is a ratio, *expressed decimally*, of the weight of a substance to the weight of an equal volume of a substance chosen as a standard, both substances having the same temperature, or the temperature of each being definitely known. Water is used as the standard for the specific gravities of liquids and solids; the most useful standard for gases—which have little or no pharmaceutical significance—is hydrogen (although sometimes air is used).

Specific gravity may be calculated by dividing the weight of a given substance by the weight of an equal volume of water. Thus, if 10 ml. of sulfuric acid weigh 18 Gm., and 10 ml. of water, under similar conditions, weigh 10 Gm., the specific gravity of the acid =

$$\frac{\text{weight of 10 ml. of sulfuric acid}}{\text{weight of 10 ml. of water}} = \frac{18 \text{ (Gm.)}}{10 \text{ (Gm.)}} = 1.8$$

Specific gravities can be expressed decimally to as many places as the accuracy of their determination warrants. In pharmaceutical work this may be two, three, or four decimal places. Since substances expand or contract at different rates when their temperatures change, variations in the specific gravity of a substance must be carefully allowed for in accurate work. In the United States Pharmacopeia the standard temperature for specific gravities is 25° C., except for that of alcohol, which is 15.56° C. by government regulation.

DENSITY VS. SPECIFIC GRAVITY

The density of a substance is a concrete number (*1.8 Gm. per ml.* in the example), while specific gravity, being a ratio between like quantities, is an abstract number (*1.8* in the example). Whereas density must vary with the table of measure, specific gravity has no dimensions and is, therefore, a constant value for each substance (when measured under controlled conditions). Thus, the density of water may be variously expressed as *1 Gm. per ml.*, or *455 gr. per f℥*, or *62½ lbs. per cu. ft.;* but the specific gravity of water is always 1.

The specific gravity of a substance and its density in the metric system are numerically equal (as a result of the definition of the gram), but they are quite different when the density is expressed in the common system.

The factor *455* (rounded off from 454.57 or 454.6 gr., the weight of 1 f℥ of water at 25° C.) is useful for calculating the approximate weight of a small volume of water measured in the apothecaries' system. But if *455* is used, the result should be expressed in no more than three significant figures. When quantities greater than a pint are involved, it is usually more convenient to convert them to their metric equivalents before calculating.

SPECIFIC GRAVITY OF LIQUIDS

To calculate the specific gravity of a liquid when its weight and volume are known:

Examples:

> *If 54.96 ml. of an oil weigh 52.78 Gm., what is the specific gravity of the oil?*

> 54.96 ml. of water weigh 54.96 Gm.

> Specific gravity of oil $= \dfrac{52.78 \text{ (Gm.)}}{54.96 \text{ (Gm.)}} = 0.9603$, *answer.*

> *If a pint of a certain liquid weighs 9250 grains, what is the specific gravity of the liquid?*

> 1 pint = 16 f℥

> 16 f℥ of water weigh 7280 grains

$$\text{Specific gravity of liquid} = \frac{9250 \ (\text{gr.})}{7280 \ (\text{gr.})} = 1.27, \ answer.$$

If 25.0 ml. of a liquid weigh 560 grains, what is the specific gravity?

25.0 ml. of water weigh 25.0 Gm.

In order to make a valid ratio, the weights must be in the same denomination.

560 gr. = 36.3 Gm.

$$\text{Specific gravity of liquid} = \frac{36.3 \ (\text{Gm.})}{25.0 \ (\text{Gm.})} = 1.45, \ answer.$$

To calculate the specific gravity of a liquid, determined with a specific gravity bottle:

In the determination of the specific gravity of a liquid by means of a *specific gravity bottle*,[1] the container is filled and weighed first with water and then with the liquid. By subtracting the weight of the empty container from the two weights, we have the *weights of equal volumes*—even though we may not know exactly what the volumes are.

Example:

A specific gravity bottle weighs 23.66 Gm. When filled with water it weighs 72.95 Gm.; when filled with another liquid it weighs 73.56 Gm. What is the specific gravity of the liquid?

73.56 Gm. − 23.66 Gm. = 49.90 Gm. of liquid

72.95 Gm. − 23.66 Gm. = 49.29 Gm. of water

$$\text{Specific gravity of liquid} = \frac{49.90 \ (\text{Gm.})}{42.29 \ (\text{Gm.})} = 1.180, \ answer.$$

To calculate the specific gravity of a liquid determined by the displacement or plummet method:

The basis for the determination of the specific gravity of a liquid by this method is *Archimedes' principle*, which states that a body immersed in a liquid displaces an amount of the liquid equal to its own volume and suffers an apparent loss in weight equal to the weight of the displaced liquid. Thus, we can weigh a plummet when suspended in water and when suspended in a liquid whose

---

[1] A container intended to be used as a specific gravity bottle, with a known capacity (commonly 10, 25, or 100 ml.) so that the weight of water it will contain is already known, is called a *pycnometer*.

specific gravity is to be determined, and by subtracting from these weights the weight of the plummet in air, we get the *weights of equal volumes of the liquids* needed in our calculation.

Example:

A glass plummet weighs 12.64 Gm. in air, 8.57 Gm. when immersed in water, and 9.12 Gm. when immersed in an oil. Calculate the specific gravity of the oil.

12.64 Gm. − 9.12 Gm. = 3.52 Gm. of displaced oil
12.64 Gm. − 8.57 Gm. = 4.07 Gm. of displaced water

Specific gravity of oil $= \dfrac{3.52 \ (\text{Gm.})}{4.07 \ (\text{Gm.})} = 0.865$, *answer.*

SPECIFIC GRAVITY OF SOLIDS

To calculate the specific gravity of a solid heavier than and insoluble in water:

The specific gravity of a solid heavier than and insoluble in water may be calculated simply by dividing the weight of the solid in air by the weight of water that it displaces when immersed in it. The weight of water displaced (apparent loss of weight in water) is equal to the *weight of an equal volume of water.*

Example:

A piece of glass weighs 38.525 Gm. in air and 23.525 Gm. when immersed in water. What is its specific gravity?

38.525 Gm. − 23.525 Gm. = 15.000 Gm. of displaced water
(weight of an equal volume of water)

Specific gravity of glass $= \dfrac{38.525 \ (\text{Gm.})}{15.000 \ (\text{Gm.})} = 2.5683$, *answer.*

To calculate the specific gravity of a solid heavier than and soluble in water:

The weights of equal volumes of any two substances are proportional to their specific gravities. Therefore, given a solid heavier than and soluble in water, we may use the method just discussed, but *substituting some liquid of known specific gravity* in which the solid is insoluble.

Example:

A crystal of a chemical salt weighs 6.423 Gm. in air and 2.873

*Gm. when immersed in an oil having a specific gravity of 0.858.
What is the specific gravity of the salt?*

6.423 Gm. − 2.873 Gm. = 3.550 Gm. of displaced oil

By the proportion:

3.550 (Gm. of oil):6.423 (Gm. of salt) =
$$0.858 \text{ (sp. gr. of oil)}:x \text{ (sp. gr. of salt)}$$
x = 1.55, *answer*.

To calculate the specific gravity of a solid lighter than and insoluble in water:

The determination of the specific gravity of a solid *lighter than* and *insoluble in water* involves the use of a sinker which is attached to the solid in order to prevent it from floating (and therefore having no apparent weight at all). The weight of the sinker in air is of no interest to us here, but its weight when immersed in water alone must be known so that the combined weight of the solid in air and the sinker in water may be calculated. By subtracting from this weight the weight of solid and sinker when immersed in water, the weight of the water displaced by the solid (and therefore the *weight of an equal volume of water*) is calculated.

Example:

A piece of wax weighs 16.35 Gm. in air, and a sinker weighs
32.84 Gm. immersed in water. When they are fastened together
and immersed in water, their combined weight is 29.68 Gm.
Calculate the specific gravity of the wax.

32.84 Gm. + 16.35 Gm. = 49.19 Gm., combined weight of
sinker in water and of wax in air

49.19 Gm. − 29.68 Gm. = 19.51 Gm., weight of water displaced by wax (*weight of equal volume of water*)

Specific gravity of wax = $\dfrac{16.35 \text{ (Gm.)}}{19.51 \text{ (Gm.)}}$ = 0.8380, *answer*.

To calculate the specific gravity of granulated solids heavier than and insoluble in water:

A specific gravity bottle can be used with crystals, powders, and other forms of solids whose volume cannot be directly measured. If such a substance is *insoluble in water*, we may weigh a portion of it, introduce this amount into the bottle, fill up the bottle with water, and weigh the mixture. The solid will displace a *volume of water equal to its own volume,* and the weight of this displaced water can be calculated.

Example:

A bottle weighs 50.0 Gm. when empty and 96.8 Gm. when filled with water. If 28.8 Gm. of a granulated metal are placed in the bottle and the bottle is filled with water, the total weight is 118.4 Gm. What is the specific gravity of the metal?

96.8 Gm. − 50.0 Gm. = 46.8 Gm., weight of water filling the bottle

46.8 Gm. + 28.8 Gm. = 75.6 Gm., combined weight of water and metal

118.4 Gm. − 50.0 Gm. = 68.4 Gm., combined weight of water and metal in bottle

75.6 Gm. − 68.4 Gm. = 7.2 Gm., weight of water displaced by metal (*weight of equal volume of water*)

Specific gravity of metal $= \dfrac{28.8 \text{ (Gm.)}}{7.2 \text{ (Gm.)}} = 4.0$, *answer.*

SPECIFIC VOLUME

Specific volume (in pharmaceutical practice limited almost exclusively to liquids) is the ratio of the volume of a substance to the volume of an equal weight of another substance taken as a standard, both having the same temperature. Water is the standard for liquids and solids.

Whereas specific gravity is a comparison of weights of equal volumes, specific volume is a comparison of volumes of equal weights. Because of this relationship, specific gravity and specific volume are *reciprocals* of each other—that is, if they are multiplied together the product is 1. Specific volume tells us how much greater (or smaller) in volume a mass is than the same weight of water. It may be calculated by dividing the volume of a given mass by the volume of an equal weight of water. Thus, if 25 Gm. of glycerin measure 20 ml., and 25 Gm. of water measure 25 ml. under the same conditions, the specific volume of the glycerin =

$$\frac{\text{volume of 25 Gm. of glycerin}}{\text{volume of 25 Gm. of water}} = \frac{20 \text{ (ml.)}}{25 \text{ (ml.)}} = 0.8$$

To calculate the specific volume of a liquid, given the volume of a specified weight:

Calculate the specific volume of a syrup 91.0 ml. of which weigh 107.16 Gm.

107.16 Gm. of water measure 107.16 ml.

Specific volume of syrup $= \dfrac{91.0 \text{ (ml.)}}{107.16 \text{ (ml.)}} = 0.850$, *answer.*

To calculate the specific volume of a liquid, given its specific gravity, and to calculate its specific gravity given its specific volume:

Since specific gravity and specific volume are reciprocals of each other, a substance that is heavier than water will have a higher specific gravity and a lower specific volume, whereas a substance that is lighter than water will have a lower specific gravity and a higher specific volume. It follows, therefore, that we may determine the specific volume of any substance by dividing 1 by its specific gravity; and we may determine the specific gravity of a substance by dividing 1 by its specific volume.

Examples:

What is the specific volume of phosphoric acid having a specific gravity of 1.71?

$\dfrac{1}{1.71} = 0.585$, *answer.*

If a liquid has a specific volume of 1.396, what is its specific gravity?

$\dfrac{1}{1.396} = 0.716$, *answer.*

Practice Problems

1. If 250 ml. of alcohol weigh 203 Gm. what is its density?

2. A piece of copper metal weighs 53.6 Gm. and has a volume of 6 ml. Calculate its density.

3. A 30 ml. sample of sulfuric acid weighs 55 Gm. Calculate its density.

4. If 125 ml. of a liquid weigh 160 Gm., what is its specific gravity?

5. If 1200 ml. of a liquid weigh 1125 Gm., what is its specific gravity?

6. If 500 ml. of ferric chloride solution weigh 650 Gm., what is its specific gravity?

7. If a liter of syrup weighs 1313 Gm., what is its specific gravity?

8. If 134 Gm. of a liquid measure 142.6 ml., what is its specific gravity?

9. One pint of hydrochloric acid weighs 558 Gm. Calculate its specific gravity.

10. If 2 f℥ of glycerin weigh 1140 grains, what is its specific gravity?

11. If 30 ml. of a certain liquid weigh 570 grains, what is its specific gravity?

12. If 1 pint of a solution weighs 825 Gm., what is its specific gravity?

13. If 25 ml. of a liquid weigh 1 avoirdupois ounce, what is its specific gravity?

14. If 5 ml. of a liquid weigh 100 grains, what is its specific gravity?

15. What is the specific gravity of a liquid, if 750 ml. weigh 670 Gm.?

16. If 46.63 Gm. of an oil measure 51.5 ml., what is its specific gravity?

17. If two gallons of syrup weigh 20 lbs., what is its specific gravity?

18. A pycnometer weighs 12.95 Gm. When filled with water, it weighs 37.96 Gm. When filled with a sample of glycerin, it weighs 43.96 Gm. Calculate the specific gravity of the glycerin.

19. A specific gravity bottle weighs 62.35 Gm. Filled with water it weighs 87.42 Gm.; filled with another liquid it weighs 91.68 Gm. What is the specific gravity of the liquid?

20. An empty bottle weighs 50.0 Gm. When filled with water, it weighs 100.0 Gm.; when filled with an oil, it weighs 94.0 Gm. Calculate the specific gravity of the oil.

21. A pycnometer weighs 21.62 Gm. Filled with water it weighs 46.71 Gm.; filled with another liquid it weighs 43.28 Gm. Calculate the specific gravity of the liquid?

22. A pycnometer weighs 32.83 Gm. Filled with water it weighs 43.96 Gm. Filled with a sample it weighs 43.17 Gm. What is the specific gravity of the sample?

23. A glass plummet weighs 14.35 Gm. in air, 11.40 Gm. when immersed in water, and 8.95 Gm. when immersed in sulfuric acid. Calculate the specific gravity of the acid.

24. A glass stopper weighs 39.625 Gm. in air, 24.625 Gm. in water, and 28.375 Gm. in ether. What is the specific gravity of the ether?

25. A piece of glass weighs 7.42 Gm. in air, 5.16 Gm. when immersed in water, and 5.64 Gm. when immersed in an unknown liquid. Calculate the specific gravity of the liquid.

26. A piece of glass weighs 23.61 Gm. in air, 17.38 Gm. when immersed in water, and 18.76 Gm. when immersed in another liquid. Calculate the specific gravity of the liquid.

27. A glass plummet weighs 318 grains in air, 147 grains when immersed in water, and 175 grains when immersed in an oil. Calculate the specific gravity of the oil.

28. A piece of metal weighs 8.624 Gm. in air and 5.615 Gm. when immersed in water. What is its specific gravity?

29. If a solid weighs 84.62 Gm. in air and 58.48 Gm. when immersed in water, what is its specific gravity?

30. A piece of metal weighs 9.300 Gm. in air and 7.600 Gm. when immersed in water. Calculate the specific gravity of the metal.

31. A piece of metal weighs 848 grains in air and 768 grains when immersed in water. Calculate its specific gravity.

32. What is the specific gravity of a solid weighing 35.555 Gm. in air and 32.333 Gm. in water?

33. A crystal of a chemical salt weighs 19.705 Gm. in air and 13.270 Gm. when immersed in alcohol. If the alcohol has a specific gravity of 0.816, what is the specific gravity of the salt?

34. A chemical crystal weighs 3.630 Gm. in air and 1.820 Gm. when immersed in an oil. If the specific gravity of the oil is 0.837, what is the specific gravity of the chemical?

35. A substance weighing 150 grains in air is found to weigh 64.75 grains when immersed in an oil. If the specific gravity of the oil is 0.870, what is the specific gravity of the substance?

36. A crystal of a certain chemical weighs 42.25 grains in air and 25.25 grains when immersed in an oil. The specific gravity of the oil is 0.921. Calculate the specific gravity of the chemical.

37. A crystal weighs 20.50 Gm. in air, and 12.25 Gm. in turpentine oil (specific gravity 0.860). What is the specific gravity of the crystal?

38. A piece of wax weighs 42.65 Gm. in air, and a sinker weighs 38.42 Gm. in water. Together they weigh 33.18 Gm. in water. Calculate the specific gravity of the wax.

39. A piece of cork weighs 154 grains in air, and a sinker weighs 921 grains in water. Together they weigh 425 grains in water. What is the specific gravity of the cork?

40. A piece of paraffin weighs 13.750 Gm. A sinker weighs 9.000 Gm. in water. When they are fastened together, they weigh 7.800 Gm. in water. What is the specific gravity of the paraffin?

41. A bottle holds 115 Gm. of water. When 20 Gm. of an insoluble powder are introduced into the bottle and it is filled with water, the contents weigh 125 Gm. What is the specific gravity of the powder?

42. An insoluble powder weighs 12 Gm. A specific gravity bottle, weighing 21 Gm. when empty, weighs 121 Gm. when filled with water. When the powder is introduced into the bottle and the bottle is filled with water, the three together weigh 130 Gm. What is the specific gravity of the powder?

43. A pycnometer holds 25 Gm. of water. When 14 Gm. of a metal are introduced into it and it is filled with water, the contents weigh 37 Gm. What is the specific gravity of the metal?

44. Calculate the specific volume of a liquid 43.61 Gm. of which measure 38.0 ml.

45. Calculate the specific volume of a liquid 73.42 Gm. of which measure 81.5 ml.

46. If 120 Gm. of acetone measure 150 ml., what is its specific volume?

47. If olive oil has a specific gravity of 0.912, what is its specific volume?

48. The specific gravity of alcohol is 0.815. What is its specific volume?

49. What is the specific volume of sulfuric acid having a specific gravity of 1.826?

50. If chloroform has a specific gravity of 1.476, what is its specific volume?

51. What is the specific gravity of a liquid having a specific volume of 0.825?

52. If a liquid has a specific volume of 1.316, what is its specific gravity?

CHAPTER IX

WEIGHTS AND VOLUMES OF LIQUIDS

THE weights of equal volumes and the volumes of equal weights of liquids are proportional to their specific gravities. To calculate, therefore, the *weight of a given volume* or the *volume of a given weight* of a liquid, its specific gravity must be known.

When specific gravity is used as a factor in a calculation, the result should contain no more significant figures than the number in the factor.

Because of the simple relationship between the units in the metric system, such problems are simply and easily solved when only metric quantities are involved, but they become more complex when units of the common systems are used.

CALCULATIONS OF WEIGHT

To calculate the weight of a liquid when given its volume and specific gravity:

The *weight of any given volume* of a liquid of known specific gravity can be calculated by this proportion:

$$\begin{pmatrix}1 \text{ (specific grav-} \\ \text{ity of water)}\end{pmatrix} : \begin{pmatrix}\text{Specific grav-} \\ \text{ity of liquid}\end{pmatrix} = \begin{pmatrix}\text{Weight of equal} \\ \text{volume of water}\end{pmatrix} : x$$

x = weight of liquid

And from this we may derive a useful equation:

Weight of liquid =

Weight of equal volume of water $\times$ Specific gravity of liquid

Examples:

What is the weight of 3620 ml. of alcohol having a specific gravity of 0.820?

3620 ml. of water weigh 3620 Gm.

3620 Gm. $\times$ 0.820 = 2968 Gm., *answer.*

What is the weight of 4 f℥ of paraldehyde having a specific gravity of 0.990?

4 f℥ of water weigh 455 gr. × 4 or 1820 gr.

1820 gr. × 0.990 = 1802 gr., or (retaining only significant figures) 1800 gr., *answer.*

What is the weight, in Gm., of 2 f℥ of a liquid having a specific gravity of 1.118?

In this type of problem it is generally best to convert the given volume to its metric equivalent first and then to solve the problem in the metric system.

2 × 29.57 ml. = 59.14 ml.

59.14 ml. of water weigh 59.14 Gm.

59.14 Gm. × 1.118 = 66.12 Gm., *answer.*

What is the weight, in grains, of 50 ml. of ether having a specific gravity of 0.715?

In problems of this type it is generally best to solve the problem in the metric system and then to convert the weight to the common system.

50 ml. of water weigh 50 Gm.

50 Gm. × 0.715 = 35.75 Gm. = 551 gr., *answer.*

CALCULATIONS OF VOLUME

To calculate the volume of a liquid when given its weight and specific gravity:

The *volume of any given weight* of a liquid of known specific gravity can be calculated by this proportion:

$$\begin{pmatrix} \text{Specific grav-} \\ \text{ity of liquid} \end{pmatrix} : \begin{pmatrix} 1 \text{ (specific grav-} \\ \text{ity of water)} \end{pmatrix} = \begin{pmatrix} \text{Volume of equal} \\ \text{weight of water} \end{pmatrix} : x$$

x = volume of liquid

And the derived equation will be:

$$\text{Volume of liquid} = \frac{\text{Volume of equal weight of water}}{\text{Specific gravity of liquid}}$$

Examples:

What is the volume of 492 Gm. of nitric acid with a specific gravity of 1.40?

492 Gm. of water measure 492 ml.

$$\frac{492 \text{ ml.}}{1.40} = 351 \text{ ml.}, \textit{answer.}$$

What is the volume, in minims, of 1 oz. of a perfume oil having a specific gravity of 0.850?

1 oz. = 437.5 gr.

437.5 gr. of water measure $\frac{437.5}{455}$ f℥ or 462 ℳ

$$\frac{462 \text{ ℳ}}{0.850} = 544 \text{ or } 540 \text{ ℳ}, \textit{answer.}$$

Or:

1 oz. = 28.35 Gm.

28.35 Gm. of water measure 28.35 ml.

$$\frac{28.35 \text{ ml.}}{0.850} = 33.25 \text{ ml.} = 541 \text{ or } 540 \text{ ℳ}, \textit{answer.}$$

What is the volume, in f℥, of 1 lb. of methyl salicylate with a specific gravity of 1.185?

1 lb. = 454 Gm.

454 Gm. of water measure 454 ml.

$$\frac{454 \text{ ml.}}{1.185} = 383.1 \text{ ml.} = 12.96 \text{ f℥, or (with 3-figure}$$
accuracy), 13.0 f℥, *answer.*

What is the volume, in pints, of 50 lb. of glycerin having a specific gravity of 1.25?

50 lb. = 454 × 50 = 22700 Gm.

22700 Gm. of water measure 22700 ml.

$$\frac{22700 \text{ ml.}}{1.25} = 18160 \text{ ml.} = 38.4 \text{ pints}, \textit{answer.}$$

What is the volume, in f℥, of 1600 Gm. of a liquid with a specific gravity of 1.314?

1600 Gm. of water measure 1600 ml.

$$\frac{1600 \text{ ml.}}{1.314} = 1217.7 \text{ ml.} = 41.17 \text{ f℥}, \textit{answer.}$$

8

To calculate the cost of a given volume of a liquid bought by weight:

Examples:

What is the cost of 1000 ml. of glycerin, specific gravity 1.249, bought at 50 cents per lb.?

1000 ml. of water weigh 1000 Gm.

Weight of 1000 ml. of glycerin = 1000 Gm. × 1.249 = 1249 Gm.

1 lb. = 454 Gm.

454 (Gm.):1249 (Gm.) = $0.50:x

x = $1.38, *answer.*

What is the cost of 2 f℥ of cassia oil, specific gravity 1.055, bought at $3.50 per lb.?

2 f℥ = 59.14 ml.

59.14 ml. of water weigh 59.14 Gm.

Weight of 59.14 ml. of oil = 59.14 Gm. × 1.055 = 62.39 Gm.

1 lb. = 454 Gm.

454 (Gm.):62.39 (Gm.) = $3.50:x

x = $0.48, *answer.*

What is the cost of 1 pint of chloroform, specific gravity 1.475, bought at $0.70 per lb.?

1 pint = 473 ml.

473 ml. of water weigh 473 Gm.

Weight of 473 ml. of chloroform = 473 Gm. × 1.475 = 697.7 Gm.

1 lb. = 454 Gm.

454 (Gm.):697.7 (Gm.) = $0.70:x

x = $1.08, *answer.*

Practice Problems

1. What is the weight of 100 ml. of hydrochloric acid having a specific gravity of 1.16?

2. What is the weight of 300 ml. of glycerin having a specific gravity of 1.25?

3. What is the weight, in grams, of 14 ml. of mercury having a specific gravity of 13.6?

4. How many grams do 225 ml. of sulfuric acid weigh if its specific gravity is 1.83?

5. What is the weight, in kilograms, of 5 liters of sulfuric acid with a specific gravity of 1.84?

6. What is the weight of 650 ml. of chloroform having a specific gravity of 1.475?

7. If the specific gravity of alcohol is 0.812, what is the weight, in kilograms, of 10 liters?

8. What is the weight, in grains, of 4 f℥ of glycerin having a specific gravity of 1.25?

9. If the specific gravity of alcohol is 0.812, what is the weight, in grains, of 3 f℥ ?

10. What is the weight, in grams, of 240 ℧ of chloroform having a specific gravity of 1.475?

11. What is the weight, in pounds, of 5 pints of nitric acid having a specific gravity of 1.42?

12. What is the weight, in grams, of 1 pint of chloroform having a specific gravity of 1.475?

13. What is the weight, in grams, of 8 f℥ of an oil with a specific gravity of 0.870?

14. Calculate the weight, in grams, of 10 pints of hydrochloric acid having a specific gravity of 1.155.

15. What is the weight, in kilograms, of 1 gallon of syrup having a specific gravity of 1.313?

16. What is the weight, in grams, of 1 pint of a mixture of equal parts of alcohol (specific gravity 0.812) and glycerin (specific gravity 1.25)?

17. What is the weight, in grains, of 95 ml. of chloroform having a specific gravity of 1.476?

18. How many grains do 500 ml. of alcohol (specific gravity 0.812) weigh?

19. What is the weight, in pounds, of 4370 ml. of a syrup with a specific gravity of 1.37?

20. What is the weight, in pounds, of 1 liter of glycerin having a specific gravity of 1.25?

21. What is the volume, in milliliters, of 100 Gm. of an acid having a specific gravity of 1.71?

22. What is the volume, in milliliters, of 227 Gm. of a liquid having a specific gravity of 1.230?

23. How many milliliters does 1 Kg. of sulfuric acid with a specific gravity of 1.83 measure?

24. What is the volume of 1000 Gm. of mercury having a specific gravity of 13.6?

25. A formula calls for 425 Gm. of hydrochloric acid with a specific gravity of 1.155. How many milliliters of the acid should be used?

26. What is the volume of 650 Gm. of ferric chloride solution with a specific gravity of 1.30?

27. A formula for 1000 ml. of a preparation calls for 800 Gm. of cottonseed oil with a specific gravity of 0.920. How many milliliters of cottonseed oil should be used in preparing 5 liters of the formula?

28. A formula for a vanishing cream contains 750 Gm. of glycerin. How many milliliters of glycerin (specific gravity 1.25) should be used?

29. What is the volume, in milliliters, of 1 kilo of peppermint oil with a specific gravity of 0.908?

30. What is the volume, in milliliters, of a liniment containing 1 lb. of chloroform (specific gravity 1.475) and 5 lb. of methyl salicylate (specific gravity 1.180)?

31. What is the volume, in minims, of 60 grains of an acid solution having a specific gravity of 1.08?

32. What is the volume, in fluidounces, of $\frac{1}{2}$ lb. of ether with a specific gravity of 0.714?

33. What is the volume, in pints, of 9 lb. of sulfuric acid having a specific gravity of 1.83?

34. Calculate the volume, in fluidounces, of 1 lb. of an oil with a specific gravity of 0.904?

35. What is the volume, in pints, of 40 lb. of a liquid with a specific gravity of 1.32?

36. What is the volume, in pints, of 10 lb. of peppermint oil having a specific gravity of 0.904?

37. What is the cost of 10 liters of a liquid (specific gravity 1.20) bought at 88 cents per lb.?

38. What is the cost of 3 liters of chloroform (specific gravity 1.475) bought at 70 cents per lb.?

39. What is the cost of 4 f℥ of ether (specific gravity 0.715) bought at $1.00 per lb.?

40. What is the cost of 1 pint of oleic acid (specific gravity 0.895) bought at $2.50 per Kg.?

41. What will 10 gallons of glycerin (specific gravity 1.25) cost at 45 cents per lb.?

42. A formula for a mouth rinse contains 1.6 ml. of cinnamon oil per 1000 ml. If the cinnamon oil (specific gravity 1.050) is bought at $2.75 per lb., calculate the cost of the oil required to prepare 5 gallons of the mouth rinse.

43. A perfume oil has a specific gravity of 0.960 and costs $5.75 per Kg. What is the cost of 4 f℥ ?

44. A prescription calls for 0.3 Gm. of syrupy phosphoric acid (specific gravity 1.71). How many milliliters should be used in compounding the prescription?

45. A formula for 1000 Gm. of a soft soap contains 380 Gm. of a vegetable oil. If the oil has a specific gravity of 0.890, how many milliliters should be used in preparing 10 lb. of the soft soap?

46. A cosmetic formula calls for 500 Gm. of peach kernel oil (specific gravity 0.910) per 1000 Gm. of finished product. How many milliliters of the oil should be used in preparing 5000 Gm. of the formula?

47. A sunscreen lotion contains 5 Gm. of menthyl salicylate (specific gravity 1.045) per 100 ml. How many milliliters of menthyl salicylate should be used in preparing 1 gallon of the lotion?

48.	White Wax	12.5 Gm.
	Mineral Oil	60.0 Gm.
	Lanolin	2.5 Gm.
	Sodium Borate	1.0 Gm.
	Rose Water	24.0 Gm.

How many milliliters of mineral oil having a specific gravity of 0.860 should be used in preparing 5 lb. of the above formula?

49.

Stearic Acid	14.0 Gm.
Triethanolamine	0.7 Gm.
Cetyl Alcohol	3.0 Gm.
Sodium Lauryl Sulfate	0.5 Gm.
Propylene Glycol	5.0 Gm.
Distilled Water	76.8 ml.

How many milliliters of triethanolamine (specific gravity 1.125) and how many milliliters of propylene glycol (specific gravity 1.035) should be used in preparing 2500 Gm. of the above formula?

CHAPTER X

PERCENTAGE PREPARATIONS

PERCENTAGE

The term *per cent* and its corresponding sign (%) mean "by the hundred" or "in a hundred," and *percentage* means "rate per hundred"; so *50 per cent* (or *50%*) and *a percentage of 50* are equivalent expressions. A per cent may also be expressed as a *ratio*, represented as a common or decimal fraction. For example, *50%* means *50 parts in 100* of the same kind, and may be expressed as $\frac{50}{100}$ or *0.50*. Per cent, therefore, is simply another fraction of such frequent and familiar use that its numerator is expressed, but its denominator is left understood. It should be noted that per cent is always an abstract quantity, and that, as such, it may be applied to anything.

For the purposes of computation, per cents are usually changed to equivalent decimal fractions. This is done by dropping the % sign and dividing the expressed numerator by *100*. Thus, *12.5%* = *12.5:100*, or *0.125*, and *0.05%* = *0.05:100*, or *0.0005*. We must not forget that in the reverse process (changing a decimal to a per cent) the decimal is multiplied by *100* and the % sign is affixed.

Percentage is an essential part of the arithmetic of pharmacy. The pharmacist encounters it constantly and uses it as a convenient means of expressing the concentration of a solute in a solution, of the amount of active material in a drug or preparation, or of the quantity of an ingredient in a mixture.

PERCENTAGE SOLUTIONS

Percentage, as it applies to solutions, has a very special meaning. It was pointed out above that percentage expresses *parts per 100 parts*. Obviously, then, in a *true percentage solution* the *parts* of the percentage would represent *grams* of a solute in *100 Gm.* of solution. In general practice, however, the dispensing pharmacist most frequently encounters a different kind of percentage solution, one in which the *parts* of the percentage represent *grams* of a solute in

(119)

100 ml. of solution. In order to avoid the possibility of any mis-interpretation of the meaning of the term "percentage solution," the *United States Pharmacopeia* states that:

"Percentage concentrations of solutions are expressed as follows:

"*Per cent weight in weight*—(w/w) expresses the number of grams of an active constituent in 100 grams of solution.

"*Per cent weight in volume*—(w/v) expresses the number of grams of an active constituent in 100 milliliters of solution, and is used in prescription practice regardless of whether water or some other liquid is the solvent.

"*Per cent volume in volume*—(v/v) expresses the number of milliliters of an active constituent in 100 milliliters of solution.

"When *per cent* is used in prescriptions without qualification, it means: for mixtures of solids, per cent weight in weight; for solutions of solids in liquids, per cent weight in volume; for solutions of liquids in liquids, per cent volume in volume; and for solutions of gases in liquids, per cent weight in volume. For example, a 1 per cent solution is prepared by dissolving 1 gram of a solid or 1 milli-liter of a liquid in sufficient of the solvent to make 100 milliliters of the solution. A solution of approximately the same strength may be prepared by apothecary weight and measure by dissolving 4.5 grains of a solid or 4.8 minims of a liquid in sufficient of the solvent to make 1 fluidounce of the solution.

"In dispensing prescriptions, slight changes in volume owing to variations in room temperatures may be disregarded."[1]

PERCENTAGE WEIGHT-IN-VOLUME

One way of making all weight-in-volume solutions conform to this official interpretation would be to convert all common and apothecaries' weights to grams and all volumes to milliliters before expressing percentage strength. But, as suggested by the *Pharma-copeia*, such a procedure is not required.

For, if *1 gram* in *100 milliliters of solution* is taken as the only "correct" strength of a 1% (w/w) solution, this means that 1 gram of solute is contained in a volume of solution *that would weigh 100 grams if, like water, the solution had a specific gravity of 1*—if, in other words, each milliliter of solution weighed *1 gram*. Hence, to make a solution of the same strength by any system of measure, we have only to dissolve *1* weight unit of solute in sufficient solvent to make a volume that would weigh *100* of those weight units if the solution were pure water.

A solution so compounded, then, would contain not only *1 Gm.*

[1] U.S.P. XV, 1955. General Notices, page 12.

in every *100 ml.* (the volume of *100 Gm.* of water) but likewise approximately *4.55* grains[1] in every fluidounce (the volume of *455 grains* of water at 25° C.). Therefore, we may look upon a *weight-in-volume* solution as a kind of *weight-in-weight* solution in disguise: the percentage strength being based after all upon a comparison of parts by weight, but the weight of the solution being arbitrarily calculated from its designated volume as if it had a specific gravity of *1*.

To calculate the weight of the active ingredient in a specified volume of solution, given its percentage weight-in-volume:

Taking water to represent any solvent, we may prepare weight-in-volume percentage solutions which are equivalent in strength

[1] "Disregarding the difference between cubic centimeter and milliliter, which is so small that it does not affect the equivalents used, this quantity was derived as follows:

    1 cubic centimeter of water at 4° C. weighs 1 gram
       1 fluidounce = 29.573 cubic centimeters
          1 gram = 15.4324 grains
Using these equivalents
    100 cc. : 29.573 cc.   = 1 Gm. : x
                   x = 0.29573 Gm.
    1 Gm. : 0.29573 Gm. = 15.4324 gr. : y
                   y = 4.5638 grains

"This would be the number of grains of a solid in 1 fluidounce of a 1 per cent solution if the liquid were measured at 4° C., but percentage solutions are generally prepared at or near the official temperature of 25° C., and any volume of a liquid weighs slightly less at 25° C. than it does at 4° C. The effect of this is that a theoretical 1% solution, containing 4.5638 grains of a chemical in 1 fluidounce at 4° C., will contain less than this weight in 1 fluidounce if it were prepared at 4° C. and the fluidounce is measured at 25° C. The quantities are approximately proportional to the quantities of water in fluidounces measured at each of the respective temperatures. The correction of this slight difference can be made by the following methods:

    1 fluidounce of water weighs 456.38 grains in vacuum at 4° C.
    1 fluidounce of water weighs 454.57 grains in air at 25° C.

Using these numbers, we have this proportion:
    456.38 : 454.57 = 4.5638 : z
               z = 4.5457 grains in 1 fluidounce of a 1 per cent
                      solution at 25° C.

"In this correction, water is taken to represent any solvent, and the small amount of solvent displaced by the solid is disregarded. This can be done without introducing an appreciable error for any ordinary percentage solution, because the total difference is so small.

"The number of grains in one fluidounce of a 1 per cent weight-in-volume solution may be rounded off to 4.5, 4.55, or 4.546, to attain different degrees of accuracy in preparing such solutions."

(Quoted from "The Calculation of Percentage Solutions in the U.S.P. XI" by Dr. Theodore J. Bradley, *American Druggist*, July, 1936.)

when calculated by either the metric or the apothecaries' system if we use the following rules:

Rule 1.   In the metric system, multiply the required number of milliliters by the percentage strength, expressed as a decimal, to obtain the number of grams of solute in the solution. *The volume in milliliters represents the weight in grams of the solution if it were pure water.*

Volume in ml. × % (expressed as a decimal) = Gm. of solute

Rule 2.   In the apothecaries' system multiply the *weight* of a fluidounce of water (455 grains) by the percentage strength, expressed as a decimal, and by the number of fluidounces to obtain the number of grains of solute in the solution.

455 × % (expressed as a decimal) × vol. in f℥ = gr. of solute

Or, as suggested by the *Pharmacopeia,*

4.5 × % (expressed as a whole number) × vol. in f℥ = gr. of solute

Examples:

How many grams of dextrose are required to prepare 4000 ml. of a 5% solution?

4000 × 0.05 = 200 Gm., *answer.*

℞	Potassium Permanganate	0.02%
	Distilled Water ad	250.0
	Sig. As directed.	

How many grams of potassium permanganate should be used in compounding the prescription?

0.02% = 0.0002

250 × 0.0002 = 0.050 Gm., *answer.*

How many grains of mild silver protein should be used in preparing 4 f℥ of a 10% solution?

455 × 0.10 × 4 = 182 gr., *answer.*

Or,

4.5 × 10 × 4 = 180 gr., *answer.*

℞	Atropine Sulfate	2%
	Distilled Water q.s. ad	℥iv
	Sig. Use in the eye.	

How many grains of atropine sulfate should be used in compounding the prescription?

$\text{℥iv} = \frac{1}{2} \text{ f℥}$

$455 \times 0.02 \times \frac{1}{2} = 4.55 \text{ gr.,}$ *answer.*

Or,

$4.5 \times 2 \times \frac{1}{2} = 4.5 \text{ gr.,}$ *answer.*

To calculate the percentage weight-in-volume of a solution, given the weight of the solute and the volume of the solution:

It should be remembered that the volume, in milliliters, of the solution represents the weight, in grams, of the solution if it were pure water.

Examples:

What is the percentage strength (w/v) of a solution of urea, if 80 ml. contain 12 Gm.?

80 ml. of water weigh 80 Gm.

By the proportion:

80 (Gm.):12 (Gm.) = 100 (%):x

x = 15%, *answer.*

What is the percentage strength (w/v) of a solution of strong silver protein, if 45.5 grains are dissolved in enough distilled water to make 8 f℥?

8 f℥ of water weigh 3640 gr.

By the proportion:

3640 (gr.):45.5 (gr.) = 100 (%):x

x = 1.25%, *answer.*

To calculate the volume of a solution, given its percentage strength weight-in-volume and the weight of the solute:

Examples:

How many milliliters of a 3% solution can be made from 27 Gm. of boric acid?

By the proportion:

3 (%):100 (%) = 27 (Gm.):x

x = 900 Gm., weight of the solution if it were water

Volume in ml. = 900 ml., *answer.*

How many fluidounces of a 10% solution can be made from 182 grains of colloidal silver iodide?

By the proportion:

10 (%):100 (%) = 182 (gr.):x

x = 1820 gr., weight of solution if it were water

Volume in f℥ = $\frac{1820}{455}$ f℥ = 4 f℥, *answer.*

PERCENTAGE VOLUME-IN-VOLUME

Liquids are usually measured by volume, and the percentage strength indicates the number of parts by volume of the active ingredient that are contained in the total volume of the solution considered as 100 parts by volume. If there is any possibility of misinterpretation, this kind of percentage should be specified: *e.g., 10% (v/v).*

To calculate the volume of the active ingredient in a specified volume of a solution, given its percentage strength volume-in-volume:

Examples:

> ℞   Liquefied Phenol   2.5%
>   Boric Acid Solution ad   240.0 ml.
>   Sig. For external use.

How many milliliters of liquefied phenol should be used in compounding the prescription?

Volume in ml. × % (expressed as a decimal) = ml. of active ingredient
240 ml. × 0.025 = 6 ml., *answer.*

> ℞   Wintergreen Oil   5%
>   Isopropyl Alcohol ad   f℥ iv
>   Sig. Apply.

How many minims of wintergreen oil should be used in compounding the prescription?

Vol. in ♏ × % (expressed as a decimal) = vol. in ♏ of active ingredient

480 ♏ × 4 × 0.05 = 96 ♏, *answer.*

Or, as suggested by the *Pharmacopeia,*

4.8 × % (expressed as a whole number) × vol. in f℥ =
vol. in ℳ of active ingredient

4.8 × 5 × 4 = 96 ℳ, *answer.*

To calculate the percentage volume-in-volume of a solution, given the volume of active ingredient and the volume of the solution:

The required volumes may have to be calculated from given weights and specific gravities.

Examples:

In preparing 250 ml. of a certain lotion, a pharmacist used 4 ml. of liquefied phenol. What was the percentage (v/v) of liquefied phenol in the lotion?

By the proportion:

250 (ml.):4 (ml.) = 100 (%):x

x = 1.6%, *answer.*

A formula for 8 f℥ of a mouth rinse contains 10 ℳ of a flavoring oil. What is the percentage (v/v) of the oil in the mouth rinse?

8 f℥ = 3840 ℳ

By the proportion:

3840 (ℳ):10 (ℳ) = 100 (%):x

x = 0.26%, *answer.*

What is the percentage strength (v/v) of a solution of 800 Gm. of a liquid with a specific gravity of 0.800 in enough water to make 4000 ml.?

800 Gm. of water measure 800 ml.

800 ml. ÷ 0.800 = 1000 ml. of active ingredient

By the proportion:

4000 (ml.):1000 (ml.) = 100 (%):x

x = 25%, *answer.*

To calculate the volume of a solution, given the volume of the active ingredient and its percentage strength (v/v):

The volume of the active ingredient may have to be first calculated from its weight and specific gravity.

Examples:

Spearmint spirit contains 10% (v/v) of spearmint oil. What volume of the spirit will contain 75 ml. of spearmint oil?

By the proportion:

10 (%):100 (%) = 75 (ml.):x

x = 750 ml., *answer.*

Chloroform liniment contains 30% (v/v) of chloroform. How many milliliters of chloroform liniment can be prepared from 1 lb. of chloroform (sp. gr. 1.475)?

1 lb. = 454 Gm.

454 Gm. of water measure 454 ml.

454 ml. ÷ 1.475 = 308 ml. of chloroform

By the proportion:

30 (%):100 (%) = 308 (ml.):x

x = 1027 or 1030 ml., *answer.*

PERCENTAGE WEIGHT-IN-WEIGHT

Percentage weight-in-weight (*true percentage* or *percentage by weight*) indicates the number of parts by weight of active ingredient that are contained in the total weight of the solution considered as 100 parts by weight.

Liquids are not customarily measured by weight, and therefore, a weight-in-weight solution of a solid or a liquid in a liquid should be so designated: *e.g., 10% (w/w).*

To calculate the weight of the active ingredient in a specified weight of the solution, given its weight-in-weight percentage strength:

Examples:

√*How many grams of phenol should be used to prepare 240 Gm. of a 5% (w/w) solution in water?*

Weight of solution in Gm. × % (expressed as a decimal) = Gm. of solute

240 Gm. × 0.05 = 12 Gm., *answer.*

How many Gm. of a chemical are required to make 120 ml. of a 20% (w/w) solution having a specific gravity of 1.15?

120 ml. of water weigh 120 Gm.

120 Gm. × 1.15 = 138 Gm., weight of 120 ml. of solution

138 Gm. × 0.20 = 27.6 Gm. plus enough water to make
120 ml., *answer.*

★ **To calculate the weight of either active ingredient or diluent, given the weight of the other and the percentage strength (w/w) of the solution:**

The weights of active ingredient and diluent are proportional to their percentages.

Example:

How many grams of a chemical should be dissolved in 240 ml. of water to make a 4% (w/w) solution?

100% − 4% = 96% (by weight) of water

240 ml. of water weigh 240 Gm.

By the proportion:

96 (%):4 (%) = 240 (Gm.):x

x = 10 Gm., *answer.* of med. + 240 ml of H₂O

It is usually impossible to prepare a specified *volume* of a solution of given weight-in-weight percentage strength, since the volume displaced by the active ingredient cannot be known in advance. If an excess is not undesirable, we may make a volume somewhat more than that specified by taking the given volume to refer to the solvent and from this quantity calculating the weight of the solvent (the specific gravity of the solvent must be known). Using this weight, we may follow the method above to calculate the corresponding weight of the active ingredient needed.

Examples: something of this sort for bonus pts

How should you prepare 100 ml. of a 2% (w/w) solution of a chemical in a solvent having a specific gravity of 1.25?

100 ml. of water weigh 100 Gm.

100 Gm. × 1.25 = 125 Gm., weight of 100 ml. of solvent

100% − 2% = 98% (by weight) of solvent

By the proportion:

98 (%):2 (%) = 125 (Gm.):x

x = 2.55 Gm.

2.55 Gm. of chemical and 125 Gm. (or 100 ml.) of solvent,
answer.

*How should you prepare 6 f℥ of a 20% (w/w) solution of a
chemical in water?*

6 f℥ of water weigh 2730 gr.

100% − 20% = 80% (by weight) of solvent

By the proportion:

80 (%):20 (%) = 2730 (gr.):x

x = 682 gr.

682 gr. of chemical plus 6 f℥ of water, *answer.*

To calculate the percentage strength (w/w) of a solution, given the weight of the active ingredient and the weight of the solution:

If the weight of the finished solution is not given, other data must
be supplied from which it may be calculated: the weights of both
ingredients, for instance, or the volume and the specific gravity
of the solution.

Examples:

*If 1500 Gm. of a solution contain 75 Gm. of a chemical, what is
the percentage strength (w/w) of the solution?*

By the proportion:

1500 (Gm.):75 (Gm.) = 100 (%):x

x = 5%, *answer.*

*If 5 Gm. of boric acid are dissolved in 100 ml. of water, what is
the percentage strength (w/w) of the solution?*

100 ml. of water weigh 100 Gm.

100 Gm. + 5 Gm. = 105 Gm., weight of solution

By the proportion:

105 (Gm.):5 (Gm.) = 100 (%):x

x = 4.76%, *answer.*

If 1000 ml. of syrup with a specific gravity of 1.313 contain 850 Gm. of sucrose, what is its percentage strength (w/w)?

1000 ml. of water weigh 1000 Gm.

1000 Gm. × 1.313 = 1313 Gm., weight of 1000 ml. of syrup

By the proportion:

1313 (Gm.):850 (Gm.) = 100 (%):x

x = 64.7%, *answer.*

To calculate the weight of a solution, given the weight of its active ingredient and its percentage strength (w/w):

Example:

What weight of a 5% (w/w) solution can be prepared from 2 Gm. of active ingredient?

By the proportion:

5 (%):100 (%) = 2 (Gm.):x

x = 40 Gm., *answer.*

WEIGHT-IN-WEIGHT MIXTURES OF SOLIDS

Solids are usually measured by weight, and the percentage strength of a mixture of solids indicates the number of parts by weight of the active ingredient that are contained in the total weight of the mixture considered as *100 parts* by weight.

To calculate the amount of active ingredient in a specified weight of a mixture of solids, given its percentage strength (w/w):

Examples:

Rʑ   Mercury Bichloride $\frac{1}{50}\%$
       Petrolatum ad   10.0 Gm.
       Sig. For the eye.

How many milligrams of mercury bichloride should be used in compounding the prescription?

$\frac{1}{50}\% = 0.02\%$

9

10 Gm. × 0.0002 = 0.002 Gm. or 2 mg., *answer.*

℞ Chrysarobin   5%
    Petrolatum ad   ℥ ss
    Sig. Apply to affected areas.

How many grains of chrysarobin should be used in compounding the prescription?

℥ ss = 240 gr.

240 gr. × 0.05 = 12 gr., *answer.*

℞ Merbromin   2%
    Cocoa Butter ad   2.0
    Ft. suppos. tales no. vi
    Sig. One at night.

How many grams of merbromin should be used in compounding the prescription?

2 Gm. × 6 = 12 Gm., total weight of mixture

12 Gm. × 0.02 = 0.24 Gm., *answer.*

℞ Zinc Oxide   5%
    Belladonna Extract   ¼%
    Cocoa Butter ad   ℥ ss
    Ft. suppos. tales no. x
    Sig. One as directed.

How many grains of zinc oxide and how many grains of belladonna extract should be used in compounding the prescription?

℥ ss = 30 gr.

30 gr. × 10 = 300 gr., total weight of mixture

300 gr. × 0.05 = 15 gr. of zinc oxide, *and*

300 gr. × 0.0025 = 0.75 gr. = ¾ gr. of belladonna extract,
                                              answers.

RATIO STRENGTH

The concentrations of weak solutions are very frequently expressed in terms of ratio strength. Since all percentages are a ratio of parts per hundred, ratio strength is merely another way of expressing the percentage strength of solutions (and, less frequently, of mixtures of solids). For example, *5%* means *5 parts per 100* or *5:100*. Although *5 parts per 100* designates a ratio strength, it is customary to translate this designation into a ratio the first figure of which is *1;* thus, *5:100 = 1:20*.

When a ratio strength, for example *1:1000*, is used to designate a concentration, it is to be interpreted as follows:

For solids in liquids—1 gram of solute in *1000 milliliters* of solution or *1 grain* of solute in a volume of solution represented by that of *1000 grains* of water.

For liquids in liquids—1 milliliter of active ingredient in *1000 milliliters* of solution or *1 minim* of active ingredient in *1000 minims* of solution.

For solids in solids—1 gram of active ingredient in *1000 grams* of mixture or *1 grain* of active ingredient in *1000 grains of mixture*.

The ratio and percentage strengths of any solution or mixture of solids are proportional, and either is easily converted to the other by the use of proportion.

To calculate ratio strength, given the percentage strength:

Example:

Express 0.02% as a ratio strength.

0.02% = 0.02 parts per 100

By the proportion:

0.02 (parts):100 (parts) = 1 (part):x (parts)

x = 5000

Ratio strength = 1:5000, *answer.*

To calculate percentage strength, given the ratio strength:

Example:

Express 1:4000 as a percentage strength.

By the proportion:

4000 (parts):1 (part) = 100 (%):x

x = 0.025%, *answer.*

To calculate the ratio strength of a solution, given the weight of solute in a specified volume of solution:

Example:

A certain injectable contains 2 mg. of a drug per ml. of solution. What is the ratio strength (w/v) of the solution?

2 mg. = 0.002 Gm.

By the proportion:

0.002 (Gm.):1 (Gm.) = 1 (ml.):x

x = 500 ml.

Ratio strength = 1:500, *answer.*

What is the ratio strength (w/v) of a solution made by dissolving two tablets, each containing 0.125 Gm. of mercury bichloride, in enough water to make 500 ml.?

0.125 Gm. × 2 = 0.250 Gm. of mercury bichloride

By the proportion:

0.250 (Gm.):500 (Gm.) = 1 (ml.):x

x = 2000 ml.

Ratio strength = 1:2000, *answer.*

To solve problems involving ratio strength:

In solving problems in which the calculations are based on ratio strength, it is sometimes convenient to translate the problem into one based on percentage strength and to solve it according to the rules and methods discussed under percentage solutions and percentage mixtures of solids.

Examples:

How many grams of potassium permanganate should be used in preparing 500 ml. of a 1:2500 solution?

1:2500 = 0.04%

500 × 0.0004 = 0.2 Gm., *answer.*

Or,

1:2500 means 1 Gm. in 2500 ml. of solution

By the proportion:

2500 (ml.):500 (ml.) = 1 (Gm.):x

x = 0.2 Gm., *answer.*

℞   Sol. Mercury Oxycyanide
        1:5000   120.0
    Sig. Use as eye wash.

How many milligrams of mercury oxycyanide should be used in compounding the prescription?

1:5000 = 0.02%

120 × 0.0002 = 0.024 Gm. or 24 mg., *answer.*

Or,

1:5000 means 1 Gm. in 5000 ml. of solution

By the proportion:

5000 (ml.):120 (ml.) = 1 (Gm.):x

x = 0.024 Gm. or 24 mg., *answer.*

How many grains of mercuric chloride are required to prepare f℥viii of a 1:4000 solution?

1:4000 = 0.025%

4.5 × 0.025 × 8 = 0.9 gr., *answer.*

Or,

1:4000 means 1 gr. in a volume of solution represented by that of 4000 gr. of water

8 f℥ of water weigh 3640 gr.

By the proportion:

4000 (gr.):3640 (gr.) = 1 (gr.):x

x = 0.9 gr., *answer.*

℞   Eserine Salicylate   1:400
    Ophthalmic Base ad   8.0 Gm.
    Sig. Apply to the eye.

How many milligrams of eserine salicylate should be used in compounding the prescription?

1:400 = 0.25%

8 Gm. × 0.0025 = 0.020 Gm. or 20 mg., *answer.*

Or,

1:400 means 1 Gm. in 400 Gm. of ointment

By the proportion:

400 (Gm.):8 (Gm.) = 1 (Gm.):x

x = 0.020 Gm. or 20 mg., *answer.*

℞   Atropine Sulfate   1:200
    Petrolatum ad   ℨ ii
    Sig. Apply to the eye.

How many grains of atropine sulfate should be used in compounding the prescription?

1:200 ⇒ 0.5%

℥ ii = 120 gr.

120 gr. × 0.005 = 0.6 gr., *answer*.

Or,

1:200 means 1 gr. in 200 gr. of ointment

By the proportion:

200 (gr.):120 (gr.) = 1 (gr.):x

x = 0.6 gr., *answer*.

Practice Problems

1. How many grams of mercuric chloride are required to prepare 250 ml. of a 5% (w/v) solution?

2. How many grams of boric acid are there in 30 ml. of a 2% (w/v) solution?

3. How many grams of phenol are required to prepare 480 ml. of a $\frac{1}{10}$% (w/v) solution?

4. ℞   Sol. Ferrous Sulfate
          2%   125.0
      Sig. Use as directed.

How many grams of ferrous sulfate should be used in compounding the prescription?

5. ℞   Sol. Strong Silver Protein
          0.5%   60 ml.
      Sig. Apply externally.

How many grams of strong silver protein should be used in compounding the prescription?

6. ℞   Histamine Phosphate Solution
          0.01%   15.0
      Sig. Use as directed.

How many milligrams of histamine phosphate should be used in compounding the prescription?

7. ℞ Sol. Sodium Thiosulfate
                25%   180.0
       Sig. For external use.

How many grams of sodium thiosulfate should be used in compounding the prescription?

8. ℞ Sol. Colloidal Silver Iodide   10%
       Sol. Ephedrine Sulfate   3%
                      aa   ad   30.0
       Sig. For the nose.

How many grams of colloidal silver iodide and how many grams of ephedrine sulfate should be used in compounding the prescription?

9. ℞ Sol. Mercury Oxycyanide
                $\frac{1}{40}$%   30.0
       Sig. Use in the eye.

How many milligrams of mercury oxycyanide should be used in prescription compounding?

10. ℞ Potassium Permanganate   0.01%
        Distilled Water ad   250.0
        Sig. For irrigation.

How many milligrams of potassium permanganate should be used in compounding the prescription?

11. How many grains of silver nitrate will be required to prepare f℥iv of a 0.25% (w/v) solution?

12. How many grains of gentian violet should be used in preparing f℥ii of a $\frac{1}{2}$% (w/v) solution?

13. ℞ Phenol   5%
        Glycerin ad   ℥ii
        Sig. Ear drops.

How many grains of phenol should be used in compounding the prescription?

14. ℞ Sol. Potassium Iodide
                100%   ℥i
       Sig. Ten drops in water a.c.

How many grains of potassium iodide should be used in compounding the prescription?

15. ℞   Cocaine   0.5%
        Mineral Oil ad   ℥ss
        Sig. Nasal spray.

How many grains of cocaine should be used in compounding the prescription?

16. ℞   Sulfathiazole Sodium   2%
        Distilled Water ad   ℥iv
        Sig. Use as directed.

How many grains of sulfathiazole sodium should be used in compounding the prescription?

17. ℞   Silver Nitrate   0.02%
        Distilled Water ad   ℥xvi
        Sig. For irrigation.

How many grains of silver nitrate should be used in compounding the prescription?

18. ℞   Pilocarpine Nitrate   4%
        Distilled Water ad   ℥ii
        Sig. Use in right eye.

How many grains of pilocarpine nitrate should be used in compounding the prescription?

19. ℞   Sol. Resorcinol   2%
        Sol. Boric Acid   5%
            aa q.s. ad   ℥vi
        Sig. Apply externally.

How many grains of resorcinol and how many grains of boric acid should be used in compounding the prescription?

20. ℞   Iodine   5%
        Liquid Petroxolin ad   ℥ii
        Sig. Apply.

How many grains of iodine should be used in compounding the prescription?

21. A formula for a mouth rinse contains $\frac{1}{10}$% (w/v) of zinc chloride. How many grams of zinc chloride should be used in preparing 25 liters of the mouth rinse?

22. If 425 Gm. of sucrose are dissolved in enough water to make 500 ml., what is the percentage strength (w/v) of the solution?

23. If 2 liters of a solution of iodine in alcohol contain 7 Gm. of iodine, what is the percentage strength (w/v) of the solution?

24. ℞ Potassium Permanganate   0.25
       Distilled Water ad   1000.
       Sig. Use as directed.

Calculate the percentage strength of the solution.

25. ℞ Phenacaine Hydrochloride   0.06
       Boric Acid   0.3
       Distilled Water ad   15.0
       Sig. One drop in left eye.

Calculate the percentages of phenacaine hydrochloride and of boric acid in the prescription.

26. ℞ Potassium Chlorate   ℥ iiss
       Water ad   ℥ vi
       Sig. Use as a gargle.

What is the percentage strength of the solution?

27. ℞ Zinc Sulfate   gr. ii
       Boric Acid   gr. xx
       Distilled Water ad   ℥ i
       Sig. Eye drops.

Calculate the percentages of zinc sulfate and of boric acid in the prescription.

28. If 1 gallon of a solution contains 18.2 gr. of potassium permanganate, what is the percentage strength of the solution?

29. If 1 pt. of an elixir contains ℥ iv of sodium thiocyanate, what is the percentage strength of the elixir?

30. How many liters of $\frac{1}{40}$% (w/v) solution can be prepared from 60 Gm. of mercuric cyanide?

31. How many milliliters of 2% (w/v) solution can be made from $\frac{1}{8}$ oz. of cocaine hydrochloride?

32. How many milliliters of a $\frac{1}{10}$% (w/v) solution can be prepared from 1 Gm. of atropine sulfate?

33. How many liters of a 2% (w/v) iodine tincture can be made from 123 Gm. of iodine?

34. How many milliliters of a 10% (w/v) solution can be made from $\frac{1}{4}$ oz. of silver nucleinate?

35. How many milliliters of a 0.9% (w/v) sodium chloride solution can be made from 1 lb. of sodium chloride?

36. How many milliliters of a $\frac{1}{10}$% (w/v) solution of mercury bichloride can be prepared from 20 tablets, each containing 0.47 Gm.?

37. How many fluidounces of a $\frac{1}{3}$% (w/v) solution can be prepared from 75 grains of scopolamine hydrobromide?

38. A certain formula contains $\frac{1}{5}\%$ (v/v) of amaranth solution. How many milliliters of amaranth solution should be used in preparing 5 liters of the formula?

39. Peppermint Spirit contains 10% (v/v) of peppermint oil. How many milliliters of peppermint oil should be used in preparing 1 gallon of the spirit?

40. A sunscreen lotion contains 5% (v/v) of menthyl salicylate. How many milliliters of menthyl salicylate should be used in preparing 5 pints of the lotion?

41. A certain menstruum is to contain 15% (v/v) of glycerin. How many milliliters of glycerin should be used in preparing 5 gallons of the menstruum?

42. How many milliliters of wintergreen oil should be used to prepare 150 ml. of a 2.5% (v/v) solution in alcohol?

43. Chloroform liniment contains 30% (v/v) of chloroform. How many milliliters of chloroform should be used in preparing 5 pints of the liniment?

44. ℞   Liquefied Phenol   2%
       Calamine Lotion ad   480 ml.
       Sig. Apply to affected areas.

How many milliliters of liquefied phenol should be used in compounding the prescription?

45. ℞   Mercury Bichloride   0.1%
       Resorcin Monoacetate   3.0%
       Isopropyl Alcohol ad   250 ml.
       Sig. For the scalp.

How many grams of mercury bichloride and how many milliliters of resorcin monoacetate should be used in compounding the prescription?

46. ℞   Liquefied Phenol   0.5%
       Zinc Oxide   5.0%
       Lime Water ad   ℥iv
       Sig. Apply.

How many minims of liquefied phenol and how many grains of zinc oxide should be used in compounding the prescription?

47. ℞   Formic Acid Spirit   2.5%
       Isopropanol ad   ℥viii
       Sig. For the scalp.

How many minims of formic acid spirit should be used in compounding the prescription?

48. A physician writes a prescription for f℥ iv of a collyrium to contain $\frac{1}{10}$% of zinc sulfate and 2% of adrenalin solution. How many grains of zinc sulfate and how many minims of adrenalin solution should be used in compounding the prescription?

49. ℞ Adrenalin Solution 0.02%
     Neo-Silvol Solution 10% aa ad ℥ iv
     Sig. Use in the nose.

How many minims of a 0.1% Adrenalin Solution and how many grains of Neo-Silvol should be used in compounding the prescription?

50. ℞ Coal Tar   gr. xlviii
     Zinc Oxide
     Starch aa   gr. xxxxx
     Lanolin
     Hydrophilic Petrolatum aa   ℥ ss
     Sig. Apply to affected areas.

Calculate the percentage of the first ingredient in the finished product.

51. If 1.32 ml. of liquefied phenol are dissolved in enough water to make 60 ml., what is the percentage strength (v/v) of the solution?

52. One (1) gallon of a certain lotion contains 946 ml. of benzyl benzoate. Calculate the percentage (v/v) of benzyl benzoate in the lotion.

53. Lavender Spirit contains 12.5 ml. of lavender oil in 250 ml. Calculate the percentage strength (v/v) of the spirit.

54. A formula for 1 liter of an elixir contains 0.25 ml. of a flavoring oil. What is the percentage (v/v) of the flavoring oil in the elixir?

55. If f℥ iii of a solution contain 300 minims of an active ingredient, what is the percentage strength (v/v) of the solution?

56. ℞ Chloroform   ℥ ss
     Sodium Citrate   ℥ ss
     Tolu Syrup ad   ℥ xvi
     Sig. Take as directed.

Calculate the percentage (v/v) of chloroform and the percentage (w/v) of sodium citrate in the prescription?

57. Belladonna leaf contains 0.3% of alkaloids. How many milligrams of alkaloids are contained in 100 ml. of belladonna tincture (10%)?

58. ℞   Coal Tar Solution   15.0
        Glycerin   30.0
        Boric Acid Solution ad   240.0
        Sig. Apply.

If coal tar solution contains the equivalent of 20% of active material, what percentage of the material is represented in the finished product?

59. ℞   Precipitated Sulfur   ℥ss
        Alcohol   ℥iss
        Calamine Lotion ad   ℥iv
        Sig. Apply locally.

Calculate the percentage (v/v) of alcohol in the finished product.

60. ℞   Zinc Sulfate   0.03
        Tetracaine Solution 2%   5.0
        Boric Acid Solution ad   30.0
        Sig. One drop o.d. as directed.

Calculate the percentage of tetracaine in the finished product.

61. A liniment contains 15% (v/v) of methyl salicylate. How many milliliters of the liniment can be made from 120 ml. of methyl salicylate?

62. How many milliliters of 6.5% (v/v) cinnamon spirit can be prepared from 25 ml. of cinnamon oil?

63. How many grams of a chemical are required to make 750 Gm. of a 0.25% (w/w) solution?

64. How many grams of tannic acid are required to prepare 375 Gm. of a 5% (w/w) solution in glycerin?

65. How many grams of sucrose must be dissolved in 475 ml. of water to make a 65% (w/w) solution?

66. How many grams of a chemical are required to prepare 1 liter of a 25% (w/w) solution having a specific gravity of 1.10?

67. A sample of ferrous iodide syrup contains 5.3% (w/w) of ferrous iodide. How many grams of ferrous iodide will 5000 ml. of the syrup (specific gravity 1.370) contain?

68. How many grams of tannic acid must be dissolved in 320 ml. of glycerin having a specific gravity of 1.25 to make a 20% (w/w) solution?

69. How should you prepare 250 Gm. of a 4% (w/w) solution in a solvent having a specific gravity of 0.910?

70. How should you prepare f℥ii of a 25% (w/w) solution of a chemical in water?

71. How should you prepare f℥iii of a 15% (w/w) solution of mild silver protein?

72. How many grains of boric acid must be dissolved in f℥iv of water to make a 4% (w/w) solution?

73. How many grams of a chemical should be dissolved in 180 ml. of water to make a 10% (w/w) solution?

74. If 3.1 Gm. of a chemical are dissolved in 13.9 ml. of water, what is the percentage strength (w/w) of the solution?

75. What is the percentage strength (w/w) of a solution made by dissolving 62.5 Gm. of potassium chloride in 187.5 ml. of water?

76. A ferric chloride solution has a specific gravity of 1.300 and contains 374 Gm. of iron in 2290 ml. Calculate the percentage strength (w/w) of the solution.

77. If 198 Gm. of dextrose are dissolved in 1000 ml. of water, what is the percentage strength (w/w) of the solution?

78. Twenty (20) Gm. of tannic acid are dissolved in 64 ml. of glycerin having a specific gravity of 1.25. Calculate the percentage (w/w) of tannic acid in the solution.

79. What weight of a 20% (w/w) solution can be made from 5 Gm. of a chemical?

80. How many grams of a 7% (w/w) solution can be prepared from $\frac{1}{4}$ lb. of a chemical?

81. How many grams of zinc oxide are required to prepare 5 lb. of a 10% ointment?

82. ℞ Menthol $\frac{1}{4}$%
       Phenol $\frac{1}{2}$%
       Lassar's Paste ad   30.0 Gm.
       Sig. Apply to hands.

How many milligrams of menthol and of phenol should be used in compounding the prescription?

83. ℞ Silver Nucleinate   5%
       Petrolatum ad   ℥ss
       Sig. Apply to eyes.

How many grains of silver nucleinate should be used in compounding the prescription?

84. ℞   Gentian Violet Ointment   ℥i
           0.5%
        Sig. Apply.

How many grains of gentian violet should be used in compounding the prescription?

85. ℞   Salicylic Acid   2%
        Menthol $\frac{1}{4}$%
        Talc ad   60 Gm.
        Sig. Dust on.

How many grams of salicylic acid and how many milligrams of menthol should be used in compounding the prescription?

86. ℞   Sodium Perborate   4%
        Soluble Saccharin   0.2%
        Calcium Carbonate ad   ℥ii
        Sig. Tooth powder.

How many grains of sodium perborate and of soluble saccharin should be used in compounding the prescription?

87. One liter of purified water is mixed with 5 lb. of wool fat. Calculate the percentage (w/w) of purified water in the finished product.

88. Salicylic Acid   5%
    Camphor   8%
    Menthol   1%
    Starch   36%
    Boric Acid   50%

How many grams of each ingredient should be used in preparing 5 lb. of the foot powder?

89. ℞   Procaine Hydrochloride   1%
        Cocoa Butter ad   2.0
        Ft. suppos. tales no. xii
        Sig. One at night. ⟶ each depository contains 2 Gm.

How many grams of procaine hydrochloride should be used in compounding the prescription?

90. ℞   Scopolamine Hydrobromide Ointment
              $\frac{1}{3}$%   4.0
        Sig. For the eye.

How many milligrams of scopolamine hydrobromide should be used in compounding the prescription?

91. ℞   Ammoniated Mercury   10%
        White Petrolatum ad   ℥iv
        Sig. Apply to lesions.

How many grains of ammoniated mercury should be used in compounding the prescription?

92. You are directed to mix an ounce of Whitfield's Ointment (6% salicylic acid) and two ounces of Lassar's Zinc Paste with Salicylic Acid (2% salicylic acid) with enough white petrolatum to make four ounces. What is the percentage of salicylic acid in the finished product?

93. ℞   Salicylic Acid   ℥ss
        Boric Acid Ointment
        Zinc Oxide Ointment aa   ℥ss
        Sig. Apply.

Calculate the percentage of salicylic acid in the finished product.

94. ℞   Zinc Oxide
        Calamine
        Starch aa   6.0
        Wool Fat
        Hydrophilic Petrolatum aa   60.0
        Sig. Apply.

What is the percentage of zinc oxide in the finished product?

95. A pharmacist incorporates 24 grains of ammoniated mercury into ℥i of a 5% ammoniated mercury ointment. Calculate the percentage strength of the finished product.

96. ℞   Coal Tar   5%
           in
        $\left(\begin{array}{l}\text{Diglycol Stearate } 5\% \\ \text{Petrolatum} \qquad 95\%\end{array}\right)$
        Disp. 240 Gm.
        Sig. Apply to affected areas.

How many Gm. of diglycol stearate should be used in compounding the prescription?

97. ℞   Salicylic Acid
        Zinc Oxide aa   ℥ss
        Lanolin   ℥iii
        Petrolatum   ℥vi
        Sig. Apply as directed.

Calculate the percentage of salicylic acid in the finished product.

98. Express each of the following as a percentage strength:
    - (a) 1:1500
    - (b) 1:10,000
    - (c) 1:250
    - (d) 1:400
    - (e) 1:3300
    - (f) 1:4000

99. Express each of the following as a ratio strength:
    - (a) 0.125%
    - (b) 2.5%
    - (c) 0.80%
    - (d) 0.6%
    - (e) $\frac{1}{3}$%
    - (f) $\frac{1}{20}$%

100. Express each of the following concentrations as a ratio strength:
    - (a) 2 mg. of active ingredient in 2 ml. of solution
    - (b) 0.275 mg. of active ingredient in 5 ml. of solution
    - (c) 2 Gm. of active ingredient in 250 ml. of solution
    - (d) 1 mg. of active ingredient in 0.5 ml. of solution

101. Strophanthin Injection contains 0.5 mg. of strophanthin per ml. Express this concentration as a ratio strength.

102. Thirty (30) ml. of distilled water yield 0.30 mg. of total solids. Express this amount of total solids as a ratio strength.

103. At 15° C., Calcium Hydroxide Solution contains 170 mg. of calcium hydroxide in 100 ml. Express this concentration as a ratio strength.

104. You are directed to preserve a sample of petrolatum by using 10 mg. of tocopherol per kilo of petrolatum. Express the amount of preservative as a ratio strength.

105. ℞   Tab. Potassium Permanganate   0.2
         Disp. tales no. C
         Sig. Four tablets to Oii of water.

    Express the concentration, as a ratio strength, of the solution prepared according to the directions of the prescriber.

106. Preserved water is prepared by dissolving 0.04% of a mixture of 65 parts of methylparaben and 35 parts of propylparaben in distilled water. Express the concentration of methylparaben as a ratio strength.

107. A solution of sodium fluoride contains 500 mcg. of sodium fluoride per half liter. Express this concentration as a ratio strength.

108. Given a solution of potassium permanganate prepared by dissolving four 0.325 Gm. tablets in enough distilled water to make 650 ml., calculate (a) the ratio strength and (b) the percentage strength of the solution.

109. How many grams of a chemical should be used to prepare 500 ml. of a 1:2000 (w/v) solution?

110. How many grains of a chemical are required to make 1 pint of a 1:400 (w/v) solution?

111. ℞ Potassium Permanganate Solution
      1:8000   240 ml.
      Sig. For irrigation.

How many milligrams of potassium permanganate should be used in compounding the prescription?

112. ℞ Silver Nitrate   1:10,000
      Distilled Water q.s. ad   480 ml.
      Sig. Use as directed.

How many grams of silver nitrate should be used in compounding the prescription?

113. ℞ Sol. Atropine Sulfate
      1:2000   30 ml.
      Sig. One drop in each feeding.

How many grams of atropine sulfate should be used in compounding the prescription?

114. ℞ Solution Corrosive Sublimate
      1:5000   ℥xvi
      Sig. Use as directed.

How many milligrams of corrosive sublimate should be used in compounding the prescription?

115. ℞ Sol. Mercury Oxycyanide
      1:5000
      Rose Water aa ad   60.0
      Sig. Eye wash.

How many milligrams of mercury oxycyanide should be used in compounding the prescription?

116. How many milliliters of a 1:4000 solution can be made from $\frac{1}{8}$ oz. of potassium permanganate?

117. ℞ Phenacaine Hydrochloride   1:100
      Mercury Bichloride   1:3000
      Ophthalmic Base ad   10 Gm.
      Sig. Apply to right eye.

How many grams of phenacaine hydrochloride and of mercury bichloride should be used in compounding the prescription?

10

118. ℞   Hydrastine   1:1500
         White Petrolatum ad   5.0
         Sig. For the eye.

How many milligrams of hydrastine should be used in compounding the prescription?

119. ℞   Eserine Alkaloid   1:400
         Hydrophilic Petrolatum ad   ℥ii
         Sig. Apply as directed.

How many grains of eserine alkaloid should be used in compounding the prescription?

CHAPTER XI

DILUTION AND CONCENTRATION

In the previous chapter we have considered problems arising from the quantitative relationship, in given solutions or mixtures, between the active ingredients and the total amounts of solution or mixture, or between the ingredients themselves.

Problems of a slightly different character arise when given solutions or mixtures are *diluted* (by the addition of diluent, or by admixture with solutions or mixtures of lower strength) or are *concentrated* (by the addition of active ingredient, or by admixture with solutions or mixtures of greater strength, or by evaporation of the diluent).

Such problems sometimes seem complicated and difficult. But the complication proves to be nothing more than a series of steps required in the calculation, and the difficulty usually vanishes as each step, in itself, proves to be a simple matter.

Very often a problem can be solved in several ways. The best way is not necessarily the shortest: the best way is the one that clearly is grasped and that leads to the correct answer.

These two rules, wherever they may be applied, will greatly simplify the calculations:

(1) When ratio strengths are given, convert them to percentage strengths before setting up a proportion. It is very much more troublesome to calculate with a ratio like $\frac{1}{10}:\frac{1}{500}$ than with the equivalent *10 (%):0.2 (%)*.

(2) Whenever proportional parts enter into a calculation, reduce them to lowest terms. Instead of calculating with a ratio like *75 (parts):25 (parts)*, simplify it to *3 (parts):1 (part)*.

RELATIONSHIP BETWEEN STRENGTH AND TOTAL QUANTITY

If a mixture of a given percentage or ratio strength is diluted to twice its original quantity, its active ingredient will be contained in twice as many parts of the whole, and its strength therefore will be reduced by one-half. Contrariwise, if a mixture is concentrated by evaporation to one-half its original quantity, the active ingredient (assuming that none was lost by evaporation) will be contained in one-half as many parts of the whole, and the strength will be doubled. So, if 50 ml. of a solution containing 10 Gm. of active ingredient with a strength of 20% or 1:5 (w/v) are diluted to 100 ml., the original volume is doubled, but the original strength is now reduced by one-half to 10% or 1:10 (w/v). And if by evaporation of the solvent the volume of the solution is reduced to 25 ml. or one-half the original quantity, the 10 Gm. of the active ingredient now indicate a strength of 40% or 1:2.5 (w/v).

It turns out, then, that *if the amount of active ingredient remains constant, any change in the quantity of a solution or mixture of solids is inversely proportional to the percentage or ratio strength;* that is, the percentage or ratio strength decreases as the quantity increases, and conversely.

This relationship is generally true for all mixtures except volume-in-volume and weight-in-volume solutions containing components that contract when mixed together.

DILUTION AND CONCENTRATION OF LIQUIDS

To calculate the percentage or ratio strength of a solution made by diluting or concentrating (by evaporation) a solution of given quantity and strength:

Examples:

> *If 500 ml. of a 15% (w/v) solution are diluted to 1500 ml., what will be the percentage strength (v/v)?*

By the proportion:

$$1500 \text{ (ml.)} : 500 \text{ (ml.)} = 15 \text{ (\%)} : x$$

$$x = 5\%, \text{ } answer.$$

Or,

> 500 ml. of 15% (v/v) solution contain 75 ml. of active ingredient

By the proportion:

$$1500 \text{ (ml.)} : 75 \text{ (ml.)} = 100 \text{ (\%)} : x$$

$$x = 5\%, \text{ } answer.$$

> *If 20 ml. of a 1:200 (w/v) solution of a chemical are diluted to 500 ml., what is the ratio strength (w/v)?*

$$1:200 = 0.5\%$$

By the proportion:

500 (ml.):20 (ml.) = 0.5 (%):x

x = 0.02% = 1:5000, *answer.*

Or,

By the proportion:

$$500 \text{ (ml.)}:20 \text{ (ml.)} = \frac{1}{200} :x$$

$$x = \frac{1}{5000} = 1:5000, \text{ } answer.$$

Or,

20 ml. of a 1:200 solution contain 0.1 Gm. of chemical

By the proportion:

0.1 (Gm.):1 (Gm.) = 500 (ml.):x

x = 5000 ml.

Ratio strength = 1:5000, *answer.*

If 8 ℥ of a 1:2000 (w/v) solution of a chemical are diluted to 1 quart, what will be the ratio strength (w/v)?

1 quart = 32 f℥

1:2000 = 0.05%

By the proportion:

32 (f℥):8 (f℥) = 0.05 (%):x

x = 0.0125% = 1:8000, *answer.*

Or,

By the proportion:

$$32 \text{ (f℥)}:8 \text{ (f℥)} = \frac{1}{2000} :x$$

$$x = \frac{1}{8000} = 1:8000, \text{ } answer.$$

If a syrup containing 65% (w/v) of sugar is evaporated to 85% of its volume, what per cent (w/v) of sugar will it contain?

Any convenient amount of the syrup—say, 100 ml.—may be used in the calculation. If we evaporate 100 ml. of the syrup to 85% of its volume, we shall have 85 ml.

By the proportion:

85 (ml.):100 (ml.) = 65 (%):x

x = 76.47% or 76%, *answer.*

To calculate the amount of solution of desired strength that can be made by diluting or concentrating (by evaporation) a specified quantity of a solution of given strength:

Examples:

How many grams of 10% (w/w) ammonia water can be made from 1800 Gm. of 28% (w/w) ammonia water?

By the proportion:

10 (%):28 (%) = 1800 (Gm.):x

x = 5040 Gm., *answer.*

Or,

1800 Gm. of 28% ammonia water contain 504 Gm. of ammonia (100%)

By the proportion:

10 (%):100 (%) = 504 (Gm.):x

x = 5040 Gm., *answer.*

How many milliliters of a 1:5000 (w/v) solution of potassium permanganate can be made from 50 ml. of a 0.5% solution?

1:5000 = 0.02%

By the proportion:

0.02 (%):0.5 (%) = 50 (ml.):x

x = 1250 ml., *answer.*

Or,

By the proportion:

$$\frac{1}{5000} : \frac{1}{200} = 50 \text{ (ml.)}:x$$

x = 1250 ml., *answer.*

Or,

50 ml. of a 1:5000 solution contain 0.25 Gm. of potassium permanganate

By the proportion:

1 (Gm.):0.25 (Gm.) = 5000 (ml.):x

x = 1250 ml., *answer.*

If 10 f℥ of a 30% (w/v) solution are to be evaporated so that the solution will have a strength of 50% (w/v), what will be its volume?

By the proportion:

50 (%):30 (%) = 10 (f℥):x

x = 6 f℥, *answer.*

STOCK SOLUTIONS

Stock solutions are solutions of known concentration that are frequently prepared by the pharmacist for convenience in dispensing. They are usually strong solutions from which weaker ones may be conveniently made; and, when correctly prepared, they enable the pharmacist to obtain small quantities of medicinal substances that are to be dispensed in solution.

Stock solutions are invariably prepared on a weight-in-volume basis, and their concentration is expressed as a ratio strength or, less frequently, as a percentage strength.

To calculate the amount of a solution of given strength that must be used to prepare a solution of desired amount and strength:

Examples:

How many milliliters of a 1:400 (w/v) stock solution should be used to make 4 liters of a 1:2000 (w/v) solution?

4 liters = 4000 ml.

1:400 = 0.25%   1:2000 = 0.05%

By the proportion:

0.25 (%):0.05 (%) = 4000 (ml.):x

x = 800 ml., *answer.*

Or,

By the proportion:

$$\frac{1}{400} : \frac{1}{2000} = 4000 \text{ (ml.)} : x$$

x = 800 ml., *answer.*

How many fluidounces of a 1:400 (w/v) stock solution should be used in preparing 1 gallon of a 1:2000 (w/v) solution?

1 gallon = 128 f℥

1:400 = 0.25%   1:2000 = 0.05%

By the proportion:

0.25 (%):0.05 (%) = 128 (f℥):x

x = 25⅗ f℥, *answer.*

  R̸ Sol. Potassium Permanganate
          1:5000   200 ml.
      Sig. Use as directed.

How many milliliters of a 2% stock solution of potassium permanganate should be used in compounding the prescription?

1:5000 = 0.02%

By the proportion:

2 (%):0.02 (%) = 200 (ml.):x

x = 2 ml., *answer.*

Check:

2% stock solution   1:5000 solution
  2 × 0.02 ⟶ 0.04 Gm. ⟵ 200 × 0.0002
                 potassium
              permanganate

  R̸ Solution Mercury Bichloride
          0.025%   250.0
      Sig. As directed.

How many milliliters of a 1:400 stock solution of mercury bichloride should be used in compounding the prescription?

1:400 = 0.25%

By the proportion:

0.25 (%):0.025 (%) = 250 (ml.):x

x = 25 ml., *answer.*

R̲ Atropine Sulfate   0.5%
    Distilled Water ad   10.0 ml.
    Sig. Use in eye.

How many milliliters of a 1:50 stock solution of atropine sulfate should be used in compounding the prescription?

1:50 = 2%

By the proportion:

2 (%):0.5 (%) = 10 (ml.):x

x = 2.5 ml., *answer.*

Or,

10 × 0.005 = 0.050 Gm. of atropine sulfate needed

1:50 means 1 Gm. in 50 ml. of stock solution

By the proportion:

1 (Gm.):0.050 (Gm.) = 50 (ml.):x

x = 2.5 ml., *answer.*

R̲ Atropine Sulfate   gr. iss
    Distilled Water ad   ℥ii
    Sig. For the eyes.

How many minims of a 1:50 stock solution of atropine sulfate should be used in compounding the prescription?

1:50 = 2%

1 f℥ (480 minims) of stock solution contains 4.5 × 2 × 1 or 9 gr.

By the proportion:

9 (gr.):1.5 (gr.) = 480 (𝔐):x

x = 80 𝔐, *answer.*

R̲ Pilocarpine Nitrate   1%
    Distilled Water ad   ℥i
    Sig. Use in right eye.

A stock solution contains 3 gr. of pilocarpine nitrate per fluidrachm. How many minims should be used in compounding the prescription?

4.5 × 1 × 1 = 4.5 gr. of pilocarpine nitrate needed

The stock solution contains 3 gr. per f℥i (60 ℳ)

By the proportion:

3 (gr.):4.5 (gr.) = 60 (ℳ):x

x = 90 ℳ, *answer.*

To calculate the quantity of active ingredient in any specified amount of solution when given the strength of the diluted portion of the solution:

From the strength of the diluted portion we may calculate the *quantity* of *active ingredient* that the undiluted portion must have contained and then by proportion we may calculate how much active ingredient must be present in any other amount of the stock solution.

Examples:

How much silver nitrate should be used in preparing 100 ml. of a solution such that 5 ml. diluted to a liter will yield a 1:5000 solution?

1 liter = 1000 ml.

1:5000 means 1 Gm. of silver nitrate in 5000 ml. of solution

By the proportion:

5000 (ml.):1000 (ml.) = 1 (Gm.):x

x = 0.2 Gm. of silver nitrate in 1000 ml. (1 L.) of diluted solution (1:5000), which is also the amount in 5 ml. of the stronger (stock) solution.

By the proportion:

5 (ml.):100 (ml.) = 0.2 (Gm.):x

x = 4 Gm., *answer.*

How many grains of mercuric chloride should be used to prepare f℥viii of a solution such that f℥i diluted to a pint will yield a 1:5000 solution?

1:5000 = 0.02%

1 pt. = 16 f℥

4.5 × 0.02 × 16 = 1.44 gr. of mercuric chloride in 1 pint of 1:5000 solution, which is also the amount in f℥i of stock solution.

f℥ viii = 64 f℥

By the proportion:

1 (f℥):64 (f℥) = 1.44 (gr.):x

x = 92 gr., *answer*.

> ℞ Corrosive Sublimate Solution 240.0 ml.
> Make sol. such that 15 ml. diluted to
> 500 ml. will equal a 1:5000 solution.
> Sig. ℥iv in one pint of warm water.

How many grams of corrosive sublimate should be used in compounding the prescription?

1:5000 means 1 Gm. in 5000 ml. of solution

By the proportion:

5000 (ml.):500 (ml.) = 1 (Gm.):x

x = 0.1 Gm. of corrosive sublimate in 500 ml. of 1:5000 solution, which is also the amount in 15 ml. of the stock solution.

By the proportion:

15 (ml.):240 (ml.) = 0.1 (Gm.):x

x = 1.6 Gm., *answer*.

To calculate the amount of diluent that should be added to a solution of given strength and quantity to make a solution of specified lower strength:

When given the quantity and strength of a solution, we may easily determine how much diluent should be added to reduce its strength as desired by first using proportion to calculate the quantity of weaker solution that can be made and then subtracting from this the original quantity.

Examples:

> *How much water should be added to 150 ml. of a 1:500 (w/v) stock solution of a chemical to make a 1:2000 (w/v) solution?*

    1:500 = 0.2 %   1:2000 = 0.05 %

By the proportion:

    0.05 (%):0.2 (%) = 150 (ml.):x

    x = 600 ml. of 0.05 % solution

    600 ml. − 150 ml. = 450 ml., *answer.*

> *How many fluidounces of water should be added to 6 f℥ of an 8 % (w/v) solution to make a 3 % (w/v) solution?*

By the proportion:

    3 (%):8 (%) = 6 (f℥):x

    x = 16 f℥ of 3 % solution

    16 f℥ − 6 f℥ = 10 f℥, *answer.*

If we are not given the strength of the original solution, but the quantity of active ingredient it contains, the simplest procedure is to calculate directly what must be the amount of solution of the strength desired if it contains this quantity of active ingredient; then by subtraction of the given original amount, as above, we may determine the required amount of diluent.

Examples:

> *How many milliliters of water should be added to 250 ml. of a solution containing 0.35 Gm. of a chemical to make a 1:4000 (w/v) solution?*

By the proportion:

    1 (Gm.):0.35 (Gm.) = 4000 (ml.):x

    x = 1400 ml. of 1:4000 (w/v) solution containing 0.35 Gm. of the chemical.

    1400 ml. − 250 ml. = 1150 ml., *answer.*

> ✳ *How much water should be added to 250 ml. of a 5 % (w/v) solution of potassium permanganate to make a solution such that 5 ml. diluted to 500 ml. will give a 1:5000 solution?*

    1:5000 means 1 Gm. in 5000 ml. of solution

By the proportion:

5000 (ml.):500 (ml.) = 1 (Gm.):x

x = 0.1 Gm. of potassium permanganate in 500 ml. of 1:5000 solution, which is also the amount in 5 ml. of stock solution.

250 × 0.05 = 12.5 Gm. of potassium permanganate in 250 ml. of 5% solution

By the proportion:

0.1 (Gm.):12.5 (Gm.) = 5 (ml.):x

x = 625 ml.

625 ml. − 250 ml. = 375 ml., *answer*.

DILUTION OF ALCOHOL

Since there is a noticeable contraction in volume when alcohol and water are mixed, we cannot calculate the volume of water needed to dilute alcohol to a desired volume-in-volume strength. But this contraction does not affect the *weights* of the components, and hence the *weight of water* (and from this, the *volume*) needed to dilute alcohol to a desired *weight-in-weight* strength may be calculated.

To solve miscellaneous problems involving dilution of alcohol:

Examples:

How much water should be mixed with 5000 ml. of 85% (w/v) alcohol to make 50% (v/v) alcohol?

By the proportion:

50 (%):85 (%) = 5000 (ml.):x

x = 8500 ml.

Therefore, use 5000 ml. of 85% (v/v) alcohol and enough water to make 8500 ml., *answer*.

℞	Boric Acid	1.0 Gm.
	Alcohol 70%	30.0 ml.
	Sig. Ear drops.	

How many milliliters of 95% (v/v) alcohol and how much water should be used in compounding the prescription?

By the proportion:

95 (%):70 (%) = 30 (ml.):x

x = 22 ml.

Therefore, use 22 ml. of 95% (v/v) alcohol and enough water to make 30 ml., *answer*.

How much water should be added to 4000 Gm. of 90% (w/w) alcohol to make 40% (w/w) alcohol?

By the proportion:

40 (%):90 (%) = 4000 (Gm.):x

x = 9000 Gm., weight of 40% (w/w) alcohol equivalent to 4000 Gm. of 90% (w/w) alcohol

9000 Gm. − 4000 Gm. = 5000 Gm. or 5000 ml., *answer*.

★ DILUTION OF ACIDS ★

The strength of an official undiluted (*concentrated*) acid is expressed as percentage weight-in-weight. For example, in the statement "Sulfuric Acid contains 94 to 98% of H_2SO_4," the percentages refer to *percentages by weight*. But the strengths of the official *diluted* acids are expressed as percentage weight-in-volume. For example, Diluted Hydrochloric Acid is an aqueous solution containing, in each 100 ml., not less than 9.5 Gm. and not more than 10.5 Gm. of HCl.

It is necessary, therefore, to consider the specific gravity of concentrated acids in calculating the volume to be used in preparing a desired quantity of a diluted acid.

To calculate the volume of a concentrated acid required to prepare a desired quantity of a diluted acid:

Examples:

How many milliliters of 96% (w/w) sulfuric acid having a specific gravity of 1.84 are required to make 1000 ml. of diluted sulfuric acid 10% (w/v)?

1000 × 0.10 = 100 Gm. of H_2SO_4 (100%) in 1000 ml. of

10% (w/v) acid

By the proportion:

96 (%):100 (%) = 100 (Gm.):x

x = 104 Gm. of 96% acid

104 Gm. of water measure 104 ml.

104 (ml.) ÷ 1.84 = 56.5 ml., *answer.* *q s. 1000 ml*

R̸ Phosphoric Acid   500 ml.
      $\frac{1}{4}$%
      Sig. For bladder irrigation.

How many milliliters of 85% (w/w) phosphoric acid having a specific gravity of 1.71 should be used in compounding the prescription?

500 × 0.0025 = 1.25 Gm. of H_3PO_4 (100%) in 500 ml. of $\frac{1}{4}$% (w/v) solution

By the proportion:

85 (%):100 (%) = 1.25 (Gm.):x

x = 1.47 Gm. of 85% acid

1.47 Gm. of water measure 1.47 ml.

1.47 (ml.) ÷ 1.71 = 0.86 ml., *answer.*

DILUTION AND CONCENTRATION OF SOLIDS

To solve miscellaneous problems involving dilution and concentration of solids:

Examples:

How many grams of opium containing 15% (w/w) of morphine and how many grams of lactose should be used to prepare 150 Gm. of opium containing 10% (w/w) of morphine?

By the proportion:

15 (%):10 (%) = 150 (Gm.):x

x = 100 Gm. of 15% opium, *and*

150 Gm. − 100 Gm. = 50 Gm. of lactose, *answers.*

If some moist crude drug contains 7.2% (w/w) of active ingredient and 21.6% of water, what will be the percentage (w/w) of active ingredient after the drug is dried?

100 Gm. of moist drug would contain 21.6 Gm. of water and would therefore weigh 78.4 Gm. after drying.

By the proportion:

78.4 (Gm.):100 (Gm.) = 7.2 (%):x

x = 9.2%, *answer.*

℞   Ammoniated Mercury Ointment   120.0
          2%
     Sig. Apply.

How many grams of 5% ammoniated mercury ointment and how many grams of white petrolatum (diluent) should be used in compounding the prescription?

By the proportion:

5 (%):2 (%) = 120 (Gm.):x

x = 48 Gm. of 5% ointment, *and*

120 Gm. − 48 Gm. = 72 Gm. of white petrolatum, *answers.*

℞   Ophthalmic Zinc Oxide Ointment   ℥ii
          3%
     Sig. Apply to lids.

How many grains of 20% zinc oxide ointment and how many grains of ophthalmic base should be used in compounding the prescription?

℥ii = 120 gr.

By the proportion:

20 (%):3 (%) = 120 (gr.):x

x = 18 gr. of 20% ointment, *and*

120 gr. − 18 gr. = 102 gr. of ophthalmic base, *answers.*

How many grams of coal tar should be added to 3200 Gm. of 5% coal tar ointment to prepare an ointment containing 20% of coal tar?

3200 (Gm.) $\times$ 0.05 = 160 Gm. of coal tar in 3200 Gm. of 5% ointment

3200 Gm. − 160 Gm. = 3040 Gm. of base (diluent) in 3200 Gm. of 5% ointment

In the 20% ointment the diluent will represent 80% of the total weight.

By the proportion:

80 (%):20 (%) = 3040 (Gm.):x

x = 760 Gm. of coal tar in the 20% ointment

But since the 5% ointment already contains 160 Gm. of coal tar,

760 Gm. − 160 Gm. = 600 Gm., *answer.*

A much simpler method of solving the problem above can be used if we mentally translate it to read:

How many grams of coal tar should be added to 3200 Gm. of coal tar ointment containing 95% diluent to prepare an ointment containing 80% diluent?

By the proportion:

80 (%):95 (%) = 3200 (Gm.):x

x = 3800 Gm. of ointment containing 80% diluent and 20% coal tar

3800 Gm. − 3200 Gm. = 600 Gm., *answer.*

For another simple method, using alligation alternate, see page 170.

How many milliliters of water should be added to 150 Gm. of wool fat to prepare hydrous wool fat containing 25% of water?

100% − 25% = 75% wool fat in hydrous wool fat

By the proportion:

75 (%):100 (%) = 150 (Gm.):x

x = 200 Gm. of hydrous wool fat

200 Gm. − 150 Gm. = 50 Gm. or ml. of water, *answer.*

11

A more direct solution:

$$75 \; (\%) : 25 \; (\%) = 150 \; (Gm.) : x$$

x = 50 Gm. or ml. of water, *answer.*

TRITURATIONS

Triturations are dilutions of potent medicinal substances prepared by mixing finely powdered medicaments with finely powdered lactose in a definite proportion by weight. Officially, triturations are made according to the general formula: *dilute one part by weight of the medicinal substance with nine parts by weight of lactose.* They are, therefore, *10%* or *1:10 (w/w)* mixtures.

These dilutions offer to the dispensing pharmacist a means of obtaining conveniently and accurately small quantities of potent substances.

To calculate the quantity of a trituration required to obtain a given amount of a medicinal substance:

Examples:

How many grams of a 1:10 trituration of mercuric iodide are required to obtain 25 mg. of mercuric iodide?

10 Gm. of trituration contain 1 Gm. of mercuric iodide

25 mg. = 0.025 Gm.

By the proportion:

$$1 \; (Gm.) : 0.025 \; (Gm.) = 10 \; (Gm.) : x$$

x = 0.25 Gm., *answer.*

How many grains of 1:10 trituration of strychnine sulfate are needed to obtain $\frac{1}{10}$ gr. of strychnine sulfate?

10 gr. of trituration contain 1 gr. of strychnine sulfate

By the proportion:

$$1 \; (gr.) : \tfrac{1}{10} \; (gr.) = 10 \; (gr.) : x$$

x = 1 gr., *answer.*

     ℞   Atropine Sulfate   gr. $\frac{1}{120}$
          Aspirin   gr. v
          Ft. cap. tales no. xv
          Sig. One capsule as directed.

How many grains of 10% trituration of atropine sulfate should be used to obtain the atropine sulfate needed in the prescription?

$\frac{1}{120}$ gr. $\times$ 15 = $\frac{15}{120}$ or $\frac{1}{8}$ gr. of atropine sulfate needed

10% trituration contains 1 gr. of atropine sulfate in 10 gr.

By the proportion:

1 (gr.): $\frac{1}{8}$ (gr.) = 10 (gr.): x

x = $1\frac{1}{4}$ gr., *answer.*

ALLIGATION

Alligation is an arithmetical method of solving problems that involve the mixing of solutions or mixtures of solids possessing different percentage strengths.

ALLIGATION MEDIAL

Alligation medial is a method by which the "weighted average" percentage strength of a mixture of two or more substances whose quantities and concentrations are known may be quickly calculated. The percentage strength, expressed as a whole number, of each component of the mixture is multiplied by its corresponding quantity, and the sum of the products is divided by the sum of the quantities to give the percentage strength of the mixture—provided, of course, that the quantities have been expressed in a common denomination, whether of weight or of volume.

To calculate the percentage strength of a mixture that has been made by mixing two or more components of given percentage strengths:

Examples:

What is the percentage (v/v) of alcohol in a mixture of 3000 ml. of 40% (v/v) alcohol, 1000 ml. of 60% (v/v) alcohol, and 1000 ml. of 70% (v/v) alcohol?

$$
\begin{array}{rcl}
40 \times 3000 &=& 120000 \\
60 \times 1000 &=& 60000 \\
70 \times 1000 &=& 70000 \\
\hline
\end{array}
$$

Totals: 5000   250000

250000 ÷ 5000 = 50%, *answer.*

What is the percentage of zinc oxide in an ointment prepared by mixing 200 Gm. of 10% ointment, 50 Gm. of 20% ointment, and 100 Gm. of 5% ointment?

$$10 \times 200 = 2000$$
$$20 \times 50 = 1000$$
$$5 \times 100 = 500$$

Totals: 350   3500

$3500 \div 350 = 10\%$, *answer.*

In some problems the addition of a solvent or vehicle must be considered. It is generally best to consider the diluent as of zero percentage strength as in the following problem.

℞	Terpin Hydrate Elixir	60.0
	Chloroform Spirit	10.0
	Hydriodic Acid Syrup ad	120.0
	Sig. 4 ml. for cough.	

Terpin hydrate elixir contains 40% (v/v) of alcohol and chloroform spirit contains 90% (v/v) of alcohol. What is the percentage (v/v) of alcohol in the prescription?

$$40 \times 60 = 2400$$
$$90 \times 10 = 900$$
$$0 \times 50 = 0$$

Totals: 120   3300

$3300 \div 120 = 27.5\%$, *answer.*

ALLIGATION ALTERNATE

Alligation alternate is a method by which we may calculate the number of parts of two or more components of a given strength when they are to be mixed to prepare a mixture of desired strength. A final proportion permits us to translate relative parts to any specific denomination.

The strength of a mixture must lie somewhere between the strengths of its components—that is, the mixture must be somewhat stronger than its weakest component and somewhat weaker than its strongest; and, as already indicated, the strength of the mixture is always a "weighted" average: it lies nearer to that of its weaker or stronger components depending upon the relative amounts involved.

This "weighted" average can be found by means of an extremely simple scheme, as illustrated in the diagram below.

To find the relative amounts of solutions or other substances of different strengths that should be used to make a mixture of required strength:

Examples:

In what proportion should alcohols of 95% and 50% strengths be mixed to make 70% alcohol?

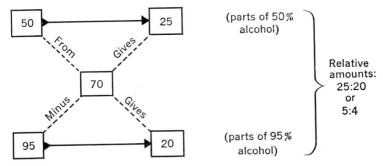

Note that the difference between the *desired strength* (70%) and the *strength of the weaker component* (50%) indicates the *number of parts of the stronger* to be used (20 parts); and the difference between the *strength of the stronger component* (95%) and the *desired strength* (70%) indicates the *number of parts of the weaker* to be used (25 parts).

The result can be shown to be correct by *alligation medial:*

$$95 \times 20 = 1900$$
$$50 \times 25 = 1250$$

Totals: 45   3150

$$3150 \div 45 = 70\%$$

The customary layout of alligation alternate, used in the examples below, is a convenient simplification of the diagram.

In what proportion should 15% boric acid ointment be mixed with white petrolatum to produce a 2% boric acid ointment?

15%		2 parts of 15% ointment
	2%	
0%		13 parts of white petrolatum

Relative amounts: 2:13, *answer.*

Check: 15 × 2 = 30
            0 × 13 = 0

Totals: 15   30

       30 ÷ 15 = 2%

A hospital pharmacist wants to use three lots of ichthammol ointment containing 5%, 20%, and 50% of ichthammol. In what proportion should they be mixed to prepare a 10% ichthammol ointment?

Here the one lot containing *less* (5%) than the *required percentage* (10%) must be *linked to each of the lots* containing *more* (20% and 50%) than the required percentage. The two amounts of the weakest lot are then added together to get the total number of parts of this lot needed when both the stronger lots are included in the final mixture.

5%		10 + 40 = 50 parts of 5 % ointment
20%	10%	5 parts of 20% ointment
50%		5 parts of 50% ointment

Relative amounts: 50:5:5 or 10:1:1, *answer.*

Check: 5 × 10 =   50
                  20 × 1 =   20
                  50 × 1 =   50

Totals: 12   120

        120 ÷ 12 = 10%

There are, of course, other answers, for the two stronger lots may be mixed first in any proportions desired, yielding a mixture that may then be mixed with the weakest lot in a proportion giving the desired strength.

In what proportions may a manufacturing pharmacist mix 3%, 5%, 15%, and 20% zinc oxide ointments to produce a 10% ointment?

Each of the weaker lots is paired with one of the stronger to give the desired strength; and since we may pair them in two ways, we may get two sets of correct answers.

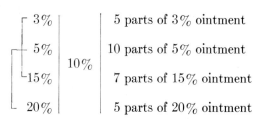

3%		10 parts of 3% ointment
5%	10%	5 parts of 5% ointment
15%		5 parts of 15% ointment
20%		7 parts of 20% ointment

Relative amounts: 10:5:5:7, *answer.*

Check: $3 \times 10 = 30$
$5 \times 5 = 25$
$15 \times 5 = 75$
$20 \times 7 = 140$

Totals: 27   270

$270 \div 27 = 10\%$

Or,

3%		5 parts of 3% ointment
5%	10%	10 parts of 5% ointment
15%		7 parts of 15% ointment
20%		5 parts of 20% ointment

Relative amounts: 5:10:7:5, *answer.*

Check: $3 \times 5 = 15$
$5 \times 10 = 50$
$15 \times 7 = 105$
$20 \times 5 = 100$

Totals: 27   270

$270 \div 27 = 10\%$

How many milliliters of 5% (w/v) mild silver protein solution and how many milliliters of 25% (w/v) mild silver protein solution are required to make 500 ml. of a 10% (w/v) solution?

5%		15 parts of 5% solution
	10%	
25%		5 parts of 25% solution

Relative amounts: 15:5, or 3:1 with a total of 4 parts

By the proportions:

4 (parts):3 (parts) = 500 (ml.):x

x = 375 ml. of 5% solution, *and*

4 (parts):1 (part) = 500 (ml.):y

y = 125 ml. of 25% solution, *answers*.

℞ Phenobarbital   2.5
   Iso-Alcoholic Elixir   480.0
   Sig. 4 ml. at bedtime.

A concentration of 30% of alcohol is required to keep the pheno-barbital in solution. How many milliliters of high alcoholic elixir (78%) and how many milliliters of low alcoholic elixir (10%) should be used in compounding the prescription?

78%		20 parts of high alcoholic elixir
	30%	
10%		48 parts of low alcoholic elixir

Relative amounts: 20:48, or 5:12 with a total of 17 parts

By the proportions:

17 (parts):5 (parts) = 480 (ml.):x

x = 141 ml. of high alcoholic elixir, *and*

17 (parts):12 (parts) = 480 (ml.):y

y = 339 ml. of low alcoholic elixir, *answers*.

To calculate the quantity of a solution or mixture of given strength that should be mixed with a specified quantity of another solution or mixture of given strength to make a solution or mixture of desired strength:

Examples:

How many grams of a drug containing 12.9% of alkaloids should be mixed with 300 Gm. of 8.9% drug to make a 10.5% mixture

$$
\begin{array}{c|c|l}
8.9\% & & 2.4 \text{ parts of } 8.9\% \text{ drug} \\
& 10.5\% & \\
12.9\% & & 1.6 \text{ parts of } 12.9\% \text{ drug}
\end{array}
$$

Relative amounts: 2.4:1.6 or 3:2

By the proportion:

3 (parts):2 (parts) = 300 (Gm.):x

x = 200 Gm., *answer.*

How many milliliters of water should be mixed with 25 Gm. of 30% (w/w) sulfuric acid and 50 Gm. of 60% (w/w) sulfuric acid to make 10% (w/w) acid?

$$
\begin{aligned}
30 \times 25 &= 750 \\
60 \times 50 &= 3000 \\
\hline
\text{Totals: } 75 \quad & 3750
\end{aligned}
$$

3750 ÷ 75 = 50% (w/w) strength of 3750 Gm. of a mixture of 30% and 60% acids.

$$
\begin{array}{c|c|l}
50\% & & 10 \text{ parts of } 50\% \text{ mixture} \\
& 10\% & \\
0\% & & 40 \text{ parts of water}
\end{array}
$$

Relative amounts: 10:40, or 1:4

By the proportion:

1 (part):4 (parts) = 75 (Gm.):x

x = 300 Gm., or 300 ml., *answer.*

Check:
$$
\begin{aligned}
50 \times 75 &= 3750 \\
0 \times 300 &= 0 \\
\hline
375 \quad & 3750
\end{aligned}
$$

3750 ÷ 375 = 10%

How many grams of petrolatum should be mixed with 250 Gm. of 10% and 750 Gm. of 20% tannic acid ointments to prepare a 5% ointment?

$$
\begin{aligned}
10 \times 250 &= 2500 \\
20 \times 750 &= 15000 \\
\hline
\text{Totals: } 1000 \quad & 17500
\end{aligned}
$$

$$17500 \div 1000 = 17.5\% \text{ of tannic acid in } 1000$$
Gm. of a mixture of 10% and 20% ointments.

17.5%		5 parts of 17.5% mixture
	5%	
0%		12.5 parts of petrolatum

Relative amounts: 5:12.5, or 2:5

By the proportion:

2 (parts):5 (parts) = 1000 (Gm.):x

x = 2500 Gm., *answer.*

Check: $17.5 \times 1000 = 17500$
          $0 \times 2500 = \qquad 0$

        Totals: 3500   17500

$$17500 \div 3500 = 5\%$$

To calculate the amount of active ingredient that must be added to increase the strength of a mixture of given amount and strength:

Examples:

Compare the solution of the following problem by use of alligation alternate with other methods used on pp. 160–161.

How many grams of coal tar should be added to 3200 Gm. of 5% coal tar ointment to prepare an ointment containing 20% of coal tar?

Coal tar (active ingredient) = 100%

5%		80 parts of 5% ointment
	20%	
100%		15 parts of 100% coal tar

Relative amounts: 80:15, or 16:3

By the proportion:

16 (parts):3 (parts) = 3200 (Gm.):x

x = 600 Gm., *answer.*

Check: $5 \times 3200 = 16000$
       $100 \times 600 = 60000$

        Totals: 3800   76000

$$76000 \div 3800 = 20\%$$

How many grams of ichthammol should be added to 400 Gm. of a 10% ointment of ichthammol to make a 20% ointment?

Ichthammol (active ingredient) = 100%

10%			80 parts of 10% ointment
	20%		
100%			10 parts of ichthammol

Relative amounts: 80:10, or 8:1

By the proportion:

8 (parts):1 (part) = 400 (Gm.):x

x = 50 Gm., *answer.*

Check: 10 × 400 = 4000
            100 × 50 = 5000

Totals: 450   9000

9000 ÷ 450 = 20%

SPECIFIC GRAVITY OF MIXTURES

The methods of alligation medial and alligation alternate may be used in solving problems concerning the specific gravities of different quantities of liquids of known specific gravities—provided that there is no change in volume when the liquids are mixed, and that they are measured in a common denomination of *volume.*

To calculate the specific gravity of a mixture given the specific gravities of its ingredients:

Example:

What is the specific gravity of a mixture of 1000 ml. of syrup with a specific gravity of 1.300, 400 ml. of a glycerin with a specific gravity of 1.250, and 1000 ml. of an elixir with a specific gravity of 0.950?

1.300 × 1000 = 1300
1.250 × 400 = 500
0.950 × 1000 = 950

Totals: 2400   2750

2750 ÷ 2400 = 1.146, *answer.*

To calculate the relative or specific amounts of ingredients of given specific gravities required to make a mixture of desired specific gravity:

Examples:

In what proportion must glycerin with a specific gravity of 1.25 and water be mixed to give a liquid having a specific gravity of 1.10?

1.25		0.10 parts of glycerin
	1.10	
1.00		0.15 parts of water

Relative amounts: 0.10:0.15 or 2:3, *answer.*

How many milliliters of each of two liquids with specific gravities of 0.875 and 0.950 should be used to prepare 1500 ml. of a liquid having a specific gravity of 0.925?

0.875		0.025 or 25 parts of liquid with specific gravity of 0.875
	0.925	
0.950		0.050 or 50 parts of liquid with specific gravity of 0.950

Relative amounts: 25:50, or 1:2 with a total of 3 parts

By the proportions:

3 (parts):1 (part) = 1500 (ml.):x

x = 500 ml. of liquid with specific gravity of 0.875, *and*

3 (parts):2 (parts) = 1500 (ml.):y

y = 1000 ml. of liquid with specific gravity of 0.950, *answers.*

Practice Problems

1. If 250 ml. of a 1:800 (v/v) solution are diluted to 1000 ml., what will be the ratio strength (v/v)?

2. If 1 pint of a 1:500 (w/v) solution is diluted to 24 f℥, what will be the ratio strength (w/v)?

3. If 400 ml. of a 20% (w/v) solution are diluted to 2 liters, what will be the percentage strength (w/v)?

4. If 55 ml. of an 18% (w/v) solution are diluted to 330 ml., what will be the percentage strength (w/v)?

5. If a solution containing 10.5% (w/w) of a chemical is evaporated to 70% of its weight, what per cent (w/w) of the chemical will it then contain?

6. If a solution containing 60% (v/v) of active ingredient is evaporated to 80% of its volume, what will be its percentage strength (v/v)?

7. What is the strength of a sodium chloride solution obtained by evaporating 800 Gm. of a 10% (w/w) solution to 250 Gm.?

8. How many grams of 10% (w/w) phosphoric acid can be made from 1 kilogram of 85% (w/w) acid?

9. How many milliliters of 0.45% (w/v) sodium hypochlorite solution can be prepared from 800 ml. of an 11.25% (w/v) solution?

10. How many milliliters of 50% (v/v) solution can be prepared by diluting 800 ml. of 95% (v/v) solution?

11. How many milliliters of 10% (w/v) solution can be made from 50 ml. of 85% (w/v) solution?

12. To what volume must 500 ml. of a 10% (w/v) solution of a chemical be evaporated to become a 16% (w/v) solution?

13. To what weight must 1360 Gm. of a 12% (w/w) acid solution be evaporated to become a 30% (w/w) solution?

14. How many gallons of 70% (v/v) alcohol can be made from 10 gallons of 95% (v/v) alcohol?

15. How many pounds of 10% (w/w) sulfuric acid can be made from 9 lb. of 94% (w/w) sulfuric acid?

16. How many grams of 5% (w/w) zinc chloride solution can be made from 25 ml. of a 50% (w/w) solution having a specific gravity of 1.55?

17. How many milliliters of normal saline solution (0.9% w/v) can be prepared from 250 ml. of 25% (w/v) salt solution?

18. How many milliliters of a 1:1000 mercury bichloride solution can be prepared from 100 ml. of a 1:50 solution?

19. How many milliliters of a 1:8000 potassium permanganate solution can be prepared from 20 ml. of a 1% solution?

20. If 200 Gm. of cinchona, assaying 5% (w/w) of alkaloids, are required to make 1000 ml. of cinchona tincture, how many milliliters of

the tincture can be made from 5 lb. of cinchona containing 6.5% (w/w) of alkaloids?

21. How many fluidounces of 6% (w/v) solution can be made from 2 f℥ of 36% (w/v) solution?

22. How many milliliters of a 1:50 (w/v) stock solution of a chemical should be used to prepare 1 liter of a 1:4000 (w/v) solution?

23. How many milliliters of a 2.5% (w/v) stock solution of potassium permanganate should be used in preparing 5 liters of a 1:5000 (w/v) solution?

24. How many milliliters of water should be added to 5 liters of a 50% solution of dextrose to reduce the concentration to 30%?

25. A certain product contains Aerosol OT in a concentration of 1:20,000. How many milliliters of a ½% solution of Aerosol OT should be used in preparing 4 liters of the product?

26. ℞   Copper Sulfate   0.5%
        Glycerin   25.0%
        Purified Water ad   60.0
        Sig. One drop o.d.

How many milliliters of a 20% solution of copper sulfate in glycerin and how many milliliters of glycerin should be used in compounding the prescription?

27. ℞   Zinc Sulfate   gr. ⅛
        Boric Acid   gr. v
        Distilled Water ad   ℥i
        Sig. gtt. i o.u. p.r.n.

How many milliliters of a 3% solution of boric acid should be used to obtain the boric acid needed in the prescription?

28. ℞   Opium Tincture   10.0
        Glycerin   20.0
        Dil. Lead Subacet. Sol.
        Rose Water aa ad   120.0
        Sig. For external use.

Diluted lead subacetate solution contains 0.75% (w/v) of lead (as lead subacetate). How many milliliters of lead subacetate solution containing 22.5% (w/v) of lead (as lead subacetate) should be used in compounding the prescription?

29. ℞   Iodine   0.2%
        Eucalyptol   0.5%
        Mineral Oil ad   ℥i
        Sig. For the nose.

A stock solution of iodine (4 gr. per ℥i) and a stock solution of eucalyptol (4℥ per ℥i) are available. How many minims of each solution should be used in compounding the prescription?

30. How many milliliters of a 1:50 stock solution of mercuric chloride should be used in preparing 250 ml. of a 0.02% solution?

31. One pint of a stock solution contains 12 gr. of mercuric chloride. How much of this solution should be used to make 8 f℥ of a 1:5000 solution?

32. Eight fluidounces of a stock solution contain 120 gr. of a chemical. How many minims of the stock solution should be used to make 1 pint of a 1:5000 solution?

33. How many milliliters of a 1:200 stock solution of atropine sulfate are required to prepare 60 ml. of a 0.025% solution?

34. ℞ Potassium Permanganate Solution   500 ml.
        1:8000
     Sig. As directed.

How many milliliters of a 5% stock solution of potassium permanganate should be used in compounding the prescription?

35. ℞ Atropine Sulfate   0.015
     Distilled Water ad   30.0
     Sig. Use as directed.

How many milliliters of a 1:50 stock solution of atropine sulfate should be used in compounding the prescription?

36. ℞ Solution of Zinc Sulfate   ℥ii
        0.2%
     Sig. For the eye.

A stock solution contains 5 gr. of zinc sulfate per fluidrachm. How many minims of the stock solution should be used to obtain the zinc sulfate needed for the prescription?

37. ℞ Potassium Permanganate Solution   1000 ml.
        0.025%
     Sig. For external use.

How many milliliters of a 1:40 stock solution of potassium permanganate should be used in compounding the prescription?

38. ℞ Sol. Adrenalin   ℥iv
        1:2500
     Sig. Use as directed.

How many minims of a 1:1000 adrenalin solution should be used in compounding the prescription?

39. ℞   Histamine Phosphate Solution   15.0
            1:10000
        Sig. Use as directed.

If the prescription is to be prepared from a solution containing 0.275 mg. of histamine phosphate per milliliter, how many milliliters should be used in compounding?

40. ℞   Pilocarpine Nitrate Solution   ℥ i
            0.2%
        Sig. As directed.

A stock solution of pilocarpine nitrate contains 1 gr. per f℥i. How many minims of the stock solution should be used in compounding the prescription?

41. ℞   Coal Tar Solution   15.0
        Glycerin   15.0
        Witch Hazel   20.0
        Boric Acid Sol. 2% ad   250.0
        Sig. Apply externally.

How many milliliters of 5% boric acid solution and how much water should be used in compounding the prescription?

42. ℞   Sol. Epinephrine Hydrochloride   ℥ii
            1:5000
        Sol. Colloidal Silver Iodide ad   ℥i
            5%
        Sig. For the nose.

How many minims of a 1:1000 epinephrine hydrochloride solution should be used in compounding the prescription?

43. ℞   Phenol   1.2
        Boric Acid Sol. 2%   90.0
        Coal Tar Solution   12.0
        Calamine Lotion ad   240.0
        Sig. Apply.

How many milliliters of 5% boric acid solution and how much water should be used in compounding the prescription?

44. A physician writes for an ophthalmic suspension to contain 100 mg. of cortisone acetate in 8 ml. of normal saline solution. The

pharmacist has on hand a 2.5% suspension of cortisone acetate in normal saline solution. How many milliliters of this suspension and how many milliliters of normal saline solution should he use in compounding the prescription?

45. ℞ Aluminum Acetate Solution
        1:8
     Alcohol 70% aa ad   120.0
     Sig. Apply locally as directed.

How many milliliters of aluminum acetate solution should be used in compounding the prescription?

46. The formula for a mouth wash calls for 0.05% by volume of methyl salicylate. How many minims of a 12% (v/v) stock solution of methyl salicylate in alcohol will be needed to prepare a quart of the mouth wash?

47. ℞ Atropine Sulfate   gr. $\frac{1}{200}$
     Distilled Water ad   ℨ ss
     Disp. ℥ i
     Sig. ℨ ss at night.

The atropine sulfate is to be obtained from a stock solution containing $\frac{4}{5}$ grain per fluidounce. How many minims of the stock solution should be used?

48. How many grams of silver nitrate are required to make 250 ml. of a solution such that 8 ml. diluted to one liter will give a 1:5000 solution?

49. ℞ Potassium Permanganate q.s.
     Distilled Water ad   1000.0
     Sig. 4 ml. diluted to 500 ml. will yield a 1:10000 solution.

(a) How many grams of potassium permanganate should be used?

(b) How many milliliters of a 2.5% stock solution of potassium permanganate should be used to obtain the potassium permangate needed in (a)?

50. How many grains of mercuric chloride should be used in preparing 6 f℥ of a solution such that f℥ i diluted to a pint will give a 1:8000 solution?

51. ℞ Potassium Permanganate q.s.
     Distilled Water ad   ℥ xvi
     Sig. f℥ ii diluted to a pint = 1:5000 solution.

How many grains of potassium permanganate should be used in compounding the prescription?

12

52. How many grains of potassium permanganate should be used in preparing a half pint of a solution such that a half drachm diluted to half a quart will equal a 1:2000 solution?

53. How many grams of copper sulfate are required to make 125 ml. of a solution such that 4 ml. diluted to 500 ml. will give a 1:3000 solution?

54. ℞   Silver Nitrate   q.s.
        Distilled Water ad 480.0 ml.
        Sig. 15 ml. diluted to a liter will equal a 1:8000 solution.

How many grams of silver nitrate should be used in compounding the prescription?

55. How much atropine sulfate would you use in making 10 fluidounces of a solution of such strength that ℥i diluted to four fluidounces will give a solution containing $\frac{1}{150}$ gr. in each teaspoonful?

56. Calculate the quantity of chemicals required to make 16 fluidounces of an aqueous solution so that 1 fluidounce added to 3 fluidounces of water will represent 1:500 of ephedrine sulfate and 1:3000 of chlorobutanol.

57. A hospital pharmacist has on hand 500 ml. of a 2% stock solution of mercury bichloride. How many milliliters of water should he add to the stock solution to make a solution such that 10 ml. diluted to 500 ml. will yield a 1:5000 solution?

58. ℞   Potassium Permanganate   q.s.
        Distilled Water ad   ℥ii
        Sig. Dilute as directed.

How much potassium permanganate should be used to make a solution which will yield a 1:5000 solution when the 2 fluidounces are added to 30 fluidounces of distilled water?

59. How many milliliters of water should be added to 1500 ml. of a 1:2500 (w/v) solution to make a 1:4000 (w/v) solution?

60. How much water should be added to a pint of a 1:2000 (w/v) solution to make a 1:2500 (w/v) solution?

61. How much water should be added to a liter of 1:3000 (w/v) solution to make a 1:8000 (w/v) solution?

62. How much water should be added to 1 liter of a solution containing 2.5 Gm. of a chemical to make a 1:2000 solution?

63. How much water should be added to 250 Gm. of 95% (w/w) sulfuric acid to make 10% (w/w) acid?

64. To what volume should 500 ml. of a 2% mercuric chloride solution be diluted to make a solution such that 10 ml. diluted to 800 ml. will equal a 1:8000 solution?

65. How much water should be added to 2500 ml. of 83% (v/v) alcohol to prepare 50% (v/v) alcohol?

66. How much water should be mixed with 3000 ml. of 94 %(v/v) alcohol to make 30% (v/v) alcohol?

67. How many milliliters of water should be mixed with 3000 Gm. of 83% (w/w) alcohol to make 70% (w/w) alcohol?

68. How many milliliters of water should be mixed with 1200 Gm. of 65% (w/w) alcohol to make 45% (w/w) alcohol?

69. ℞   Methyl Salicylate   30.0
         Chloroform Liniment   30.0
         Alcohol 80% ad   120.0
         Sig. Apply to parts.

How many milliliters of 95% (v/v) alcohol and how much water should be used in compounding the prescription?

70. ℞   Castor Oil   5.0
         Formic Acid Spirit   35.0
         Alcohol 85%   200.0
         Sig. For the scalp.

How many milliliters of 95% (v/v) alcohol and how much water should be used in compounding the prescription?

71. How many milliliters of 95% (w/w) sulfuric acid having a specific gravity of 1.820 should be used in preparing 2 liters of 10% (w/v) acid?

72. How many milliliters of 37% (w/w) hydrochloric acid having a specific gravity of 1.18 should be used in preparing 1000 ml. of 10% (w/v) acid?

73. The formula for Hydriodic Acid Syrup is:
         Diluted Hydriodic Acid   140 ml.
         Sucrose   450 Gm.
         Water ad   1000 ml.

Diluted hydriodic acid contains 10 Gm. of HI in each 100 ml. How many milliliters of a 19% (w/w) solution of HI, specific gravity 1.200, should be used in preparing 4000 ml. of hydriodic acid syrup?

74. ℞   Sol. Phosphoric Acid   120.0
            0.04%
        Sig. For irrigation.

How many milliliters of syrupy phosphoric acid, 85% (w/w), specific gravity 1.71, should be used in compounding the prescription?

75. How many milliliters of 28% (w/w) ammonia water having a specific gravity of 0.89 should be used in preparing 2000 ml. of 10% (w/w) ammonia water with a specific gravity of 0.96?

76. How many milliliters of 92% (w/w) alcohol having a specific gravity of 0.816 should be used in preparing 5 liters of 40% (w/w) alcohol with a specific gravity of 0.939?

77. How many milliliters of 26° Baumé (28% w/w) ammonia solution are required to prepare 500 ml. of 5% (w/v) ammonia solution?

$$Specific \ gravity = \frac{140}{130 + °B.}$$

78. How many milliliters of 85% (w/w) phosphoric acid having a specific gravity of 1.712 are required to prepare 2500 ml. of a 10% (w/w) acid having a specific gravity of 1.057?

79. In compounding a prescription for 500 ml. of diluted phosphoric acid, a pharmacist used 50 ml. of 85% phosphoric acid with a specific gravity of 1.71. What was the percentage strength (w/v) of the finished product?

80. Ferrous Iodide Syrup contains 7.5 Gm. of ferrous iodide in each 100 ml. How many milliliters of a 47.5% (w/w) solution of ferrous iodide (sp. gr. 1.95) should be used in preparing 10 liters of the syrup?

81. The formula for 1000 ml. of Aromatic Ammonia Spirit calls for 90 ml. of diluted ammonia solution. How many milliliters of a 27% (w/w) solution of ammonia, sp. gr. 0.90, should be used to prepare the diluted ammonia solution required for making 10 liters of the spirit? Diluted ammonia solution contains 9.5% (w/v) of ammonia.

82. ℞   Lactic Acid 25%   250.0
        Sig. 15 ml. in two quarts of water.

How many milliliters of lactic acid, 87% (w/w), sp. gr. 1.205, should be used in compounding the prescription?

83. Fifty (50) ml. of strong ammonia solution, 27.5% (w/w), sp. gr. 0.90, are diluted with 250 ml. of alcohol, sp. gr. 0.82. What is the concentration of ammonia in the resulting product, calculated on a w/w basis? On a w/v basis?

84. A sample of opium contains 28% of moisture and 10% of morphine. How many grams of morphine could be obtained from 350 Gm. of the dry opium?

85. How many grams of lactose should be added to 75 Gm. of belladonna extract assaying 1.50% (w/w) of alkaloids to reduce its strength to 1.40% (w/w)?

86. ℞   Scarlet Red Ointment   ℥ ii
        2%
Sig. Apply.

How many grains of 10% scarlet red ointment and how many grains of petrolatum should be used in compounding the prescription?

87. ℞   Yellow Mercuric Oxide Ointment   10 Gm.
        $\frac{1}{4}$%
Sig. Apply to eyelids.

How many grams of 10% ointment of yellow mercuric oxide and how many grams of petrolatum should be used in compounding the prescription?

88. How many grams of sulfathiazole should be added to 3400 Gm. of a 10% sulfathiazole cream to prepare one containing 15% of sulfathiazole?

89. How many grams of petrolatum should be added to 250 Gm. of a 25% ichthammol ointment to make a 5% ointment?

90. ℞ Zinc Oxide   1.5
       Hydrophilic Petrolatum   2.5
       Distilled Water   5.0
       Hydrophilic Ointment ad   30.0
       Sig. Apply to affected areas.

How much zinc oxide should be added to the product in order to make an ointment containing 10% of zinc oxide?

91. ℞ Coal Tar   5%
       Bentonite Base ad   50.0
       Sig. Apply as directed.

In compounding, a pharmacist prepared 50 Gm. of the base and added to it 2.5 Gm. of coal tar. Calculate the concentration of coal tar in the finished product.

92. How much lactose and how much strychnine sulfate should be used to make ℥iv of a 1:10 trituration of strychnine sulfate?

93. A prescription calls for 0.005 Gm. of atropine sulfate. How much of a 1:10 trituration should be used to obtain the atropine sulfate?

94. ℞   Red Mercuric Iodide   gr. $\frac{1}{20}$
        Lactose   q.s.
        Ft. tal. tab. no. 60
        Sig. As directed.

How much of a 1:10 trituration of red mercuric iodide should be used in compounding the prescription?

95. How many grains of a 1:12 trituration of strychnine sulfate will be required to obtain $\frac{2}{3}$ gr. of strychnine sulfate?

96. If f℥iv of a prescription contain $\frac{1}{160}$ gr. of atropine sulfate per teaspoonful, how many grains of a 10% trituration of atropine sulfate should be used in compounding the prescription?

97. How many milligrams of 1:10 trituration of strychnine sulfate are required to obtain 0.5 mg. of strychnine sulfate?

98. ℞   Atropine Sulfate Tablets   0.000065
        Disp. tales no. 50
        Sig. One in each feeding.

How much of a 1:10 trituration of atropine sulfate should be used in compounding the prescription?

99. ℞   Tabs. Atropine Sulf.   gr. $\frac{1}{500}$
        Disp. such no. xxx
        Sig. As directed.

How many grains of a 10% trituration of atropine sulfate should be used in compounding the prescription?

100. ℞   Atropine Sulfate   gr. $\frac{1}{120}$
         Calcium Carbonate   gr. x
         Ft. pulv. no. xv
         Sig. One powder as directed.

How many grains of a 1:10 trituration of atropine sulfate should be used in compounding the prescription?

101. ℞   Strychnine Sulfate   0.00065
         Iron and Ammonium Citrate   0.5
         Ft. caps. tales no. 20
         Sig. One capsule b.i.d.

How many grains of a 10% trituration of strychnine sulfate should be used in compounding the prescription?

102. ℞   Atropine Sulfate   0.130 mg.
         Acetylsalicylic Acid   0.3
         Ft. pulv. tal. no. 20
         Sig. One b.i.d.

How many milligrams of a 1:10 trituration of atropine sulfate should be used in compounding the prescription?

103. ℞   Sol. Atropine Sulfate   f℥xvi
         (Each teaspoonful = $\frac{1}{320}$ gr.)
         Sig. ℥i in water as directed.

How many grains of a 10% trituration of atropine sulfate should be used in compounding the prescription?

104. ℞   Strychnine Sulfate   0.0013
         Iron & Ammonium Citrate   0.5
         Aromatic Elixir ad   8.0
         D.T.D. no. xv
         Sig. 8 ml. in aq. b.i.d.

If the strychnine sulfate is available only as a 10% trituration, how much of the trituration should be used in compounding the prescription?

105. In preparing a 10% trituration of atropine sulfate, a pharmacist used the contents of an original $\frac{1}{8}$ oz. bottle and enough lactose to make ℥x. What percentage of error did he incur?

106. What is the percentage of alcohol in a mixture of 900 ml. of 45% alcohol, 500 ml. of 60% alcohol, 300 ml. of 75% alcohol, and 600 ml. of 35% alcohol?

107. Four equal amounts of cinchona, containing 4.5%, 6.5%, 8%, and 10% of total alkaloids, respectively, were mixed. What was the percentage strength of the mixture?

108. What is the percentage of alcohol in a lotion containing 1500 ml. of witch hazel (14% alcohol), 2000 ml. of glycerin, and 5000 ml. of 50% alcohol?

109. A pharmacist mixes 200 Gm. of 10% ichthammol ointment, 450 Gm. of 5% ichthammol ointment, and 1000 Gm. of petrolatum (diluent). What is the percentage of ichthammol in the finished product?

110. What is the percentage of alcohol in a mixture of 150 ml. of a tincture containing 20% of alcohol, 35 ml. of a fluidextract containing 65% of alcohol, 50 ml. of a tincture containing 50% of alcohol, and enough aromatic elixir (22% of alcohol) to make 1000 ml.?

111. A preparation contains one fluidrachm of a tincture containing 25% of alcohol, four fluidrachms of a fluidextract containing 80% of alcohol, 60 minims of a tincture containing 50% of alcohol, two fluidrachms of a tincture containing 85% of alcohol, and enough of an elixir containing 15% of alcohol to make eight fluidounces. What is the percentage of alcohol in the preparation?

112. A pharmacist mixes 2500 Gm. of 10% sulfuric acid, 1500 Gm. of 5% sulfuric acid, and 2500 Gm. of 20% sulfuric acid. Calculate the percentage strength of the finished product.

113. ℞   Chloroform Spirit   50.0 ml.   (88% alcohol)
       Aromatic Elixir   150.0 ml.   (22% alcohol)
       Terpin Hydrate Elixir   300.0 ml.   (40% alcohol)
       Sig. 4 ml. for cough.

Calculate the percentage of alcohol in the prescription.

114. ℞   Witch Hazel   250.0   (14% alcohol)
       Alcohol   200.0   (95% alcohol)
       Boric Acid Sol. ad   1000.0
       Sig. Apply externally.

Calculate the percentage of alcohol in the prescription.

115. ℞   Aconite Fluidextract   90.0   (60% alcohol)
       Alcohol   160.0   (95% alcohol)
       Chloroform   250.0
       Soap Liniment ad   2000.0   (60% alcohol)
       Sig. Apply.

Calculate the percentage of alcohol in the prescription.

116. In what proportion should 95% alcohol be mixed with 30% alcohol to make 70% alcohol?

117. In what proportion should solutions of 0.38% (w/v) and 1.2% (w/v) be mixed to make a 0.5% (w/v) solution?

118. In what proportion should two lots of crude drug containing respectively 1.7% (w/w) and 2.8% (w/w) of active ingredient be mixed to make a mixture containing 2.1% (w/w) of the active ingredient?

119. In what proportion should 3% and 10% ammoniated mercury ointments be mixed to prepare a 5% ointment?

120. In what proportion should 10% (w/w) ammonia solution be mixed with 28% (w/w) ammonia solution to produce a 15% (w/w) ammonia solution?

121. In what proportion should 1.5% and 30% hydrogen peroxide solutions be mixed to prepare a 3% hydrogen peroxide solution?

122. In what proportion should a 20% zinc oxide ointment be mixed with white petrolatum to produce a 3% zinc oxide ointment?

123. The menstruum for the extraction of a vegetable drug is 70% alcohol. In what proportion may 50%, 60%, and 95% alcohol be mixed in order to prepare a menstruum of the desired concentration?

124. In what proportion may three lots of opium, containing 8%, 12%, and 14% of morphine, be mixed to produce a 10% opium?

125. In what proportion may 3%, 5%, and 15% ointments be mixed to produce a 10% ointment?

126. Three lots of a ground drug contain 1.5%, 2.5% ,and 3.0% of total alkaloids. In what proportion may they be used to make a mixture containing 1.7% of total alkaloids?

127. In what proportion may 3%, 5%, 7%, and 15% zinc oxide ointments be mixed to produce a 10% ointment?

128. In what proportion may lots of crude drug containing 6% (w/w), 10% (w/w), 13% (w/w), and 16% (w/w) of active ingredient be mixed to make a mixture containing 13.5% (w/w) of the active ingredient?

129. How many milliliters of 10% (w/v) solution should be mixed with 300 ml. of 92.5% (w/v) solution to make a 20% (w/v) solution?

130. How many grams of a drug containing 14% (w/w) of active ingredient should be mixed with 600 Gm. of 7% (w/w) drug to make a 9.5% (w/w) mixture?

131. ℞ Belladonna Tincture   60.0
        Iso-Alcoholic Elixir ad   240.0
        Sig. 4 ml. t.i.d.

Belladonna tincture contains 65% of alcohol. How many milliliters of high alcoholic elixir (78%) and how many of low alcoholic elixir (10%) should be used in compounding the prescription?

132. ℞ Compound Gentian Tincture   90 ml.
        Iso-Alcoholic Elixir ad   180 ml.
        Sig. 4 ml. in water a.c.

Compound gentian tincture contains 45% of alcohol. How many milliliters of high alcoholic elixir (78%) and how many milliliters of low alcoholic elixir (10%) should be used in compounding the prescription?

133. How many grams of petrolatum and how many grams of 25% zinc oxide ointment should be used to prepare 2500 Gm. of a 3% ointment?

134. What is the percentage of iodine in a mixture of 3 liters of 7% (w/v) iodine solution, 10 pints of 2% (w/v) solution, and 2270 ml. of 3.5% (w/v) solution?

135. A manufacturing pharmacist has four lots of ichthammol ointment, containing 5%, 10%, 25%, and 50% of ichthammol. How many grams of each may he use to prepare 4800 Gm. of a 20% ichthammol ointment?

136. How many grams of 50% ichthammol ointment should be mixed with 250 Gm. of 15% ointment to make a 20% ichthammol ointment?

137. How many grams of ammoniated mercury should be mixed with 700 Gm. of 5% ammoniated mercury ointment, 200 Gm. of 2% ointment, and 100 Gm. of 1% ointment to make a 10% ointment?

138. How much water must be added to a mixture of 300 Gm. of 65%, 250 Gm. of 35%, and 100 Gm. of 15% acid to produce a 10% acid?

139. How many grams of 3%, 5%, 8%, and 15% boric acid ointments may be mixed to prepare 2500 Gm. of a 10% boric acid ointment?

140. How many milliliters of 5%, 8%, 15%, and 20% (w/v) solutions of a chemical may be used to make 5000 ml. of a 10% (w/v) solution?

141. How many milliliters of water should be added to 2640 Gm. of Phenol, U.S.P., containing 98% of phenol, to prepare Liquefied Phenol, U.S.P., containing 88% of phenol?

142. How many milliliters of water should be added to 500 Gm. of lanolin (25% w/w of water) to prepare a product containing 40% (w/w) of water?

143. How many grams of ichthammol should be added to 750 Gm. of 10% ichthammol ointment to make an ointment containing 15% of ichthammol?

144. How many grams of boric acid should be added to 1000 Gm. of 5% boric acid ointment to make a 20% boric acid ointment?

145. How many grams of petrolatum should be added to 250 Gm. of 20% sulfathiazole ointment to make a 5% sulfathiazole ointment?

146. How many grams of coal tar should be added to 2700 Gm. of a greaseless ointment base to prepare a 10% ointment of coal tar?

147. How many grams of tannic acid should be added to 200 Gm. of a 5% tannic acid ointment to make a 20% ointment?

148. A sample of lanolin weighing 5 lb. is found to contain 35% of water. How much wool fat must be added to it to reduce the water content to 25%?

149. You have on hand 500 ml. of a 12% and 1 liter of a 6% solution of sodium hypochlorite. How many milliliters of water should be added to a mixture of the two solutions to prepare a solution containing 0.5% of sodium hypochlorite?

150. If wool fat absorbs twice its weight of water, how much additional water will be absorbed by 4000 Gm. of hydrous wool fat containing 25% of water?

151. You have on hand 800 Gm. of a 5% coal tar ointment and 1200 Gm. of a 10% coal tar ointment. (a) If the two ointments are mixed, what is the concentration of coal tar in the finished product? (b) How many grams of coal tar should be added to the product to obtain an ointment containing 15% of coal tar?

152. What is the specific gravity of a mixture containing 1000 ml. of water, 500 ml. of glycerin having a specific gravity of 1.25, and 1500 ml. of alcohol having a specific gravity of 0.81? (Assume that there is no contraction on mixing the liquids.)

153. The formula for Formic Acid Spirit is as follows:

Formic Acid	40 ml.
Water	225 ml.
Alcohol	735 ml.

The specific gravity of formic acid is 1.060 and the specific gravity of the alcohol is 0.800. Calculate the specific gravity of the spirit.

154. How many milliliters of each of two liquids with specific gravities respectively of 1.58 and 1.12 should be mixed to make 1000 ml. of a mixture with a specific gravity of 1.38?

155. How many milliliters of a liquid with a specific gravity of

1.48 and of a liquid with a specific gravity of 0.71 should be mixed to prepare 100 ml. of a mixture with a specific gravity of 1.05?

156. How many milliliters of a syrup having a specific gravity of 1.350 should be mixed with 3000 ml. of one having a specific gravity of 1.250 to obtain a product having a specific gravity of 1.310?

CHAPTER XII

ISOTONIC SOLUTIONS

WHEN a solvent passes through a semipermeable membrane from a dilute solution into a more concentrated one with the result that the concentrations tend to become equalized, the phenomenon is known as *osmosis*. The pressure responsible for this phenomenon is called *osmotic pressure*, and it proves to be caused by and to vary with the solute.

If the solute is a non-electrolyte, its solution will contain only molecules, and the osmotic pressure of the solution will vary only with the concentration of the solute. If, on the other hand, the solute is an electrolyte, its solution will contain ions, and the osmotic pressure of the solution will vary not only with the concentration but also with the degree of ionization of the solute. Obviously then, ionizable substances, having a relatively greater number of particles in solution, should exert a greater osmotic pressure than could undissociated molecules.

Like osmotic pressure, the other colligative properties of solutions, namely, vapor pressure, boiling point, and freezing point, depend upon the number of particles in solution. These properties, therefore, are related, and a change in any one of them will produce corresponding changes in the others.

Among the recent results of the accumulating knowledge of the colligative properties of solutions is the growing medical conviction that many solutions designed to be mixed with body fluids should have the same osmotic pressure—in other words, should be made *isotonic* with those fluids—for greater comfort, efficacy, and safety. Solutions of lower osmotic pressure than that of a body fluid are *hypotonic*, whereas those having a higher osmotic pressure are *hypertonic*. Blood and the fluids of the eye and nose have so far been principally concerned, and of these the pharmacist is most likely to be asked to make eye preparations, or *collyria*, isotonic with lachrymal fluid.

Various methods have been proposed for calculating this problem, the simplicity of which is concealed under a mass of theory that is unfamiliar to many pharmacists. Available figures involved vary

(189)

from close approximations (*e. g.*, molecular weights) to arbitrary guesses (*e. g.*, the degree of dissociation of many new medicinals in solution), and it seems quite unnecessary to carry calculations out to third and fourth place "accuracy" as sometimes attempted.

The first thing we need is a convenient procedure for making any simple solution isotonic with another of known tonicity. Theoretically, any one of the colligative properties of solutions could be used as a basis for determining tonicity. Practically and most conveniently, a comparison of freezing points may be used for this purpose. For some time, −0.56° C. and −0.80° C. were generally accepted as the freezing points for blood serum and lachrymal fluid, respectively. At the present time, there seems to be strong evidence to indicate that the freezing point of lachrymal fluid is the same as that of blood, and most investigators now agree that the figure, −0.56° C., represents the freezing point of both fluids. Now it happens that when one gram molecular weight of any non-electrolyte—that is, a substance with negligible dissociation, such as boric acid—is dissolved in 1000 Gm. of water, the freezing point of the solution is about 1.86° C. below the freezing point of pure water. By simple proportion, therefore, we may calculate the weight of any non-electrolyte that should be dissolved in each 1000 Gm. of water if the solution is to be isotonic with the body fluids.

Boric acid, for example, has a molecular weight of 61.8, and hence (in theory) 61.8 Gm. in 1000 Gm. of water should produce a freezing point of −1.86° C. Therefore:

By the proportion:

1.86 (° C.):0.56 (° C.) = 61.8 (Gm.):x

x = 18.6 Gm.

In short, 18.6 Gm. of boric acid in 1000 Gm. of water, having a weight-in-volume strength of approximately 1.85%, should make a solution isotonic with lachrymal fluid.

With electrolytes, the problem is not quite so simple. Since osmotic pressure depends rather upon the number than upon the kind of particles, substances that dissociate have a tonic effect that increases with the degree of dissociation, and the greater the dissociation, the smaller the quantity required to produce any given osmotic pressure. Sodium chloride in weak solutions is about 85% dissociated, each 100 molecules yielding 185 particles, or 1.85 times as many particles as are yielded by 100 molecules of a non-electrolyte. This dissociation factor, commonly symbolized by the letter i, must be included in the proportion when we seek to determine the strength of an isotonic solution of sodium chloride (molecular weight, 58.5):

By the proportion:

[1.86 (° C.) × 1.85]:0.56 (° C.) = 58.5 (Gm.):x

x = 9.52 Gm.

Hence, 9.52 Gm. of sodium chloride in 1000 Gm. of water should make a solution isotonic with blood or lachrymal fluid. At 4° C. this solution should have a weight-in-volume strength of approximately 0.95%; but at normal temperature the volume of water would be somewhat greater, and a *0.90% (w/v)* sodium chloride solution is taken to be isotonic with the body fluids.

Simple isotonic solutions, then, may be calculated by this general formula:

$$\frac{0.56 \times \text{molecular weight}}{1.86 \times \text{dissociation } (i)} = \text{Gm. of solute per 1000 Gm. of water}$$

The value of i for many a medicinal salt has not been experimentally determined. Some salts (such as zinc sulfate, with only some 40% dissociation and an i value therefore of 1.4) are exceptional; but most medicinal salts approximate the dissociation of sodium chloride in weak solutions, and if the number of ions is known we may use the following values, lacking better information:

Non-electrolytes and substances
of slight dissociation: 1.0
Substances that dissociate into 2 ions: 1.8
Substances that dissociate into 3 ions: 2.6
Substances that dissociate into 4 ions: 3.4
Substances that dissociate into 5 ions: 4.2

A special problem arises when a prescription directs us to make a solution isotonic by adding the proper amount of some substance other than the active ingredient or ingredients. Given a 0.5% (w/v) solution of sodium chloride, we may easily calculate that 0.9 Gm. − 0.5 Gm. = 0.4 Gm. of additional sodium chloride should be contained in each 100 ml. if the solution is to be made isotonic with a body fluid. But how much sodium chloride should be used in preparing 100 ml. of a 1% (w/v) solution of atropine sulfate, which is to be made isotonic with lachrymal fluid? The answer depends upon *how much sodium chloride is in effect represented by the atropine sulfate.*

The relative tonic effect of two substances—that is, the quantity of one that is the equivalent in tonic effect to a given quantity of the other—may be calculated if the quantity of one having a certain effect in a specified quantity of solvent be divided by the quantity of the other having the same effect in the same quantity of solvent. For example, we have calculated above that 1.85 Gm. of boric acid per 100 Gm. of water and that 0.95 Gm. of sodium chloride per 100 Gm. of water are both instrumental in making an aqueous solution isotonic with lachrymal fluid. But if 1.85 Gm. of boric acid is the tonicic equivalent of 0.95 Gm. of sodium chloride, then 1 Gm. of boric acid must be the equivalent of 0.95 Gm. ÷ 1.85 Gm. = 0.52 Gm. of sodium chloride. And similarly, 1 Gm. of sodium chloride must be the tonicic equivalent of 1.85 Gm. ÷ 0.95 Gm. = 1.90 Gm. of boric acid.

We have seen that there is one quantity of any substance that should in theory have a constant tonic effect if dissolved in 1000 Gm. of water: this is one gram molecular weight of the substance divided by its i or relative dissociation value. Hence, the relative quantity of sodium chloride that is the tonicic equivalent of a quantity of boric acid may be calculated by these ratios:

$$\frac{58.5 \div 1.8}{61.8 \div 1.0} \text{ or } \frac{58.5 \times 1.0}{61.8 \times 1.8}$$

and we may formulate a convenient rule: *quantities of two substances that are tonicic equivalents are proportional to the molecular weights of each multiplied by the i value of the other.*

To return to the problem involving 1 Gm. of atropine sulfate in 100 ml. of solution:

Molecular weight of sodium chloride = 58.5; $i = 1.8$
Molecular weight of atropine sulfate = 695; $i = 2.6$

By the proportion:

$(695 \times 1.8):(58.5 \times 2.6) = 1 \text{ (Gm.)}:x$
x = 0.12 Gm. of sodium chloride represented by 1 Gm. of atropine sulfate

Since a solution isotonic with lachrymal fluid should contain the equivalent of 0.9 Gm. of sodium chloride in each 100 ml. of solution, the difference to be added must be 0.90 Gm. − 0.12 Gm. = 0.78 Gm. of sodium chloride.

The Table on pages 204–206 gives the sodium chloride equivalents of each of the substances listed. These values were calculated according to the rule stated above. If the number of grams (or grains) of a substance included in a prescription be multiplied by its sodium chloride equivalent, the amount of sodium chloride represented by that substance is determined.

The procedure for the *calculation of isotonic solutions with sodium chloride equivalents* may be outlined as follows:

Step 1.   Calculate the amount (in Gm. or gr.) of sodium chloride represented by the ingredients in the prescription. This may be done by multiplying the amount (in Gm. or gr.) of each substance by its sodium chloride equivalent.

Step 2.   Calculate the amount (in Gm. or gr.) of sodium chloride, alone, that would be contained in an isotonic solution of the volume specified in the prescription—namely, *the amount of sodium chloride in a 0.9% solution of the specified volume.* (Such a solution would contain 0.009 Gm. per ml., or 4.1 gr. per f℥.)

Step 3.   Subtract the amount of sodium chloride represented by the ingredients in the prescription (Step 1) from the amount of sodium chloride, alone, that would be represented in the specified volume of an isotonic solution (Step 2). The answer represents the amount (in Gm. or gr.) of sodium chloride to be added to make the solution isotonic.

Step 4.   If an agent other than sodium chloride, such as boric acid, dextrose, sodium or potassium nitrate, is to be used to make a solution isotonic, divide the amount of sodium chloride (Step 3) by the sodium chloride equivalent of the other substance.

To calculate the dissociation (i) factor of an electrolyte:

Examples:

Zinc sulfate is a 2-ion electrolyte, dissociating 40% in a certain concentration. Calculate its dissociation (i) factor.

On the basis of 40% dissociation, 100 particles of zinc sulfate will yield:

	40	zinc ions
	40	sulfate ions
	60	undissociated particles
or	140	particles

Since 140 particles represent 1.4 times as many particles as there were before dissociation, the dissociation (*i*) factor is 1.4, *answer.*

13

Zinc chloride is a 3-ion electrolyte, dissociating 80% in a certain concentration. Calculate its dissociation (i) factor.

On the basis of 80% dissociation, 100 particles of zinc chloride will yield:

	80	zinc ions
	80	chloride ions
	80	chloride ions
	20	undissociated particles
or	260	particles

Since 260 particles represent 2.6 times as many particles as there were before dissociation, the dissociation (*i*) factor is 2.6, *answer.*

To calculate the sodium chloride equivalent of a substance:

Remember that the sodium chloride equivalent of a substance may be calculated as follows:

$$\frac{\text{molecular weight of sodium chloride}}{i \text{ factor of sodium chloride}} \times \frac{i \text{ factor of the substance}}{\text{molecular weight of the substance}} = \text{sodium chloride equivalent}$$

Example:

Papaverine hydrochloride (molecular weight 376) is a 2-ion electrolyte, dissociating 80% in a given concentration. Calculate its sodium chloride equivalent.

Since papaverine hydrochloride is a 2-ion electrolyte, dissociating 80%, its *i* factor is 1.8.

$$\frac{58.5}{1.8} \times \frac{1.8}{376} = 0.156, \text{ or } 0.16, \text{ } answer.$$

To calculate the amount of tonicic agent required:

Examples:

℞	Pilocarpine Nitrate	0.3 Gm.
	Sodium Chloride	q.s.
	Distilled Water ad	30.0 ml.
	Ft. isoton. sol.	
	Sig. For the eye.	

How much sodium chloride should be used in compounding the prescription?

Step 1.   0.22 × 0.3 Gm. = 0.066 Gm. of sodium chloride represented by the pilocarpine nitrate

Step 2.   30 × 0.009 = 0.270 Gm. of sodium chloride in 30 ml. of an isotonic sodium chloride solution

Step 3.   0.270 Gm.   (from Step 2)
             −0.066 Gm.   (from Step 1)
             ───────
             0.204 Gm. of sodium chloride to be used, *answer.*

    ℞   Atropine Sulfate   gr. v
        Sodium Chloride   q.s.
        Distilled Water ad   ℥ i
        Ft. isoton. sol.
        Sig. One drop in right eye.

How many grains of sodium chloride should be used in compounding the prescription?

Step 1.   0.12 × 5 gr. = 0.6 gr. of sodium chloride represented by the atropine sulfate

Step 2.   455 × 1 × 0.009 = 4.1 gr. of sodium chloride in ℥ i of an isotonic sodium chloride solution

Step 3.   4.1 gr.   (from Step 2)
             −0.6 gr.   (from Step 1)
             ───────
             3.5 gr. of sodium chloride to be used, *answer.*

    ℞   Holocaine Hydrochloride   1%
        Chlorobutanol $\frac{1}{2}$%
        Boric Acid   q.s.
        Distilled Water ad   60.0
        Ft. isoton. sol.
        Sig. One drop in each eye.

How much boric acid should be used in compounding the prescription?

The prescription calls for 0.6 Gm. of holocaine hydrochloride and 0.3 Gm. of chlorobutanol.

Step 1.   0.17 × 0.6 Gm. = 0.102 Gm. of sodium chloride represented by holocaine hydrochloride

        0.18 × 0.3 Gm. = 0.054 Gm. of sodium chloride represented by chlorobutanol
                           ───────
           Total: 0.156 Gm. of sodium chloride represented by both ingredients

Step 2.   60 × 0.009 = 0.540 Gm. of sodium chloride in 60 ml. of
                      an isotonic sodium chloride solution

Step 3.   0.540 Gm.   (from Step 2)
                −0.156 Gm.   (from Step 1)
                _____

            0.384 Gm. of sodium chloride required to make the
                      solution isotonic

But since the prescription calls for boric acid:

Step 4.   0.384 Gm. ÷ 0.52 (sodium chloride equivalent of boric
             acid) = 0.738 Gm. of boric acid to be used, *answer.*

        ℞   Sol. Silver Nitrate   60.0
                1–500
             Ft. isoton. sol.
             Sig. For eye use.

    *How much sodium nitrate should be used in compounding the
    prescription?*

The prescription contains 0.120 Gm. of silver nitrate.

Step 1.   0.34 × 0.120 Gm. = 0.041 Gm. of sodium chloride repre-
                      sented by silver nitrate

Step 2.   60 × 0.009 = 0.540 Gm. of sodium chloride in 60 ml. of
                      an isotonic sodium chloride solution

Step 3.   0.540 Gm.   (from Step 2)
                −0.041 Gm.   (from Step 1)
                _____

            0.499 Gm. of sodium chloride required to make solution
                      isotonic

But the prescription requires sodium nitrate, since, in this solution,
sodium chloride is incompatible with silver nitrate.   Therefore,

Step 4.   0.499 Gm. ÷ 0.69 (sodium chloride equivalent of sodium
             nitrate) = 0.720 Gm. of sodium nitrate to be used, *answer.*

        ℞   Ingredient X   0.5
             Sodium Chloride   q.s.
             Distilled Water ad   50.0
             Ft. isoton. sol.
             Sig. Eye drops.

How much sodium chloride should be used in compounding the prescription?

Let us assume that Ingredient X is a new substance for which no sodium chloride equivalent is to be found in the Table, and that its molecular weight is 295 and its *i* factor is 2.4.

The sodium chloride equivalent of Ingredient X may be calculated as follows:

$$\frac{58.5 \times 2.4}{1.8 \times 295} = 0.26, \text{ the sodium chloride equivalent for Ingredient X}$$

Then,

Step 1.   0.26 × 0.5 Gm. = 0.130 Gm. of sodium chloride represented by Ingredient X

Step 2.   50 × 0.009 = 0.450 Gm. of sodium chloride in 50 ml. of an isotonic sodium chloride solution

Step 3.   0.450 Gm.   (from Step 2)
           −0.130 Gm.   (from Step 1)
_____
           0.320 Gm. of sodium chloride to be used, *answer.*

Practice Problems

1. Isotonic Sodium Chloride Solution contains 0.9% of sodium chloride. If the sodium chloride equivalent of boric acid is 0.52, what is the percentage strength of an isotonic solution of boric acid?

2. Procaine hydrochloride is a 2-ion electrolyte, dissociating 80% in a certain concentration. (a) Calculate its dissociation (*i*) factor. (b) Calculate its sodium chloride equivalent. (c) Calculate the freezing point of a molal solution of procaine hydrochloride.

3. The freezing point of a molal solution of a non-electrolyte is −1.86° C. What is the freezing point of an 0.1% solution of zinc chloride (136), dissociating 80%?[1]

4. The freezing point of a 5% solution of boric acid is −1.55° C. How much boric acid should be used in preparing 1000 ml. of an isotonic solution?

[1] For lack of more definite information, the student must assume that the volume of the molal solution is approximately 1 L.

5. ℞   Ephedrine Sulfate   gr. iv
        Sodium Chloride   q.s.
        Distilled Water ad   ℥ i
        Ft. isoton. sol.
        Sig. Use as directed.

How many grains of sodium chloride should be used in compounding the prescription?

6. ℞   Pilocarpine Nitrate   gr. ii
        Chlorobutanol   gr. ss
        Sodium Chloride   q.s.
        Distilled Water ad   ℥ ss
        Ft. isoton. sol.
        Sig. One drop in right eye.

How many grains of sodium chloride should be used in compounding the prescription?

7. ℞   Copper Sulfate Solution   2%
        Rose Water aa   50.0
        Sodium Chloride   q.s.
        Ft. isoton. sol.
        Sig. Use as directed.

How much sodium chloride should be used in compounding the prescription?

8. ℞   Dionin $\frac{1}{2}$%
        Scopolamine Hydrobromide $\frac{1}{3}$%
        Sodium Chloride   q.s.
        Distilled Water ad   30.0
        Ft. isoton. sol.
        Sig. Use in the eye.

How much sodium chloride should be used in compounding the prescription?

9. ℞   Pilocarpine Hydrochloride   0.210
        Nupercaine Hydrochloride   0.625
        Sodium Chloride   q.s.
        Distilled Water ad   60.0
        Ft. isoton. sol.
        Sig. One drop in eye as directed.

How much sodium chloride should be used in compounding the prescription?

10. ℞ Carbamylcholine Chloride 1.5%
      Sodium Chloride q.s.
      Distilled Water ad 10.0
      Ft. isoton. sol.
      Sig. One drop in eye to maintain miosis.

How many milligrams of sodium chloride should be used in compounding the prescription?

11. ℞ Zinc Sulfate 0.06
      Boric Acid q.s.
      Distilled Water ad 30.0
      Ft. isoton. sol.
      Sig. Drop in eyes.

How much boric acid should be used in compounding the prescription?

12. ℞ Atropine Sulfate 1%
      Boric Acid q.s.
      Distilled Water ad 30.0
      Ft. isoton. sol.
      Sig. One drop in each eye.

How much boric acid should be used in compounding the prescription?

13. ℞ Potassium Iodide gr. v
      Sodium Chloride q.s.
      Distilled Water ad ℥i
      Ft. isoton. sol.
      Sig. Use in the eye.

How many grains of sodium chloride should be used in compounding the prescription?

14. ℞ Sol. Silver Nitrate 15.0
        0.5%
      Ft. isoton. sol.
      Sig. For the eyes.

How much sodium nitrate should be used in compounding the prescription?

15. ℞ Cocaine Hydrochloride 0.150
      Sodium Chloride q.s.
      Distilled Water ad 15.0
      Ft. isoton. sol.
      Sig. One drop in left eye.

How much sodium chloride should be used in compounding the prescription?

16. ℞　Sol. Physostigmine Salicylate　　30 ml.
　　　　$\frac{1}{2}$%
　　　Ft. isoton. sol. with boric acid
　　　Sig. One drop in left eye t.i.d.

How much boric acid should be used in compounding the prescription?

17. ℞　Zinc Sulfate　　　　　　　0.12
　　　Antipyrine　　　　　　　　0.65
　　　Sodium Chloride　　　　　　q.s.
　　　Distilled Water ad　　　　60.0
　　　Ft. isoton. sol.
　　　Sig. Eye drops.

How much sodium chloride should be used in compounding the prescription?

18. ℞　Cocaine Hydrochloride　　　　　0.6
　　　Eucatropine Hydrochloride　　0.6
　　　Chlorobutanol　　　　　　　　0.1
　　　Sodium Chloride　　　　　　　q.s.
　　　Distilled Water ad　　　　　30.0
　　　Ft. isoton. sol.
　　　Sig. For the eye.

How much sodium chloride should be used in compounding the prescription?

19. ℞　Tetracaine Hydrochloride　　0.1
　　　Zinc Sulfate　　　　　　　　0.05
　　　Boric Acid　　　　　　　　　q.s.
　　　Distilled Water ad　　　　30.0
　　　Ft. isoton. sol.
　　　Sig. Drop in eye.

How much boric acid should be used in compounding the prescription?

20. ℞　Sol. Homatropine Hydrobromide　　15.0
　　　　1%
　　　Ft. isoton. sol. with boric acid.
　　　Sig. For the eyes.

How much boric acid should be used in compounding the prescription?

21. ℞ Procaine Hydrochloride   1%
      Sodium Chloride   q.s.
      Distilled Water ad   100.0
      Ft. isoton. sol.
      Sig. For injection.

How much sodium chloride should be used in compounding the prescription?

22. ℞ Eserine Salicylate   0.03
      Phenacaine Hydrochloride   0.150
      Boric Acid   q.s.
      Distilled Water ad   30.0
      Ft. isoton. sol.
      Sig. Drop in eyes.

How much boric acid should be used in compounding the prescription?

23. ℞ Tetracaine Hydrochloride   1%
      Chlorobutanol $\frac{1}{2}$%
      Sodium Chloride   q.s.
      Distilled Water ad   60.0
      Ft. isoton. sol.
      Sig. Use in the eye.

How much sodium chloride should be used in compounding the prescription?

24. ℞ Phenylephrine Hydrochloride   1.0
      Chlorobutanol   0.5
      Sodium Bisulfite   0.2
      Sodium Chloride   q.s.
      Distilled Water ad   100.0
      Ft. isoton. sol.
      Sig. Use as directed.

How many milliliters of an 0.9% solution of sodium chloride should be used in compounding the prescription?

25. ℞ Holocaine Hydrochloride $\frac{1}{2}$%
      Hyoscine Hydrobromide $\frac{1}{3}$%
      Boric Acid Solution   q.s.
      Distilled Water ad   60.0
      Ft. isoton. sol.
      Sig. For the eyes.

How many milliliters of a 5% solution of boric acid should be used in compounding the prescription?

26. ℞   Ephedrine Hydrochloride   0.5
        Chlorobutanol   0.25
        Dextrose   q.s.
        Rose Water ad   50.0
        Ft. isoton. sol.
        Sig. Nose drops.

How much dextrose should be used in compounding the prescription?

27. ℞   Dionin   5%
        Sodium Chloride   q.s.
        Distilled Water ad   ℥i
        Ft. isoton. sol.
        Sig. Use as directed in the eye.

How many grains of sodium chloride should be used in compounding the prescription?

28. ℞   Butacaine Sulfate   0.6
        Boric Acid   q.s.
        Rose Water ad   30.0
        Ft. isoton. sol.
        Sig. Eye drops.

How much boric acid should be used in compounding the prescription?

29. ℞   Scopolamine Hydrobromide $\frac{1}{3}$%
        Phenacaine Hydrochloride   1%
        Sodium Chloride   q.s.
        Distilled Water ad   15.0
        Ft. isoton. sol.
        Sig. One drop in eye.

How much sodium chloride should be used in compounding the prescription?

30. ℞   Physostigmine Salicylate $\frac{1}{4}$%
        Boric Acid   q.s.
        Distilled Water ad   60.0
        Ft. isoton. sol.
        Sig. One drop in right eye.

How many milliliters of a 3% boric acid solution should be used in compounding the prescription?

31. ℞   Tetracaine Hydrochloride   0.5%
       Sol. Epinephrine Hydrochloride   10.0
          1:1000
       Boric Acid   q.s.
       Distilled Water ad   30.0
       Ft. isoton. sol.
       Sig. Eye drops.

The solution of epinephrine hydrochloride (1:1000) is already isotonic. How much boric acid should be used in compounding the prescription?

32. ℞   Oxytetracycline Hydrochloride   0.050
       Chlorobutanol   0.1
       Sodium Chloride   q.s.
       Distilled Water ad   30.0
       Ft. isoton. sol.
       Sig. Eye drops.

Oxytetracycline hydrochloride (molecular weight 500) has an i value of 1.9. How many milligrams of sodium chloride should be used in compounding the prescription?

33. ℞   Ingredient X   gr. x
       Boric Acid   q.s.
       Distilled Water ad   ℥ i
       Ft. isoton. sol.
       Sig. For the eye.

Ingredient X (molecular weight 252) has an i value of 1.8.

How many grains of boric acid should be used in compounding the prescription?

TABLE OF SODIUM CHLORIDE EQUIVALENTS

Substance	Molecular weight	Ions	i	Sodium chloride equivalent
Alum (ammonium).12H$_2$O	453	4	3.4	0.24
Alum (potassium).12H$_2$O	474	4	3.4	0.23
Alypin hydrochloride	315	2	1.8	0.19
Ammonium chloride	53.5	2	1.8	1.09
Amphetamine sulfate	368	3	2.6	0.23
Amydricaine				
(See Alypin hydrochloride)				
Amylcaine hydrochloride	287	2	1.8	0.20
Antipyrine	188	1	1.0	0.17
Apothesine hydrochloride	298	2	1.8	0.20
Argyrol				
(See Mild silver protein)				
Atropine sulfate.H$_2$O	695	3	2.6	0.12
Benzedrine sulfate				
(See Amphetamine sulfate)				
Benzyl alcohol	108	1	1.0	0.30
Borax				
(See Sodium borate)				
Boric acid	61.8	1	1.0	0.52
Butacaine sulfate	711	3	2.6	0.12
Butyn sulfate				
(See Butacaine sulfate)				
Caffeine	194	1	1.0	0.17
Calcium chloride.2H$_2$O	147	3	2.6	0.57
Calcium gluconate.H$_2$O	448	3	2.6	0.19
Calcium lactate.5H$_2$O	308	3	2.6	0.27
Camphor	152	1	1.0	0.21
Carbachol	183	2	1.8	0.33
Carbamylcholine coloride				
(See Carbachol)				
Chloramphenicol	323	1	1.0	0.10
Chlorobutanol	177	1	1.0	0.18
Chloromycetin				
(See Chloramphenicol)				
Cocaine hydrochloride	340	2	1.8	0.17
Cupric sulfate.5H$_2$O	250	2	1.4	0.18
Dextrose (anhydrous)	180	1	1.0	0.18
Dextrose.H$_2$O	198	1	1.0	0.16
Dionin				
(See Ethylmorphine hydrochloride)				
Diothane hydrochloride	434	2	1.8	0.14
Emetine hydrochloride	554	3	2.6	0.15
Ephedrine hydrochloride	202	2	1.8	0.29
Ephedrine sulfate	429	3	2.6	0.20
Epinephrine hydrochloride	220	2	1.8	0.27
Epinephrine bitartrate	333	2	1.8	0.18
Eserine salicylate				
(See Physostigmine salicylate)				
Eserine sulfate				
(See Physostigmine sulfate)				
Ethylhydrocupreine hydrochloride	377	2	1.8	0.16

TABLE OF SODIUM CHLORIDE EQUIVALENTS

Substance	Molecular weight	Ions	i	Sodium chloride equivalent
Ethylmorphine hydrochloride.$2H_2O$ . .	386	2	1.8	0.15
Eucatropine hydrochloride	328	2	1.8	0.22
Euphthalmine hydrochloride				
(See Eucatropine hydrochloride)				
Fluorescein sodium	376	3	2.6	0.22
Glycerin	92.1	1	1.0	0.36
Holocaine hydrochloride				
(See Phenacaine hydrochloride)				
Homatropine hydrobromide	356	2	1.8	0.16
Hydroxyamphetamine hydrobromide .	232	2	1.8	0.25
Hyoscine hydrobromide				
(See Scopolamine hydrobromide)				
Hyoscine hydrochloride				
(See Scopolamine hydrochloride)				
Larocaine hydrochloride	315	2	1.8	0.19
Magnesium sulfate.$7H_2O$	247	2	1.8	0.24
Menthol	156	1	1.0	0.21
Mercuric cyanide	253	3	1.0	0.13
Mercuric oxycyanide	469	3	1.0	0.07
Mercuric succinimide	397	2	1.0	0.08
Mercury bichloride	272	3	1.0	0.12
Methenamine	140	1	1.0	0.23
Metycaine hydrochloride . . .	298	2	1.8	0.20
Mild protein silver (20% silver) . .	540 (?)	1	1.0	0.06
Morphine hydrochloride.$3H_2O$ . .	376	2	1.8	0.16
Morphine sulfate.$5H_2O$	759	3	2.6	0.11
Neo-synephrine hydrochloride				
(See Phenylephrine hydrochloride)				
Novocain				
(See Procaine hydrochloride) . .				
Nupercaine hydrochloride	380	2	1.8	0.15
Optochin				
(See Ethylhydrocupreine hydrochloride)				
Phenacaine hydrochloride	353	2	1.8	0.17
Phenobarbital Sodium	254	2	1.8	0.23
Phenylephrine hydrochloride . . .	204	2	1.8	0.29
Physostigmine salicylate	413	2	1.8	0.14
Physostigmine sulfate	649	3	2.6	0.13
Pilocarpine hydrochloride . . .	245	2	1.8	0.24
Pilocarpine nitrate	271	2	1.8	0.22
Pontocaine hydrochloride				
(See Tetracaine hydrochloride)				
Potassium biphosphate	136	2	1.8	0.43
Potassium chloride	74.6	2	1.8	0.78
Potassium iodide	166	2	1.8	0.35
Potassium nitrate	101	2	1.8	0.58
Procaine hydrochloride	273	2	1.8	0.21
Propadrine	188	2	1.8	0.31
Protargol				
(See Strong protein silver)				
Scopolamine hydrobromide.$3H_2O$ . .	438	2	1.8	0.13

TABLE OF SODIUM CHLORIDE EQUIVALENTS

Substance	Molecular weight	Ions	i	Sodium chloride equivalent
Scopolamine hydrochloride.$2H_2O$	376	2	1.8	0.16
Silver nitrate	170	2	1.8	0.34
Sodium bicarbonate	84.0	2	1.8	0.70
Sodium biphosphate	120	2	1.8	0.49
Sodium biphosphate.H_2O	138	2	1.8	0.42
Sodium bisulfite	104	3	2.6	0.81
Sodium borate.$10H_2O$	381	5	4.2	0.36
Sodium carbonate	106	3	2.6	0.80
Sodium carbonate.H_2O	124	3	2.6	0.68
Sodium chloride	58.5	2	1.8	1.00
Sodium citrate.$2H_2O$	294	4	3.4	0.38
Sodium iodide	150	2	1.8	0.39
Sodium lactate	112	2	1.8	0.52
Sodium nitrate	85.0	2	1.8	0.69
Sodium phosphate.$2H_2O$	178	3	2.6	0.47
Sodium phosphate.$7H_2O$	268	3	2.6	0.31
Sodium phosphate.$12H_2O$	358	3	2.6	0.24
Sodium sulfite	126	3	2.6	0.64
Strong protein silver (7.5% to 8.5% silver)	1350 (?)	1	1.0	0.024
Sulfadiazine sodium	272	2	1.8	0.21
Sulfanilamide	172	1	1.0	0.19
Sulfapyridine sodium	289	2	1.8	0.20
Sulfathiazole sodium (sesquihydrate)	304	2	1.8	0.19
Tannic acid	324 (?)	1	1.0	0.10
Tetracaine hydrochloride	301	2	1.8	0.19
Tutocaine hydrochloride	287	2	1.8	0.20
Urea	60.1	1	1.0	0.54
Zinc chloride	136	3	2.6	0.62
Zinc sulfate.$7H_2O$	288	2	1.4	0.16

CHAPTER XIII

CHEMICAL PROBLEMS

ATOMIC AND MOLECULAR WEIGHTS

Most chemical problems involve the use of *atomic* or *combining weights* of the elements, and the validity of their solutions depends upon the *Law of Definite Proportions*.

The *atomic weight* of an element is the ratio of the weight of its atom to the weight of an atom of another element taken as a standard. The standard chosen is the weight of an oxygen atom as 16.0000; and the relative weights of most of the important elements are either whole numbers or very nearly so.

Examples:

Element	Atomic Weight	Approximate Atomic Weight
Oxygen	16.0000	16
Hydrogen	1.0080	1
Sodium	22.997	23
Calcium	40.08	40

A table of accurate and approximate atomic weights is given on the inside back cover.

The *combining* or *equivalent weight* of an *element* is that weight of the element that will combine (or displace) one gram atomic weight of hydrogen (or the equivalent weight of some other element). For example, when hydrogen and chlorine react to form HCl, 1.0080 Gm. of hydrogen react with 35.457 Gm. of chlorine; therefore, the equivalent weight of chlorine is 35.457.

The *equivalent weight* of a *compound* is that weight of the compound that will interact with one equivalent weight of an element. Thus, HCl has an equivalent weight of 36.4650 for it contains 1.0080 Gm. of hydrogen and this is displaceable by one equivalent weight of a metal.

The *Law of Definite Proportions* states that elements invariably combine in the same proportion by weight to form a given compound.

To calculate molecular weights from atomic weights:

The *molecular weight* of an element or compound is the sum of the weights of the atoms in the molecule.

Example:

   Calculate the molecular weight of phosphoric acid, H_3PO_4.

$$H_3 \qquad\qquad P \qquad\qquad O_4$$
$$(3 \times 1.0080) + 30.975 + (4 \times 16.0000) = 97.999, answer.$$

PERCENTAGE COMPOSITION

To calculate the percentage composition of a compound:

Examples:

   Calculate the percentage composition of tribasic calcium phosphate, $Ca_3(PO_4)_2$.

$$Ca_3 \qquad\qquad 2P \qquad\qquad 2O_4$$
$$(3 \times 40.08) + (2 \times 30.975) + (8 \times 16.0000) =$$
$$120.24 \quad + \quad 61.95 \quad + \quad 128.0000 \quad = 310.19$$

By the proportions:

   $310.19:120.24 = 100(\%):x$
   $x = 38.76\%$ of calcium, *and*

   $310.19:61.95 = 100(\%):y$
   $y = 19.97\%$ of phosphorus, *and*

   $310.19:128.00 = 100(\%):z$
   $z = 41.27\%$ of oxygen, *answers.*

Check: $38.76\% + 19.97\% + 41.27\% = 100\%$

   Calculate the percentage of water in sodium phosphate,
   $Na_2HPO_4.7H_2O$.

$$Na_2 \qquad H \qquad P \qquad O_4 \qquad\qquad 7H_2O$$
$$(2 \times 22.997) + 1.0080 + 30.975 + (4 \times 16.0000) + (7 \times 18.0160) =$$
$$45.994 \quad + 1.0080 + 30.975 + \quad 64.0000 \quad + \quad 126.1120 \quad =$$
$$268.10, \text{molecular weight of sodium phosphate}$$

By the proportion:

   $268.10:126.11 = 100(\%):x$
   $x = 47.04\%$, *answer.*

To calculate the weight of a constituent, given the weight of a compound:

Approximate atomic weights may ordinarily be used in solving problems of this kind.

Example:

> *A certain solution contains 500 mg. of sodium fluoride, NaF. How many milligrams of fluorine are represented in the solution?*

    Na   F
    23 + 19 = 42

By the proportion:

    42:19 = 500 (mg.):x
    x = 226 mg., *answer.*

To calculate the weight of a compound, given the weight of a constituent:

Approximate atomic weights may ordinarily be used in solving problems of this kind.

Example:

> *A prescription calls for 200 mg. of fluorine. How many milligrams of sodium fluoride should be used in order to obtain the prescribed amount of fluorine?*

    Na   F
    23 + 19 = 42

By the proportion:

    19:42 = 200 (mg.):x
    x = 442 mg., *answer.*

CHEMICALS IN REACTIONS

To calculate the weights of pure chemicals involved in reactions:

Approximate atomic weights may ordinarily be used in solving problems of this kind.

Examples:

> *How many grams of absolute hydrochloric acid are required to neutralize 324 Gm. of anhydrous sodium carbonate?*

$$Na_2CO_3 + 2HCl = 2NaCl + H_2O + CO_2$$

    106   2(36)
              or 72
    Molecular weight of Na_2CO_3 = 106
    Molecular weight of 2HCl = 72

By the proportion:

    106:72 = 324 (Gm.):x
    x = 223 Gm., *answer.*

How many grams of iron are required to react with 100 Gm. of iodine?

$$Fe + I_2 = FeI_2$$
56   2(127)
     or 254

By the proportion:

254:56 = 100 (Gm.):x
x = 22.1 Gm., *answer.*

How many grams of p-aminobenzoic acid and how many grams of sodium bicarbonate should be used to prepare 100 Gm. of sodium p-aminobenzoate?

$$NH_2C_6H_4COOH + NaHCO_3 = NH_2C_6H_4COONa + H_2O + CO_2$$
137   84   159

By the proportions:

159:137 = 100 (Gm.):x
x = 86.2 Gm. of p-aminobenzoic acid, *and*
159:84 = 100 (Gm.):y
y = 52.8 Gm. of sodium bicarbonate, *answers.*

How many grams of anhydrous citric acid are required to react with 25 Gm. of sodium bicarbonate?

$$3NaHCO_3 + H_3C_6H_5O_7 = Na_3C_6H_5O_7 + 3H_2O + 3CO_2$$
3(84)   192
or 252

By the proportion:

252:192 = 25 (Gm.):x
x = 19 Gm., *answer.*

To calculate the weights of chemicals involved in reactions, with consideration of percentage strengths:

In solving problems of this type, it is important to remember that proportions based upon atomic and molecular weights apply only to *pure* (absolute) or *100%* chemicals. <u>If *volume-in-volume* or *weight-in-volume* strength is specified, *it must be converted to weight-in-weight strength.*</u>

Examples:

How many grams of 85% potassium hydroxide are required to react with 125 Gm. of mercuric chloride?

$$HgCl_2 + 2KOH = HgO + 2KCl + H_2O$$
$$271 \quad 2(56)$$
$$\text{or } 112$$

By the proportion:

$$271:112 = 125 \text{ (Gm.)}:x$$
$$x = 51.7 \text{ Gm. of } 100\% \text{ KOH}$$

By the proportion:

$$85(\%):100(\%) = 51.7 \text{ (Gm.)}:x$$
$$x = 60.8 \text{ Gm., } answer.$$

How many grams of potassium bicarbonate and how many milliliters of 36% acetic acid, sp. gr. 1.045, are required to prepare 200 Gm. of potassium acetate?

$$KHCO_3 + HC_2H_3O_2 = KC_2H_3O_2 + CO_2 + H_2O$$
$$100 \quad\quad 60 \quad\quad\quad 98$$

By the proportions:

$$98:100 = 200 \text{ (Gm.)}:x$$
$$x = 204 \text{ Gm. of potassium bicarbonate, } and$$
$$98:60 = 200 \text{ (Gm.)}:y$$
$$y = 122 \text{ Gm. of } 100\% \text{ acetic acid}$$
$$36(\%):100(\%) = 122 \text{ (Gm.)}:z$$
$$z = 339 \text{ Gm. of } 36\% \text{ acetic acid}$$
$$339 \text{ Gm. of water measure } 339 \text{ ml.}$$
$$\frac{339 \text{ ml.}}{1.045} = 324 \text{ ml. of } 36\% \text{ acetic acid, } answers.$$

How many milliliters of 92% (w/w) sulfuric acid with a specific gravity of 1.83 are required to neutralize 1000 ml. of 28% (w/w) ammonia water with a specific gravity of 0.90?

$$1000 \text{ ml. of water weigh } 1000 \text{ Gm.}$$
$$1000 \text{ Gm.} \times 0.90 = 900 \text{ Gm. of } 28\% \text{ ammonia water}$$

By the proportion:

$$100(\%):28(\%) = 900 \text{ (Gm.)}:x$$
$$x = 252 \text{ Gm. of } 100\% \text{ ammonia}$$
$$2NH_3 + H_2SO_4 = (NH_4)_2SO_4$$
$$2(17) \quad\quad 98$$
$$\text{or } 34$$

By the proportions:

$34:98 = 252$ (Gm.)$:x$

$x = 726$ Gm. of 100% sulfuric acid

$92(\%):100(\%) = 726$ (Gm.)$:y$

$y = 789$ Gm. of 92% sulfuric acid

789 Gm. of water measure 789 ml.

$\dfrac{789\,\text{ml.}}{1.83} = 431$ ml., *answer.*

To solve problems involving chemically equivalent quantities:

Example:

>   *The formula for a test solution calls for 234 Gm. of monohydrated sodium carbonate ($Na_2CO_3.H_2O$). Only anhydrous sodium carbonate (Na_2CO_3) is available. How much of it should be used to replace the hydrated salt?*

$Na_2CO_3.H_2O = 124$ $Na_2CO_3 = 106$

By the proportion:

$124:106 = 234$ (Gm.)$:x$

$x = 200$ Gm., *answer.*

MILLIEQUIVALENTS

To calculate milliequivalents from the equivalent weight of an element or compound:

A *milliequivalent*, abbreviated mEq, represents $\frac{1}{1000}$ of the equivalent weight of an element or compound.

Examples:

>   *What is the concentration, in mg. per ml., of a solution containing 2 mEq of potassium chloride, KCl, per ml.?*

Molecular weight of $KCl = 74.5$

Equivalent weight of $KCl = 74.5$

1 mEq of $KCl = \frac{1}{1000} \times 74.5$ Gm. $= 0.0745$ Gm. $= 74.5$ mg.

2 mEq of $KCl = 74.5$ mg. $\times 2 = 149$ mg. per ml., *answer.*

>   *What is the concentration, in Gm. per ml., of a solution containing 4 mEq of calcium chloride, $CaCl_2.2H_2O$, per ml.?*

Molecular weight of $CaCl_2.2H_2O = 147$

Equivalent weight of $CaCl_2.2H_2O = \frac{147}{2} = 73.5$

1 mEq of $CaCl_2.2H_2O = \frac{1}{1000} \times 73.5$ Gm. $= 0.0735$ **Gm.**
4 mEq of $CaCl_2.2H_2O = 0.0735$ Gm. $\times 4 =$
$$0.294 \text{ Gm. per ml., } \textit{answer.}$$

If 1 Gm. of an ion-exchange resin removes 1.3 mEq of sodium, how many milligrams of sodium would be removed by 8 Gm. of the resin?

Equivalent weight of Na $= 23$
1 mEq of Na $= 0.023$ Gm. or 23 mg.
1.3 mEq of Na $= 30$ mg.

By the proportion:

1 (Gm.):8 (Gm.) $= 30$ (mg.):x
x $= 240$ mg., *answer.*

SAPONIFICATION VALUE

To solve chemical problems based upon saponification value:

Saponification value refers to the number of milligrams of 100% potassium hydroxide required to saponify the free acids and esters in 1 Gm. of a fat or oil. For example, when we say that olive oil has a saponification value of 190, we mean that 190 mg. of 100% KOH are required to saponify completely 1 Gm. of olive oil.

Examples:

How many grams of 85% potassium hydroxide are required to saponify completely 100 Gm. of coconut oil having a saponification value of 260?

260 mg. $= 0.260$ Gm.

By the proportion:

1 (Gm.):100 (Gm.) $= 0.260$ (Gm.):x
x $= 26$ Gm. of 100% KOH

By the proportion:

85(%):100(%) $= 26$ (Gm.):y
y $= 30.6$ Gm., *answer.*

In a formula for soft soap, 100 Gm. of 88% potassium hydroxide are used to saponify 400 Gm. of a vegetable oil. Calculate the saponification value of the oil.

By the proportion:

$100(\%):88(\%) = 100 \text{ (Gm.)}:x$

x = 88 Gm. of 100% KOH, required to saponify 400 Gm. of the oil

By the proportion:

400 (Gm.):1 (Gm.) = 88 (Gm.):y

y = 0.220 Gm. = 220 mg. = 220, *answer*.

ACID VALUE

To solve chemical problems based on acid value:

Acid value refers to the number of milligrams of 100% potassium hydroxide required to neutralize the free fatty acids in 1 Gm. of a substance. For example, if a wax has an acid value of 22, 1 Gm. of it will require 22 mg. of 100% KOH (or the equivalent weight of some other alkali) for the neutralization of the free fatty acids.

In the formulation of cold creams and other emulsions containing waxes, the amount of alkali depends upon the acid value of the wax.

Example:

> *A cold cream formula calls for 1000 Gm. of white wax having an acid value of 20. (a) How many grams of 85% KOH should be used in formulating the cream? (b) If sodium borate ($Na_2B_4O_7.10H_2O$) is used in formulating the cream, how many grams are required?*

(a)   20 mg. = 0.020 Gm.

By the proportion:

1 (Gm.):1000 (Gm.) = 0.020 (Gm.):x

x = 20 Gm. of 100% KOH

By the proportion:

85 (%):100 (%) = 20 (Gm.):y

y = 23.5 Gm. of 85% KOH, *answer*.

(b)   Since one molecule of sodium borate gives two molecules of sodium hydroxide that can react with two atoms of hydrogen, its equivalent weight is $\frac{1}{2}$ of its molecular weight (382 ÷ 2) or 191, which is the weight equivalent to 56 Gm. of KOH (molecular weight of KOH is 56).

In (a) it was calculated that 20 Gm. of 100% KOH are required.

By the proportion:

$56:191 = 20$ (Gm.):x

x = 68.2 Gm. of sodium borate, *answer*.

WEIGHTS AND VOLUMES OF GASES

The methods by which we may calculate the volume of a given weight of any gas—or the weight of a given volume—depend on Avogadro's Law, which states that *under the same conditions of temperature and pressure, equal volumes of all gases contain the same number of molecules.*

When the molecular weight of a gas (by the oxygen table of atomic weights) is taken to indicate a number of grams, the expression is called the *mole* or the *gram-molecular weight* of that gas. By another consequence of Avogadro's Law, the gram-molecular weights of all gases have a common volume, *22.4 liters,* under standard conditions of temperature and pressure (S.T.P.)—that is, at $0°$ C. and a barometric pressure of 760 mm. This volume is shared by 2×16 or 32 Gm. of oxygen, 2×1 or 2 Gm. of hydrogen, 2×14 or 28 Gm. of nitrogen, and so on. Hence, 22.4 liters (S.T.P.) of any gaseous element or compound will weigh a number of grams equal to the number expressing its molecular weight.

To calculate the volume of a gas under standard conditions of temperature and pressure, given its weight:

Example:

What is the volume (S.T.P.) of 3.87 Gm. of hydrogen, H_2?
Molecular weight of hydrogen $= 2 \times 1 = 2$
2 Gm. of hydrogen measure 22.4 liters

By the proportion:

2 (Gm.):3.87 (Gm.) = 22.4 (L.):x

x = 43 L., *answer*.

To calculate the volume of a gas formed or used in a reaction under standard conditions of temperature and pressure:

Example:

What volume (S.T.P.) of hydrogen sulfide can be produced from 20 Gm. of iron sulfide?

$FeS + 2HCl = FeCl_2 + H_2S\uparrow$
88   34

88 Gm. of FeS yield 34 Gm. of H_2S which measure 22.4 liters

By the proportion:

88 (Gm.):20 (Gm.) = 22.4 (L.):x
x = 5.1 L., *answer.*

To calculate the weight of a chemical required to make a specified volume of a gas:

Example:

How many grams of zinc are required to make 50 liters (S.T.P.) of hydrogen?

$Zn + H_2SO_4 = ZnSO_4 + H_2\uparrow$
65   2

65 Gm. of Zn will produce 2 Gm. of hydrogen which measure 22.4 liters

By the proportion:
22.4 (L.):50 (L.) = 65 (Gm.):x
x = 145 Gm., *answer.*

To calculate the volume of a gas when corrections for temperature and pressure must be made:

In the above problems the gases were assumed to be measured at S.T.P. If, however, a gas is measured under different conditions of temperature and pressure, its volume must be recalculated to obtain its volume at S.T.P.

According to Boyle's Law, the *volume of a given mass of gas varies inversely with the pressure, when the temperature is constant.* Thus, an increase in pressure results in a decrease in the volume of a gas and a decrease in pressure results in an increase in its volume.

And according to Charles' Law, the *volume of a gas is proportional to its absolute temperature, when the pressure is constant.* A gas, under constant pressure, will expand, therefore, $\frac{1}{273}$ of its volume when heated through 1° C.

Examples:

The volume of a gas measured at 750 mm. is 380 ml. What is its volume at 760 mm., if the temperature remains constant?

By the proportion:
760 (mm.):750 (mm.) = 380 (ml.):x
x = 380 $\times \frac{750}{760}$ = 375 ml., *answer.*

The volume of a gas is 686 ml. at 70° C. What is its volume at 27° C., if the pressure remains constant?

70° C. = 343° Absolute
27° C. = 300° Absolute

By the proportion:

343 (°A.):300 (°A.) = 686 (ml.):x

x = 686 × $\frac{300}{343}$ = 600 ml., *answer.*

Since the changes in the volume of a gas due to variations in pressure and temperature are *independent* of one another, the corrections may be conveniently made together by combining the proportions used in the preceding examples.

Example:

A sample of gas measured 300 ml. at 27° C. and 740 mm. Calculate its volume at S.T.P.

27° C. = 300° Absolute
0° C. = 273° Absolute

Volume at S.T.P. = 300 × $\frac{273}{300}$ × $\frac{740}{760}$ = 266 ml., *answer.*

Practice Problems

1. Calculate the molecular weight of calcium hydroxide, $Ca(OH)_2$.

2. Calculate the molecular weight of potassium permanganate, $KMnO_4$.

3. Calculate the molecular weight of ethyl alcohol, C_2H_5OH.

4. Calculate the molecular weight of ferrous sulfate, $FeSO_4.7H_2O$.

5. Calculate the molecular weight of acetic acid, CH_3COOH.

6. Calculate the percentage composition of sodium fluoride, NaF.

7. Calculate the percentage composition of ether, $(C_2H_5)_2O$.

8. What is the percentage composition of Sodium Phosphate, U.S.P., $Na_2HPO_4.7H_2O$?

9. What is the percentage composition of Sodium Biphosphate, U.S.P., $NaH_2PO_4.H_2O$?

10. Calculate the percentage of water in dextrose, $C_6H_{12}O_6.H_2O$.

11. Calculate the quantity of water in 2000 Gm. of magnesium sulfate, $MgSO_4.7H_2O$.

12. What is the percentage of iron in ferrous carbonate, $FeCO_3$?

13. What is the percentage of copper in cupric sulfate, $CuSO_4.5H_2O$?

14. What is the percentage of iron in ferrous sulfate, $FeSO_4.7H_2O$?

15. What is the percentage of mercury in mercury bichloride, $HgCl_2$?

16. A certain solution contains 110 mg. of sodium fluoride, NaF, in each 1000 ml. How many milligrams of fluorine are represented in each 2 ml. of the solution?

17. How many grams of ferrous iodide, FeI_2, can be made from 60 Gm. of iodine under the proper conditions?

18. A prescription calls for 500 ml. of a solution such that each 4 ml. will contain 0.02 mg. of fluorine. How many milligrams of sodium fluoride should be used in compounding the prescription?

19. ℞   Sodium Fluoride   q.s.
     Distilled Water ad   500 ml.
     Sig. 2 ml. diluted to 100 ml. will give a 1:1,000,000 solution of fluorine.

How many milligrams of sodium fluoride, NaF, should be used in compounding the prescription?

20. ℞   Sodium Fluoride   q.s.
     Distilled Water ad   100 ml.
     Sig. Ten (10) drops diluted to 250 ml. yield a 1:1,000,000 solution of fluorine.

The dispensing dropper calibrates 25 drops per ml. How many milligrams of sodium fluoride should be used in compounding the prescription?

21. ℞   Sol. Sodium Fluoride   500 ml.
     (10 ml. = 1500 mcg. of fluorine)
     Sig. Dilute and use as directed.

How many grams of sodium fluoride should be used in compounding the prescription?

22. ℞   Sodium Fluoride   q.s.
     Purified Water ad   60.0
     (Five drops = 1.0 mg. of fluorine)
     Sig. Five drops daily.

The dispensing dropper calibrates 20 drops per ml. How many milligrams of sodium fluoride should be used in compounding the prescription?

23. ℞ Sodium Fluoride   q.s.
      Distilled Water ad   240.0
      Make the solution so that 12 drops contain the sodium fluoride equivalent of 0.1 mg. of fluorine.
      Sig. Twelve drops as directed.

The dispensing dropper calibrates 18 drops per ml. How much sodium fluoride should be used in compounding the prescription?

24. ℞ Histamine   1:10000
      Ft. solution.   Dispense 15.0 ml.
      Sig. Label.

Ampuls containing 0.275 mg. of histamine acid phosphate per ml. are available. How many milliliters of the ampul solution should be used to obtain the amount of histamine needed for the prescription?   Histamine acid phosphate—307
                                Histamine   —111

25. How many grams of anhydrous sodium carbonate are required to neutralize 200 Gm. of absolute hydrochloric acid?

$$Na_2CO_3 + 2HCl = 2NaCl + H_2O + CO_2$$

26. How many grams of potassium iodide are required to react with 250 Gm. of mercury bichloride?

$$HgCl_2 + 2KI = HgI_2 + 2KCl$$

27. ℞ Codeine Phosphate   0.3
      Potassium Citrate   25.0
      Aromatic Elixir ad   250.0
      Sig. Pro tuss.

Assuming that no potassium citrate is available, how many grams of potassium bicarbonate (100) and how many grams of citric acid (210) are required to prepare the potassium citrate (324) for the prescription?

$$3KHCO_3 + H_3C_6H_5O_7 = K_3C_6H_5O_7 + 3H_2O + 3CO_2$$

28. Starting with 200 Gm. of mercury bichloride, how many grams of Yellow Mercuric Oxide Ointment, containing 1% of yellow mercuric oxide, can be prepared from it?

$$HgCl_2 + 2NaOH = HgO + 2NaCl + H_2O$$

29. ℞   Potassium Citrate   100.0
          Hyoscyamus Tincture   100.0
          Peppermint Water ad   500.0
          Sig. 8 ml. b.i.d.

Assuming that no potassium citrate is available, how much potassium bicarbonate and how much citric acid should be used to prepare the potassium citrate for the prescription?

$$3KHCO_3 + H_3C_6H_5O_7 = K_3C_6H_5O_7 + 3H_2O + 3CO_2$$

30. How many grams of 36% (w/w) acetic acid are required to neutralize 650 Gm. of anhydrous sodium carbonate?

$$Na_2CO_3 + 2HC_2H_3O_2 = NaC_2H_3O_2 + 2H_2O + CO_2$$

31. How many grams of magnesium sulfate, $MgSO_4.7H_2O$ and how many grams of 95% sodium hydroxide should be used in preparing 2000 ml. of milk of magnesia containing 8% (w/v) of magnesium hydroxide?

$$MgSO_4.7H_2O + 2NaOH = Mg(OH)_2 + Na_2SO_4 + 7H_2O$$

32. ℞   Potassium Acetate   10.0
          Spearmint Water ad   120.0
          Sig. 4 ml. ex aq.

Assuming that no potassium acetate is available, how many grams of potassium bicarbonate and how many milliliters of 36% acetic acid, sp. gr. 1.050, are required to prepare the potassium acetate for the prescription?

$$KHCO_3 + HC_2H_3O_2 = KC_2H_3O_2 + CO_2 + H_2O$$

33. How many grams of 95% sodium hydroxide are required to react with 513 ml. of 85% (w/w) phosphoric acid, sp. gr. 1.71?

$$2NaOH + H_3PO_4 = Na_2HPO_4 + 2H_2O$$

34. How many grams of calcium carbonate and how many milliliters of 36% (w/w) hydrochloric acid, sp. gr. 1.18, are required to make 120 ml. of a 10% (w/v) solution of calcium chloride $(CaCl_2.2H_2O)$?

$$CaCO_3 + 2HCl = CaCl_2 + CO_2 + H_2O$$

35. How many grams of Ammonium Carbonate, U.S.P., and how many milliliters of 36% (w/w) acetic acid, sp. gr. 1.045, are needed to prepare 1000 ml. of Ammonium Acetate Solution containing 7% (w/v) of ammonium acetate?

$$NH_4HCO_3.NH_4NH_2CO_2 + 3HC_2H_3O_2 =$$
$$3NH_4C_2H_3O_2 + 2CO_2 + H_2O$$

36. How many milliliters of 36% (w/w) acetic acid, sp. gr. 1.050, are required to neutralize 1000 ml. of 10% (w/w) ammonia water, sp. gr. 0.960?

37. In preparing Benedict's Solution, you are directed to use 100 Gm. of anhydrous sodium carbonate (Na_2CO_3) in 1000 ml. of the reagent. Calculate the amount of monohydrated sodium carbonate ($Na_2CO_3.H_2O$) that should be used in preparing 5 liters of the solution.

38. In preparing Sodium Phosphate Solution, N.F., 400 Gm. of exsiccated sodium phosphate (Na_2HPO_4) are required for 1000 ml. of the product. How many grams of crystallized sodium phosphate ($Na_2HPO_4.7H_2O$) should be used in place of the exsiccated salt?

39. In preparing Magnesium Citrate Solution, 2.5 Gm. of potassium bicarbonate ($KHCO_3$) are needed to charge each bottle. If no potassium bicarbonate is available, how much sodium bicarbonate ($NaHCO_3$) should be used?

40. How much monohydrated sodium carbonate ($Na_2CO_3.H_2O$) is represented by 250 Gm. of dekahydrated sodium carbonate ($Na_2CO_3.10H_2O$)?

41. ℞ Epinephrine   2%
    Chlorobutanol   0.5%
    Sodium Bisulfite   0.2%
    Sodium Chloride   0.5%
    Distilled Water ad   100 0
    Sig. For the eyes.

How many grams of epinephrine bitartrate (333) should be used to obtain the epinephrine (183) needed in the prescription?

42. The formula for Albright's Solution "M" calls for 8.84 Gm. of anhydrous sodium carbonate (Na_2CO_3) per 1000 ml. How many grams of 95% sodium hydroxide (NaOH) should be used to replace the anhydrous sodium carbonate in preparing 5 liters of the solution?

43.   Precipitated Sulfur   50.0
        Potassium Hydroxide   10.0
        Stearic Acid   200.0
        Glycerin   40.0
        Water ad   1000.0

If potassium carbonate ($K_2CO_3.1\frac{1}{2}H_2O$) were to be used in formulating the cream, how many grams should be used to replace the potassium hydroxide (KOH)?

44. ℞   Sol. Sodium p-Aminosalicylate
         (5 ml. = 1 Gm. of p-Aminosalicylic acid)
         Disp. 1000 ml.
         Sig. 5 ml. as directed.

How many grams of p-aminosalicylic acid ($NH_2C_6H_3OH$-$COOH$) and how many grams of sodium bicarbonate ($NaHCO_3$) should be used in preparing the sodium p-aminosalicylate (NH_2C_6-$H_3OHCOONa$) needed in the prescription?

$$NH_2C_6H_3OHCOOH + NaHCO_3 = NH_2C_6H_3OHCOONa + H_2O + CO_2$$

45. Ferrous Sulfate Syrup contains 40 Gm. of ferrous sulfate ($FeSO_4.7H_2O$) per 1000 ml. How many milligrams of iron (Fe) are represented in the usual dose of 8 ml. of the syrup?

46. How many grams of sodium acid phosphate (NaH_2PO_4) should be used to replace 250 Gm. of citric acid [$C_3H_4OH(COOH)_3$] in a formula for an effervescent salt?

47. How much 42% (MgO equivalent) magnesium carbonate is required to prepare a bottle of Magnesium Citrate Solution that will contain the equivalent of 6.0 Gm. of MgO?

48. Five hundred (500) Gm. of Effervescent Sodium Phosphate contain 100 Gm. of exsiccated sodium phosphate (Na_2HPO_4). How much Sodium Phosphate, U.S.P., ($Na_2HPO_4.7H_2O$) is represented in each 10-Gm. dose of Effervescent Sodium Phosphate?

49. In preparing Sodium Phosphate Solution, N.F., 400 Gm. of exsiccated sodium phosphate (Na_2HPO_4) are required for 1000 ml. of the product. How many grams of crystallized sodium phosphate ($Na_2HPO_4.7H_2O$) may be used in place of the exsiccated salt in preparing 10 pints of the solution?

50. One thousand (1000) ml. of Sodium Phosphate Solution, N.F., contain 400 Gm. of exsiccated sodium phosphate (Na_2HPO_4). How much Sodium Phosphate, U.S.P., ($Na_2HPO_4.7H_2O$) is represented in each 8-ml. dose of the solution?

51. What is the concentration, in mg. per ml., of a solution containing 5 mEq of potassium chloride, KCl, per ml.?

52. If 2 Gm. of an ion-exchange resin remove 2.7 mEq of sodium, how many milligrams of sodium would be removed by 8 Gm. of the resin?

53. A solution contains 298 mg. of potassium chloride, KCl, per ml. Express this concentration in terms of milliequivalents of potassium chloride.

54. If 1 Gm. of an ion-exchange resin removes 0.3 mEq of sodium, how much of the resin will be required to remove 0.5 Gm. of sodium chloride, NaCl?

55. A 10-ml. ampul of potassium chloride contains 2.98 Gm. of potassium chloride (KCl). Calculate the strength of the solution in terms of mEq per ml.

56. A person is to receive 36 mg. of ammonium chloride per kilo of body weight. If the person weighs 154 lb., how many milliliters of a sterile solution of ammonium chloride (NH_4Cl) containing 0.4 mEq per ml. should be administered?

57. A sterile solution of potassium chloride (KCl) contains 2 mEq per ml. If a 20-ml. ampul of the solution is diluted to a liter with sterile distilled water, what is the percentage strength of the resulting solution?

58. A certain electrolyte solution contains, as one of the ingredients, 4.6 mEq of calcium per liter. How many grams of calcium chloride ($CaCl_2.2H_2O$) should be used in preparing 20 liters of the solution?

59. Sterile solutions of ammonium chloride containing 21.4 mg. per ml. are available commercially in 500- and 1000-ml. intravenous infusion containers. Calculate the amount, in terms of milliequivalents, of ammonium chloride (NH_4Cl) in the 500-ml. container.

60. A solution contains, in each 5 ml., 0.5 Gm. of potassium acetate ($KC_2H_3O_2$), 0.5 Gm. of potassium bicarbonate ($KHCO_3$) and 0.5 Gm. of potassium citrate ($K_3C_6H_5O_7$). How many mEq of potassium (K) are contained in each 5 ml. of the solution?

61. Coconut Oil has a saponification value of 255. How much 85% potassium hydroxide should be used to saponify completely 750 Gm. of coconut oil?

62. How much 88% potassium hydroxide should be used to saponify completely 500 ml. of a vegetable oil (specific gravity 0.850) with a saponification value of 180?

63. The saponification value of stearic acid is 208. In a vanishing cream formula containing 250 Gm. of stearic acid, how much 88% potassium hydroxide is required to saponify 20% of the stearic acid?

64. How many grams of 85% potassium hydroxide should be used to saponify completely 2000 ml. of a vegetable oil (specific gravity 0.90) having a saponification value of 190?

65. In a formula for a soft soap, 400 Gm. of 85% potassium hydroxide were used to saponify 1700 Gm. of a vegetable oil. Calculate the saponification value of the oil.

66.   Stearic Acid   200 Gm.
        Potassium Hydroxide   q.s.
        Glycerin   100 Gm.
        Water ad   1000 Gm.

If the saponification value of stearic acid is 208, how many grams of 85% potassium hydroxide should be used to saponify 25% of the stearic acid in the formula?

67.   Stearic Acid   120 Gm.
        Potassium Hydroxide   q.s.
        Propylene Glycol   50 Gm.
        Water ad   1000 Gm.

(a) If the saponification value of stearic acid is 210, how many grams of 88% potassium hydroxide should be used to saponify 30% of the stearic acid?

(b) The equivalent weight of triethanolamine is 143. How many grams of triethanolamine could be used to replace the quantity of potassium hydroxide (56) needed to saponify 30% of the stearic acid in the formula?

68.   Stearic Acid   20.0
        Liquid Petrolatum   5.0
        Triethanolamine   5.0
        Coconut Oil Soap   40.0
        Glycerin   5.0
        Water   25.0

Coconut oil soap contains 40% of coconut oil. How many grams of 85% potassium hydroxide are required to saponify the coconut oil (saponification value 255) needed to prepare the soap for 5 lb. of this formula?

69. A formula for a cold cream calls for 500 Gm. of white wax. If the sample of white wax used has an acid value of 20, how much 88% potassium hydroxide is required to neutralize the free acids contained in the wax?

70. A cold cream formula contains 1500 Gm. of white wax. The acid value of the wax is 21.

(a) How many grams of pure KOH should be used?

(b) How many grams of 85% KOH should be used?

(c) The equivalent weight of sodium borate is 191. How many grams of sodium borate should be used?

71. A formula for a cosmetic cream calls for 100 Gm. of white wax. If the sample of white wax used has an acid value of 22, how much sodium borate should be used in formulating the cream? One molecule of sodium borate (382) is equivalent to two molecules of sodium hydroxide (40). The molecular weight of potassium hydroxide is 56.

72.

Precipitated Sulfur	7.0	
White Wax	10.0	
Sodium Borate	q.s.	
Mineral Oil	60.0	
Rose Water ad	100.0	

The acid value of the white wax is 20, and the equivalent weight of sodium borate is 191. How many grams of sodium borate should be used in preparing 5 lb. of the product?

73.

Stearic Acid	20.0	
Potassium Carbonate	q.s.	
Propylene Glycol	10.0	
Lanolin	5.0	
Distilled Water ad	100.0	

How many grams of potassium carbonate ($K_2CO_3.1\frac{1}{2}H_2O$) should be used to saponify 25% of the stearic acid ($C_{17}H_{35}COOH$)? Assume the stearic acid to be 100% pure.

74. What is the volume (S.T.P.) of 75.5 Gm. of ammonia, NH_3?

75. What is the volume (S.T.P.) of 28.46 Gm. of oxygen, O_2?

76. How many liters (S.T.P.) of oxygen can be made from 100 Gm. of potassium chlorate?

$$2KClO_3 = 2KCl + 3O_2\uparrow$$

77. How many liters (S.T.P.) of sulfur dioxide can be made from 200 Gm. of sulfur?

$$S + O_2 = SO_2\uparrow$$

78. How many liters (S.T.P.) of ammonia can be made from 684 Gm. of ammonium sulfate?

$$(NH_4)_2SO_4 + CaO = CaSO_4 + H_2O + 2NH_3\uparrow$$

15

79. How many grams of potassium chlorate are required to make 60 liters (S.T.P.) of oxygen?

$$2KClO_3 = 2KCl + 3O_2\uparrow$$

80. How many grams of iron are required to make 100 liters (S.T.P.) of hydrogen?

$$Fe + H_2SO_4 = FeSO_4 + H_2\uparrow$$

81. How many grams of sodium sulfite are required to make 65 liters (S.T.P.) of sulfur dioxide?

$$Na_2SO_3 + H_2SO_4 = Na_2SO_4 + H_2O + SO_2\uparrow$$

82. The volume of a gas measured at 780 mm. is 475 ml. What is its volume at 760 mm., if the temperature is kept constant?

83. Calculate the volume of 10 Gm. of hydrogen measured under standard conditions. What would be its volume if the pressure upon the gas were diminished to 750 mm., the temperature remaining constant?

84. The volume of a gas measured at 25° C. is 540 ml. What is its volume at 0° C., if the pressure is kept constant?

85. Calculate the volume of 10 Gm. of oxygen under standard conditions. What would be its volume if the temperature of the gas were increased to 27° C., the pressure remaining constant?

86. A sample of a gas measured 1000 ml. at 27° C. and 770 mm. pressure. Calculate its volume at S.T.P.

87. Calculate the volume (S.T.P.) of a sample of oxygen that occupies 125 ml. at 30° C. and 745 mm. pressure.

APPENDIX A

THERMOMETRY

A *thermometer* is an instrument for measuring temperature, or intensity of heat. For practical purposes, a liquid such as alcohol or mercury undergoes a constant and measurable expansion or contraction with a rising or lowering of temperature. If contained in a small rigid bulb attached to a hermetically sealed extension tube, the liquid forces a column upwards in the tube upon expanding and draws the column down again upon contracting. If the tube has a uniform bore and we mark it with evenly spaced lines, we have a thermometer.

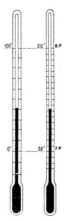

Centigrade and Fahrenheit thermometers.

Obviously, any number of degrees of temperature may be marked off between any two fixed points on the tube, and similar degrees can then be uniformly extended above and below them. Late seventeenth-century physicists suggested the constant temperatures of melting ice and of pure water boiling under normal atmospheric pressure as offering the most convenient fixed points.

In 1709, the German scientist Gabriel Fahrenheit (who improved the construction of thermometers and was the first to use mercury instead of alcohol) took for 0° the temperature of a mixture of snow and sal ammoniac (equal parts by weight). He discovered that by the scale he had marked on his thermometer, ice melted at 32° and water boiled at 212°—with a difference of 180 degrees between these two points. The *Fahrenheit thermometer* is still commonly used in the United States.

In 1742, Anders Celsius, a Swedish astronomer, suggested the convenience of a thermometer with a scale having a difference of 100 degrees between two fixed points, and the *centigrade thermometer* was devised, with 0° for the freezing and 100° for the boiling points of water.

On each thermometer, negative numbers are used to designate degrees "below" the arbitrarily selected zero.

Since 100 centigrade degrees (100°−0°) measure the same difference in temperature that is measured by 180 Fahrenheit degrees (212°−32°), each centigrade degree is the equivalent of 1.8 or $\frac{9}{5}$ the size of each Fahrenheit degree, and therefore any given rise or fall in temperature is measured by $\frac{9}{5}$ as many Fahrenheit degrees as centigrade degrees. So, we may construct a general formula for converting from one system to the other:

$$\frac{\text{Number of centigrade degrees above or below any degree centigrade}}{\text{Number of Fahrenheit degrees above or below an equivalent degree Fahrenheit}} = \frac{5}{9}$$

In other words, every 5-degree change in temperature as measured by the centigrade thermometer is a 9-degree change as measured by the Fahrenheit.

To derive a specific working proportion, it remains for us only to select points on the two thermometers that are known to be equivalent, are easy to remember, and are convenient to use in calculations.

Here are some equivalent readings above and below the melting point of ice:

0° C. = 32° F.	0° C. = 32° F.
5° C. = 41° F.	−5° C. = 23° F.
10° C. = 50° F.	−10° C. = 14° F.
15° C. = 59° F.	−15° C. = 5° F.
20° C. = 68° F.	−20° C. = −4° F.
30° C. = 86° F.	−30° C. = −22° F.
40° C. = 104° F.	−40° C. = −40° F.
50° C. = 122° F.	−50° C. = −58° F.
75° C. = 167° F.	−75° C. = −103° F.
100° C. = 212° F.	−100° C. = −148° F.
and so on.	and so on.

First or fundamental method:

Modern physicists not only have verified the hypothesis that "cold" is merely absence of heat but have established the point at which no heat would be present, called *absolute zero*. This point has been computed as approximately $-273°$ centigrade or $-459.4°$ Fahrenheit. Consequently, the temperature of absolute zero may be considered the basic point of equivalence in the two systems:

$$-273° \text{ C.} = -459.4° \text{ F.}$$

By subtracting -273 from any given number of degrees centigrade we get the number of centigrade degrees above absolute zero. But subtracting a negative number is the same as adding its positive counterpart, so we may express this operation as $C + 273$. Similarly, any number of Fahrenheit degrees above absolute zero may be expressed as $F + 459.4$.

Our general proportion can now be specifically revised:

$$\frac{C + 273}{F + 459.4} = \frac{5}{9}$$

Using this proportion, if given the value of C we could compute the corresponding value of F, and *vice versa*.

But this can scarcely be called a working formula, since the numbers involved would not permit swift calculation. There are at least two other points of equivalence that are both easy to remember and easy to use: (1) the temperature at which both thermometers happen to register the same number of degrees and (2) the temperature of melting ice.

Second method:

The temperature registered as $-40°$ centigrade happens also to be $-40°$ Fahrenheit. The difference between any number of degrees centigrade and $-40°$ C. may be expressed as $C + 40$, and the difference between any number of degrees Fahrenheit and $-40°$ F. may be expressed as $F + 40$. By our general proportion, then,

$$\frac{C + 40}{F + 40} = \frac{5}{9}$$

Since this proportion is easy to remember, it is favored by many students, who usually sum up a working procedure as follows:

(1) To convert centigrade to Fahrenheit, *add 40 to the given number of centigrade degrees, multiply by $\frac{9}{5}$, and subtract 40.*

(2) To convert Fahrenheit to centigrade, *add 40 to the given number of Fahrenheit degrees, multiply by $\frac{5}{9}$, and subtract 40.*

These rules interpret the following derived equations:

$$(1) \quad F = \tfrac{9}{5}(C + 40) - 40$$
$$(2) \quad C = \tfrac{5}{9}(F + 40) - 40$$

Third or standard method:

The method of conversion most commonly employed, since its calculations are simplest, is based on the fact that $0°$ centigrade is equivalent to $32°$ Fahrenheit. Any number of centigrade degrees above or below $0°$ C. may be expressed as $C - 0$, or simply C. Any number of Fahrenheit degrees above or below $32°$ Fahrenheit may be expressed as $F - 32$. Hence:

$$(1) \quad \frac{C}{F - 32} = \frac{5}{9}$$
$$(2) \quad C = \tfrac{5}{9}(F - 32)$$
$$(3) \quad F = 32 + \tfrac{9}{5} C$$

Perhaps a majority of scientists use equations (2) and (3), depending upon the direction of conversion, and resolve them by simple arithmetic.

Fourth and easiest method:

Here is a noteworthy fact: *no matter what specific proportion we select, if we multiply means and extremes and simplify the result we get the same working equation.*

$$(1) \quad \frac{C + 273}{F + 459.4} = \frac{5}{9}$$
$$9\,C + 2457 = 5\,F + 2297$$
$$9\,C = 5\,F - 160$$

$$(2) \quad \frac{C + 40}{F + 40} = \frac{5}{9}$$
$$9\,C + 360 = 5\,F + 200$$
$$9\,C = 5\,F - 160$$

$$(3) \qquad \frac{C}{F - 32} = \frac{5}{9}$$

$$9\,C = 5\,F - 160$$

Once the principle is understood, therefore, it would seem advisable to use this equation (by the rules of elementary algebra) for conversion in either direction. It is easy to remember; it is convenient to use; it prevents the errors that frequently arise from careless interchange of $\frac{5}{9}$ and $\frac{9}{5}$ or confusion of the minus and plus signs in the other equations.

Examples:

Convert 26° C. to Fahrenheit.

$$9\,C = 5\,F - 160$$
$$9 \times 26 = 5\,F - 160$$
$$234 + 160 = 5\,F$$
$$5\,F = 394$$
$$F = 78.8°,\ answer.[1]$$

Convert −12° C. to Fahrenheit.

$$9\,C = 5\,F - 160$$
$$9 \times -12 = 5\,F - 160$$
$$-108 + 160 = 5\,F$$
$$5\,F = 52$$
$$F = 10.4°,\ answer.$$

Convert 162° F. to centigrade.

$$9\,C = 5\,F - 160$$
$$9\,C = (5 \times 162) - 160$$
$$9\,C = 650$$
$$C = 72\tfrac{2}{9}°,\ answer.$$

Convert −62° F. to centigrade.

$$9\,C = 5\,F - 160$$
$$9\,C = (5 \times -62) - 160$$
$$9\,C = -470$$
$$C = -52\tfrac{2}{9}°,\ answer.$$

Practice Problems

1. Convert 10° C. to Fahrenheit.
2. Convert −30° C. to Fahrenheit.

[1] When centigrade degrees are converted to Fahrenheit, fractions are fifths and are customarily expressed as decimals; but when Fahrenheit degrees are converted to centigrade, fractions are ninths.

3. Convert 4° C. to Fahrenheit.

4. Convert −173° C. to Fahrenheit.

5. Convert 77° F. to centigrade.

6. Convert 240° F. to centigrade.

7. The normal temperature of the human body is 98.6° F. Express this temperature on the centigrade scale.

8. A saturated solution of sodium chloride boils at 227.1° F. What is its boiling point on the centigrade scale?

9. The range of a centigrade thermometer is −5° to 300°. What is this range on the Fahrenheit scale?

10. Liquid Petrolatum has a kinematic viscosity of 38.1 centistokes at 37.8° C. Express this temperature on the Fahrenheit scale.

11. If a reaction takes place at 71° C., at what temperature on the Fahrenheit scale will it take place?

12. If a person shows a temperature of 102.5° F. on a clinical thermometer, what temperature would he show on the centigrade scale?

13. If mercury freezes at −40° F., what is its freezing point on the centigrade scale?

14. The U.S.P. directs that in the preparation of Starch Glycerite the temperature must be kept below 144° C. What would be the reading if a Fahrenheit thermometer were used?

15. Theobroma Oil melts between 30° and 35° C. What is the range of its melting point on the Fahrenheit scale?

16. If the maximum density of water is reached at 4° C., what would this point be on the Fahrenheit scale?

17. A specific gravity determination was made at 20° C. What was the temperature on the Fahrenheit scale?

18. Oxygen can be liquefied at −119° C. Express this temperature on (a) the Fahrenheit scale and (b) the absolute scale.

19. Rabies Vaccine must be stored at a temperature between 2° and 10° C. What are these limits on the Fahrenheit scale?

20. Petrolatum melts between 38° and 50° C. What is this range on the Fahrenheit scale?

APPENDIX B

PROOF STRENGTH

It is customary to express the percentage strength of an aqueous solution of alcohol in volume-in-volume percentage, reckoned from the number of milliliters or minims or fluidounces of pure or *absolute* alcohol contained in 100 of the same unit. Consequently, if weight-in-weight percentage is specified, it should be clearly identified.

The legal and official temperature for the specific gravity of alcohol of all strengths is 60° F., or 15.56° C., at which temperature the specific gravity of absolute alcohol is 0.794.[1]

Proof spirit is an aqueous solution containing 50% (v/v) of absolute alcohol. Alcohols of other percentage strengths are said to be *above proof* or *below proof*, depending upon whether they contain more or less than 50% (v/v) of absolute alcohol.

Proof strength of alcohol is expressed by taking 50% alcohol, or proof spirit, as *100 proof*. Then 100% or *absolute* alcohol is twice as strong, or 200 proof; 25% alcohol is half as strong, or 50 proof; and, inevitably, proof strength is always numerically twice as great as percentage strength (v/v). Hence, if percentage strength (v/v) is multiplied by 2, we have the corresponding proof strength—so 35% alcohol is 70 proof, 95% alcohol is 190 proof, and so on. Conversely, if proof strength is divided by 2, we have percentage strength (v/v)—so 160 proof alcohol is of 80% (v/v) strength, 90 proof alcohol is of 45% (v/v) strength, and so on.

Alcohol and alcoholic beverages are generally measured in gallons, for purposes of taxation, whatever their percentage strengths; and for this and other reasons, a unit called the *proof gallon* is frequently used to measure, or evaluate, alcohols of given quantities and strengths. The tax on alcohol or alcoholic liquors is quoted at a definite figure per proof gallon. A *drawback* or refund of the tax paid on distilled spirits which are used in the manufacture of medicines and medicinal preparations is allowed by the government and may be obtained by eligible claimants. Like the tax on distilled spirits, the drawback is quoted at a definite rate per proof gallon.

[1] Absolute or Dehydrated Alcohol, N.F. X, must have a specific gravity of not more than 0.798 at 15.56° C.

A *proof gallon* is 1 wine gallon (a gallon by measure) of proof spirit. In other words, 1 proof gallon = 1 wine gallon of an alcohol solution containing $\frac{1}{2}$ wine gallon of absolute alcohol and having therefore a strength of 100 proof or 50% (v/v). Any quantity of alcohol containing $\frac{1}{2}$ wine gallon of absolute alcohol is said "to be the equivalent of" or "to contain" 1 proof gallon. So, 2 wine gallons of 50 proof or 25% (v/v) alcohol would contain $\frac{1}{2}$ wine gallon of absolute alcohol, and would therefore be the equivalent of 1 proof gallon; but 3 wine gallons of such a solution would contain $1\frac{1}{2}$ proof gallons.

To calculate the number of proof gallons contained in a given quantity of alcohol of specified strength:

Since a proof gallon has a percentage strength of 50 per cent (v/v), the equivalent number of proof gallons may be calculated by the formula:

$$\text{Proof gallons} = \frac{\text{Wine gallons} \times \text{Percentage strength of solution}}{50\ (\%)}$$

And since proof strength is twice percentage strength, the formula may validly be revised as follows:

$$\text{Proof gallons} = \frac{\text{Wine gallons} \times \text{Proof strength of solution}}{100\ (\text{proof})}$$

Example:

How many proof gallons are contained in 5 wine gallons of 75% (v/v) alcohol?

First method:

1 proof gallon = 1 wine gallon of 50% (v/v) strength

$$\frac{5\ (\text{wine gallons}) \times 75\ (\%)}{50\ (\%)} = 7.5 \text{ proof gallons, } answer.$$

Second method:

75% (v/v) = 150 proof

$$\frac{5\ (\text{wine gallons}) \times 150\ (\text{proof})}{100\ (\text{proof})} = 7.5 \text{ proof gallons, } answer.$$

To calculate the number of wine gallons of alcohol of specified strength equivalent to a given number of proof gallons:

$$\text{Wine gallons} = \frac{\text{Proof gallons} \times 50\ (\%)}{\text{Percentage strength of solution}}$$

$$\text{Or,} \quad \text{Wine gallons} = \frac{\text{Proof gallons} \times 100\ (\text{proof})}{\text{Proof strength of solution}}$$

Example:

> *How many wine gallons of 20% (v/v) alcohol would be the equivalent of 20 proof gallons?*

First method:

1 proof gallon = 1 wine gallon of 50% (v/v) strength

$$\frac{20 \ (\text{proof gallons}) \times 50 \ (\%)}{20 \ (\%)} = 50 \text{ wine gallons, } answer.$$

Second method:

20% (v/v) = 40 proof

$$\frac{20 \ (\text{proof gallons}) \times 100 \ (\text{proof})}{40 \ (\text{proof})} = 50 \text{ wine gallons, } answer.$$

To calculate the tax on a given quantity of alcohol of a specified strength:

Example:

> *If the tax on alcohol is quoted at $10.50 per proof gallon, how much tax would be collected upon 10 wine gallons of alcohol marked "190 proof"?*

$$\frac{10 \ (\text{wine gallons}) \times 190 \ (\text{proof})}{100 \ (\text{proof})} = 19 \text{ proof gallons}$$

$10.50 × 19 (proof gallons) = $199.50, *answer.*

Practice Problems

1. How many proof gallons are represented by 54 wine gallons of 95% (v/v) alcohol?

2. How many gallons of proof spirit are there in 25 wine gallons of a sample that contains 70% (v/v) of pure alcohol?

3. How many proof gallons are contained in 500 wine gallons of Diluted Alcohol, U.S.P., that contains 49% (v/v) of pure alcohol?

4. During a certain month, a hospital pharmacist used 54 gallons of 95% alcohol and 5 gallons of absolute (100%) alcohol. How many proof gallons did he use?

5. How many wine gallons of 60% (v/v) alcohol are the equivalent of 100 proof gallons?

6. How many wine gallons of 95% (v/v) alcohol would contain 91.2 proof gallons?

7. What number of wine gallons of 70% (v/v) alcohol would represent 5 proof gallons?

8. If a drum contains 54 wine gallons of 95% (v/v) alcohol, how much tax must be paid on it at the rate of $10.50 per proof gallon?

9. If the tax on alcohol is $10.50 per proof gallon, how much tax must be paid on 5 wine gallons of Alcohol, U.S.P., that contains 94.9% (v/v) of pure alcohol?

10. If alcohol is taxed at the rate of $10.50 per proof gallon, compute the tax on 6 wine gallons of 65% (v/v) alcohol.

11. The drawback on alcohol is $9.50 per proof gallon. If an eligible claimant has used 18 gallons of 95% alcohol, to how much drawback is he entitled?

12. A manufacturing pharmacist received a drawback of $790 on the alcohol that he used during a certain period. If the drawback on alcohol is $9.50 per proof gallon, how many wine gallons of 95% alcohol did he use?

13. The formula for an elixir calls for 4 gallons of 95% alcohol. Alcohol (95%) costs $25.00 per gallon and the drawback is $9.50 per proof gallon. Calculate the net cost of the alcohol in the formula.

14. The drawback on a quantity of 95% alcohol used in the manufacture of a certain medicinal preparation was $180.50, and the net cost of the alcohol was $67.00. If the rate of drawback is $9.50 per proof gallon, what was the original purchase price per gallon of the alcohol?

APPENDIX C

ALCOHOLOMETRIC TABLES

THE percentage strengths of mixtures of alcohol and water can be calculated from their specific gravities by reference to alcoholometric tables; and conversely, their specific gravities can be calculated from the tables when their percentage strengths are known.

It happens that alcoholometric tables, like other tables of data and of numerical figures (such as acid and alkali tables and logarithmic tables), give values of variables at certain intervals only. Consequently, when it becomes necessary to determine values between those actually given in a table, *interpolation*—a method of estimating intermediate values by proportional parts—must be used.

The alcoholometric table of the United States Pharmacopeia gives, under its several headings, *percentage strengths by volume* and *by weight* of mixtures of alcohol and water, together with the *corresponding specific gravities* at 15.56° C. and 25° C. Only two of these headings, each with its column of values, will be used to illustrate the method of interpolation in finding values of variables not given in the table. It should be noted that, in alcoholometric tables, as the percentage strength increases, the specific gravity decreases.

To find the percentage strength of alcohol when its known specific gravity is not included in the table:

Example:

> *A sample of alcohol has a specific gravity of 0.8601 at 15.56° C. By reference to the alcoholometric table, find the percentage of alcohol, by volume, in the sample.*

The known specific gravity lies between the figures 0.8608 and 0.8580 included in the table, and the difference between these figures is 0.0028. The table tells us that the per cent by volume will lie between 81 and 82, and the difference between these is 1%.

If we interpolate the known 0.8601 and the unknown x% in the table, we can calculate the value of x by proportion, and the percentage of alcohol, by volume, in the sample will be 81 + x.

$$
\left.\begin{matrix} 81 \\ \\ x \\ \\ \\ \\ 82 \end{matrix}\right\} \quad ?
\qquad
\begin{matrix} \textit{Difference} \\ = 0.0007 \end{matrix}
\left.\begin{matrix} 0.8608 \\ 0.8601 \\ \\ \\ \\ 0.8580 \end{matrix}\right.
$$

Difference = 1% ... *Difference = 0.0028*

By the proportion:

$$0.0028 : 0.0007 = 1\ (\%) : x$$
$$\text{Or, } 28 : 7 = 1\ (\%) : x$$
$$x = \tfrac{7}{28} \times 1\ (\%) = 0.25\%$$
$$81\% + 0.25\% = 81.25\%, \textit{ answer.}$$

To find the specific gravity of alcohol when its known percentage strength is not given in the table:

Example:

By reference to the alcoholometric table, find the specific gravity of a sample of alcohol whose percentage strength by volume is 86.4% at 15.56° C.

Since the percentage strength lies between 86% and 87%, the table tells us that the specific gravity lies between 0.8462 and 0.8432, and using the same procedure as in solving the preceding problem, we can find its value by proportion. But note that this value will be 0.8462 − x.

$$
\left.\begin{matrix} 86\% \\ 86.4\% \\ \\ \\ \\ 87\% \end{matrix}\right.
\begin{matrix} \textit{Difference} \\ = 0.4\% \end{matrix}
\qquad ?
\left.\begin{matrix} 0.8462 \\ x \\ \\ \\ \\ 0.8432 \end{matrix}\right.
$$

Difference = 1% ... *Difference = 0.0030*

By the proportion:

$1\ (\%):0.4\ (\%) = 0.0030:x$

$x = 0.0012$

$0.8462 - 0.0012 = 0.8450$, *answer*.

Practice Problems

1. An alcohol sample has a specific gravity of 0.9280 at 15.56° C. By referring to the alcoholometric table determine the percentage of alcohol, by volume, in the sample.

2. The specific gravity of a sample of alcohol is 0.9784 at 15.56° C. Calculate the percentage of alcohol, by volume, in the sample.

3. The specific gravity of an alcoholic distillate observed at 15.56° C. is 0.9692. By referring to the alcoholometric table determine the percentage of alcohol, by volume, in the distillate.

4. If the specific gravity of an alcoholic distillate observed at 15.56° C. is 0.9666, what is the percentage of alcohol, by volume, in the distillate?

5. A sample of alcohol has a specific gravity of 0.8425 at 15.56° C. By referring to the alcoholometric table determine its percentage strength by volume.

6. The specific gravity of an alcoholic liquid taken at 15.56° C. is 0.9813. Calculate the percentage strength by volume of the liquid.

7. By referring to the alcoholometric table determine the specific gravity of a sample of alcohol whose percentage strength is 92.3%, by volume, at 15.56° C.

8. A sample contains 12.35% of alcohol, by volume, at 15.56° C. By referring to the alcoholometric table determine the specific gravity of the sample.

9. What is the specific gravity of an alcoholic distillate that contains 25.75%, by volume, of alcohol?

10. By referring to the alcoholometric table determine the specific gravity of an alcoholic liquid whose percentage strength is 45.7%, by volume, at 15.56° C.

ALCOHOLOMETRIC TABLE

Per cent of C_2H_5OH by volume at $15.56°$ C.	Specific gravity in air at $15.56°$ C. $\overline{15.56°\ C.}$	Per cent of C_2H_5OH by volume at $15.56°$ C.	Specific gravity in air at $15.56°$ C. $\overline{15.56°\ C.}$	Per cent of C_2H_5OH by volume at $15.56°$ C.	Specific gravity in air at $15.56°$ C. $\overline{15.56°\ C.}$
		31	0.9641	66	0.8995
		32	0.9629	67	0.8972
		33	0.9617	68	0.8948
		34	0.9604	69	0.8923
0	1.0000	35	0.9590	70	0.8899
1	0.9985	36	0.9576	71	0.8874
2	0.9970	37	0.9562	72	0.8848
3	0.9956	38	0.9548	73	0.8823
4	0.9942	39	0.9533	74	0.8797
5	0.9928	40	0.9517	75	0.8771
6	0.9915	41	0.9501	76	0.8745
7	0.9902	42	0.9485	77	0.8718
8	0.9890	43	0.9469	78	0.8691
9	0.9878	44	0.9452	79	0.8664
10	0.9866	45	0.9434	80	0.8636
11	0.9854	46	0.9417	81	0.8608
12	0.9843	47	0.9399	82	0.8580
13	0.9832	48	0.9380	83	0.8551
14	0.9821	49	0.9361	84	0.8522
15	0.9810	50	0.9342	85	0.8493
16	0.9800	51	0.9322	86	0.8462
17	0.9789	52	0.9302	87	0.8432
18	0.9779	53	0.9282	88	0.8401
19	0.9769	54	0.9262	89	0.8369
20	0.9759	55	0.9241	90	0.8336
21	0.9749	56	0.9220	91	0.8303
22	0.9739	57	0.9199	92	0.8268
23	0.9729	58	0.9177	93	0.8233
24	0.9719	59	0.9155	94	0.8196
25	0.9708	60	0.9133	95	0.8158
26	0.9697	61	0.9111	96	0.8118
27	0.9687	62	0.9088	97	0.8077
28	0.9676	63	0.9065	98	0.8033
29	0.9664	64	0.9042	99	0.7986
30	0.9653	65	0.9019	100	0.7936

APPENDIX D

SOLUBILITY RATIOS

THE *solubility* of a substance is the ratio between the amount of it contained in a given amount of saturated solution (at a given temperature) and the amount of solvent therein. For instance, if 400 Gm. of saturated solution contain 100 Gm. of solute and 300 Gm. of solvent, the solubility of the active ingredient (at that temperature) is 100:300 and may be expressed as 1:3. The relative amounts of solute and solvent may be calculated from various data, such as the ratio or percentage strength of the saturated solution.

The official compendia express solubilities as 1 Gm. of solute in so many ml. of solvent (for example, *1 Gm. of sodium chloride dissolves in 2.8 ml. of water*). Solubilities may also be expressed as so many Gm. of solute in 100 ml. of a saturated solution.

To calculate the solubility of a substance:

This procedure will work for any kind of solution: (1) use the data to set up a proportion including the ratio *1:x*, *x* being the number of parts by weight containing *1* part by weight of active ingredient, and (2) if required, calculate the *volume* of *x* weight parts of solvent.

Examples:

What is the solubility of an anhydrous chemical if 100 Gm. of a saturated aqueous solution leave a residue of 25 Gm. after evaporation?

100 Gm. − 25 Gm. = 75 Gm. of water

By the proportion:

25 (Gm.):75 (Gm.) = 1 (part):x

x = 3 parts of water, indicating a solubility of 1:3, or 1 Gm. in 3 Gm. or ml. of water, *answer.*

What is the solubility of an anhydrous chemical if 100 Gm. of a saturated alcoholic solution leave a residue of 20 Gm. after evaporation? (The sp. gr. of the alcohol is 0.80.)

16

100 Gm. − 20 Gm. = 80 Gm. of alcohol

By the proportion:

20 (Gm.):80 (Gm.) = 1 (part):x

x = 4 parts of alcohol, indicating a solubility of 1:4, or
1 Gm. in 4 Gm. of alcohol

4 Gm. of water measure 4 ml.

$\dfrac{4 \text{ ml.}}{0.80}$ = 5 ml., indicating a solubility of 1 Gm. in 5 ml. of
alcohol, *answer.*

*A saturated aqueous solution contains, in each 100 ml., 25 Gm.
of a substance. The specific gravity of the solution is 1.15.
Calculate the solubility of the substance.*

100 ml. of water weigh 100 Gm.

100 Gm. × 1.15 = 115 Gm. (weight of 100 ml. of saturated
solution)

115 Gm. − 25 Gm. = 90 Gm. of water

By the proportion:

25 (Gm.):90 (Gm.) = 1 (part):x

x = 3.6 parts of water, indicating a solubility of 1:3.6, or
1 Gm. in 3.6 Gm. or ml. of water, *answer.*

*What is the solubility of the active ingredient if a saturated
aqueous solution has a strength of 20% (w/w)?*

100 parts − 20 parts = 80 parts of solvent in every 100
parts of solution

By the proportion:

20 (parts):80 (parts) = 1 (part):x

x = 4 parts of solvent, indicating a solubility of 1:4, or
1 Gm. in 4 Gm. or ml. of water, *answer.*

To determine the percentage strength (w/w) of a saturated solution when the solubility is given:

Examples:

*One Gm. of boric acid is soluble in 18 ml. of water. What is
the percentage strength (w/w) of a saturated aqueous solution?*

1 Gm. + 18 Gm. (18 ml. of water) = 19 Gm.

By the proportion:

19 (Gm.):1 (Gm.) = 100 (%):x

x = 5.26%, *answer.*

One Gm. of boric acid is soluble in 18 ml. of alcohol. What is the percentage strength (w/w) of a saturated alcoholic solution? (The specific gravity of the alcohol is 0.80.)

18 ml. of water weigh 18 Gm.

18 Gm. $\times$ 0.80 = 14.4 Gm., weight of 18 ml. of alcohol

1 Gm. + 14.4 Gm. = 15.4 Gm. of solution

By the proportion:

15.4 (Gm.):1 (Gm.) = 100 (%):x

x = 6.49%, *answer.*

Practice Problems

1. What is the solubility of a substance in water if 125 Gm. of a saturated aqueous solution yield a 20 Gm. residue upon evaporation?

2. What is the solubility of a chemical if a saturated aqueous solution has a strength of 15% (w/w)?

3. A saturated aqueous solution contains 30 Gm. of a substance in each 100 ml. The specific gravity of the solution is 1.10. Calculate the solubility of the substance.

4. One Gm. of calcium hydroxide is soluble in 630 ml. of water at 25° C. Calculate the percentage strength (w/w) of a saturated solution.

5. The solubility of potassium chlorate is 1 Gm. in 16.5 ml. of water at 25° C. What is the percentage strength (w/w) of a saturated solution?

6. A saturated aqueous solution contains, in each 500 ml., 400 Gm. of a substance. The specific gravity of the solution is 1.30. What is the solubility of the substance?

7. The solubility of a substance is 1 Gm. in 3 ml. of water. When 5 Gm. of it are dissolved in 15 ml. of water, the volume of the resulting solution is 16.8 ml. How many grams of the substance and how many milliliters of water should be used to make 200 ml. of a saturated solution?

8. One Gm. of a substance is soluble in 0.55 ml. of water. When 20 Gm. of it are dissolved in 11 ml. of water, the volume of the resulting solution is 23.5 ml.

(a) How many grams of the substance and how many milliliters of water should be used in preparing 1000 ml. of a saturated solution?

(b) Calculate the percentage strength (w/w) of the solution.

(c) Calculate the percentage strength (w/v) of the solution.

(d) What is the specific gravity of the saturated solution?

APPENDIX E

EMULSION NUCLEUS

In the preparation of emulsions by the *Continental Method* ("4-2-1 Method"), the proportions for the *nucleus* or *primary emulsion* are "fixed oil *4* parts by volume, water *2* parts by volume, and acacia *1* part by corresponding weight." The weight is measured in grams when volumes are measured in milliliters, and in apothecaries' ounces when volumes are measured in fluidounces. The mixture therefore contains one half as much water by volume as oil and one quarter as much acacia by "corresponding" weight.

When emulsions of volatile oils are prepared by this method, the proportions are "volatile oil *2* parts by volume, water *2* parts by volume, and acacia *1* part by corresponding weight."

To calculate the quantities of ingredients required for a nucleus or primary emulsion:

Examples:

R̨ Castor Oil   30%
    Acacia   q.s.
    Orange Syrup   30.0
    Water ad   250.0
    Sig. 15 ml. at night.

How much castor oil, water, and acacia are required to prepare the primary emulsion?

250 ml. × 30% = 75 ml. of castor oil required
Since castor oil is a *fixed* oil, the ratio *4-2-1* is used.

4	-	*2*	-	*1*	
75 ml.		37.5 ml.		18.75 Gm.	
oil		water		acacia	*answers.*

R̨ Cod Liver Oil   ℥ ii
    Acacia   q.s.
    Syrup   ℥ i
    Wintergreen Water ad   ℥ viii
    Sig. ʒ iv b.i.d.

How much cod liver oil, water, and acacia are required to prepare the primary emulsion?

Since cod liver oil is a *fixed* oil, the ratio *4-2-1* is used.

4	-	2	-	1	
f℥ii		f℥i		℥ss	(240 grains)
oil		water		acacia	*answers.*

R̸ Turpentine Oil 15%
   Acacia .... q.s.
   Syrup 15.0
   Water ad 120.0
   Sig. Take as directed.

How much turpentine oil, water, and acacia are required to prepare the primary emulsion?

120 ml. × 15% = 18 ml. of turpentine oil required

Since turpentine oil is a *volatile* oil, the ratio *2-2-1* is used.

2	-	2	-	1	
18 ml.		18 ml.		9 Gm.	
oil		water		acacia	*answers.*

Practice Problems

In each of the following prescriptions, calculate (a) the amount of acacia and (b) the amount of water to be used in preparing the nucleus or primary emulsion.

1. R̸ Castor Oil
      Orange Syrup aa 30.0
      Acacia .... q.s.
      Distilled Water ad 120.0
      Sig. 15 ml. at night.

2. R̸ Wild Cherry Syrup 50%
      Linseed Oil .... 20% (*A fixed oil.*)
      Acacia .... q.s.
      Water ad 250.0
      Sig. As directed.

3. R̸ Emulsion of Castor Oil .... ℥iv
      25%
      Sig. Take in two doses.

4. ℞   Cod Liver Oil   60.0
       Acacia   q.s.
       Cocoa   2.0
       Vanilla Tincture   0.5
       Syrup ad   120.0
       Sig. 8 ml. b.i.d.

5. ℞   Turpentine Oil   15.0
       Syrup   15.0
       Acacia   q.s.
       Water ad   100.0
       Sig. As directed.

6. ℞   Mineral Oil   125.0 (*A fixed oil.*)
       Acacia   q.s.
       Syrup   25.0
       Vanillin   0.01
       Alcohol   15.0
       Distilled Water ad   250.0
       Sig. Mineral Oil Emulsion.

7. ℞   Santal Oil   10.0 (*A volatile oil.*)
       Expressed Almond Oil   15.0 (*A fixed oil.*)
       Syrup   30.0
       Distilled Water ad   120.0
       Sig. Take as directed.

8. ℞   Castor Oil   20%
       Acacia   q.s.
       Tolu Balsam Syrup   50.0
       Water ad   240.0
       Sig. 8 ml. as directed.

9. ℞   Aspidium Oleoresin   4.0 (*Treat as a volatile oil.*)
       Syrup   5.0
       Vanilla Tincture   2.0
       Acacia   q.s.
       Water ad   60.0
       Sig. Take at one dose.

10. ℞   Copaiba Balsam   10.0 (*Treat as a volatile oil.*)
       Olive Oil   15.0 (*A fixed oil.*)
       Licorice Fluidextract   15.0
       Acacia   q.s.
       Water ad   120.0
       Sig. 4 ml. t.i.d.

APPENDIX F

EXPONENTIAL AND LOGARITHMIC NOTATION

EXPONENTIAL NOTATION

MANY physical and chemical measurements deal with either very large or very small numbers. Since it is difficult, in many instances, to handle conveniently numbers of such magnitude in performing even the simplest arithmetic operations in the usual manner, it is best to use exponential notation or *powers of 10* to express them. Thus, we may express *121* as *1.21 × 10²*, *1210* as *1.21 × 10³*, and *1,210,000* as *1.21 × 10⁶*. Likewise, we may express *0.0121* as *1.21 × 10⁻²*, *0.00121* as *1.21 × 10⁻³*, and *0.00000121* as *1.21 × 10⁻⁶*.

When numbers are written in this manner, the first part is called the *coefficient*, customarily written with one figure to the left of the decimal point. The second part is the *exponential factor* or *power of ten*.

The exponent represents the number of places that the decimal point has been moved—positive to the left and negative to the right—to form the exponential. Thus, when we convert *19000* to *1.9 × 10⁴*, we move the decimal point 4 places to the left; hence the exponent *4*. And when we convert *0.0000019* to *1.9 × 10⁻⁶*, we move the decimal point 6 places to the right; hence the *negative* exponent⁻⁶.

FUNDAMENTAL ARITHMETIC OPERATIONS WITH EXPONENTIALS

In the *multiplication* of exponentials, the exponents are *added*. For example, $10^2 \times 10^4 = 10^6$. In the multiplication of numbers that are expressed in exponential form, the *coefficients* are multiplied together in the usual manner and this product is then multiplied by the power of *10* found by algebraically *adding* the exponents.

Examples:

$$(2.5 \times 10^2) \times (2.5 \times 10^4) = 6.25 \times 10^6, \text{ or } 6.3 \times 10^6$$
$$(2.5 \times 10^2) \times (2.5 \times 10^{-4}) = 6.25 \times 10^{-2}, \text{ or } 6.3 \times 10^{-2}$$
$$(5.4 \times 10^2) \times (4.5 \times 10^3) = 24.3 \times 10^5 = 2.4 \times 10^6$$

In the *division* of exponentials, the exponents are *subtracted*. For example, $10^2 \div 10^5 = 10^{-3}$. And in the division of numbers that are expressed in exponential form, the *coefficients* are divided in the usual way and the result is multiplied by the power of *10* found by algebraically *subtracting* the exponents.

Examples:

$$(7.5 \times 10^5) \div (2.5 \times 10^3) = 3.0 \times 10^2$$
$$(7.5 \times 10^{-4}) \div (2.5 \times 10^6) = 3.0 \times 10^{-10}$$
$$(2.8 \times 10^{-2}) \div (8.0 \times 10^{-6}) = 0.35 \times 10^4 = 3.5 \times 10^3$$

Note that in each of the examples above the result is rounded off to the number of *significant figures* contained in the *least* accurate factor, and it is expressed with only one figure to the left of the decimal point.

In the *addition* and *subtraction* of exponentials, the expressions must be changed (by moving the decimal points) to forms having any common power of 10 and then the coefficients only are added or subtracted. The result should be rounded off to the number of *decimal places* contained in the *least* precise component, and it should be expressed with only one figure to the left of the decimal point.

Examples:

$$(1.4 \times 10^4) + (5.1 \times 10^3) =$$
$$1.4 \ \times 10^4$$
$$5.1 \times 10^3 = 0.51 \times 10^4$$

Total: 1.91×10^4, *answer.*

$$(1.4 \times 10^4) - (5.1 \times 10^3) =$$
$$1.4 \times 10^4 = 14.0 \times 10^3$$
$$5.1 \times 10^3$$

Difference: 8.9×10^3, *answer.*

$$(9.83 \times 10^3) + (4.1 \times 10^1) + (2.6 \times 10^3) =$$
$$9.83 \ \ \times 10^3$$
$$4.1 \times 10^1 = 0.041 \times 10^3$$
$$2.6 \ \ \times 10^3$$

Total: 12.471×10^3, or
$12.5 \ \ \times 10^3 = 1.25 \times 10^4$, *answer.*

Practice Problems

1. Write each of the following in exponential form:
   - (a) 12,650
   - (b) 0.0000000055
   - (c) 451
   - (d) 0.065
   - (e) 625,000,000

2. Write each of the following in the usual numerical form:
   - (a) 4.1×10^6
   - (b) 3.65×10^{-2}
   - (c) 5.13×10^{-6}
   - (d) 2.5×10^5
   - (e) 8.6956×10^3

3. Find the product:
   - (a) $(3.5 \times 10^3) \times (5.0 \times 10^4)$
   - (b) $(8.2 \times 10^2) \times (2.0 \times 10^{-6})$
   - (c) $(1.5 \times 10^{-6}) \times (4.0 \times 10^6)$
   - (d) $(1.5 \times 10^3) \times (8.0 \times 10^4)$
   - (e) $(7.2 \times 10^5) \times (5.0 \times 10^{-3})$

4. Find the quotient:
   - (a) $(9.3 \times 10^5) \div (3.1 \times 10^2)$
   - (b) $(3.6 \times 10^{-4}) \div (1.2 \times 10^6)$
   - (c) $(3.3 \times 10^7) \div (1.1 \times 10^{-2})$

5. Find the sum:
   - (a) $(9.2 \times 10^3) + (7.6 \times 10^4)$
   - (b) $(1.8 \times 10^{-6}) + (3.4 \times 10^{-5})$
   - (c) $(4.9 \times 10^2) + (2.5 \times 10^3)$

6. Find the difference:
   - (a) $(6.5 \times 10^6) - (5.9 \times 10^4)$
   - (b) $(8.2 \times 10^{-3}) - (1.6 \times 10^{-3})$
   - (c) $(7.4 \times 10^3) - (4.6 \times 10^2)$

LOGARITHMIC NOTATION

We have seen that exponential notation allows us to express any number as a *coefficient times a whole-number power of 10*—as when we interpret *150* to mean *1.5 × 10²*—and that this system of notation offers us a convenient shorthand, as it were, for expressing and manipulating very large or very small numbers.

Still another system, called *common logarithmic notation*, goes the exponential system one better. In common logarithmic notation *every number is expressed simply as a power of 10*—not with absolute precision, but with sufficient accuracy for any given purpose—and we may multiply any two numbers so expressed, or divide one by the other, by the simple process of adding or subtracting their exponents.

The *exponent* that indicates *to what power 10 must be raised to equal approximately a given number* is called the *common logarithm* of that number.

It follows that the logarithm of *10* or of any integral power of *10*, is always a positive or negative integer:

$$\log 10 \text{ (or } 1 \times 10^1) = 1$$
$$\log 100 \text{ (or } 1 \times 10^2) = 2$$
$$\log 1000 \text{ (or } 1 \times 10^3) = 3$$

and so on;

$$\log 1 \text{ (or } 1 \times 10^0) = 0$$
$$\log 0.1 \text{ (or } 1 \times 10^{-1}) = -1$$
$$\log 0.01 \text{ (or } 1 \times 10^{-2}) = -2$$

and so on. And if these were the only numbers in existence, no Table of Logarithms should be needed; for, given a number, say *1,000,000* (or 1×10^6), if we know the system we can readily supply its logarithm: *6*; or, given the logarithm *6*, we can readily reconstruct the number it represents: *1,000,000*.

But any number *not* in the *10's* series must contain a certain *excess* over some power of *10*—as *150* contains 10^2 plus an excess of *50*. Therefore, the logarithm of such a number always consists of a positive or negative whole-number exponent *plus* a positive decimal-fraction exponent (carried to as many decimal places as suit our purpose). As it turns out, the power of *10* that approximates *150* (or *1.5* $\times$ *10²*) is $10^{2.1761}$, and therefore *log 150 = 2.1761*.

The *whole-number exponent* is called the *characteristic*. It accounts for the integral power of *10* contained in the given number and hence serves to locate the *decimal point* in that number. If a number is given in ordinary notation, you can find the characteristic by converting it to exponential notation, in which the characteristic appears as a power of *10*.

The *decimal-fraction exponent* is called the *mantissa*. You can find the mantissa in a table of logarithms. The mantissa represents the *significant figures* in the given number, regardless of the location of the decimal point. In other words, given the sequence *610*, a four-place table will tell you that the mantissa is *7853*, whether the number be *61.0*, or *6.10*, or *0.00610*.

Compare this series of logarithms with the logarithms of the *10's* series given above:

Characteristics ⎫
Mantissas ⎬

$\log 6.10$ (or 6.10×10^0) $= \overbrace{0.7853}$
$\log 61.0$ (or 6.10×10^1) $= 1.7853$
$\log 610$ (or 6.10×10^2) $= 2.7853$
$\log 6100$ (or 6.10×10^3) $= 3.7853$

and so on; and

$\log 0.610$ (or 6.10×10^{-1}) $= \bar{1}.7853$
$\log 0.0610$ (or 6.10×10^{-2}) $= \bar{2}.7853$
$\log 0.00610$ (or 6.10×10^{-3}) $= \bar{3}.7853$

and so on. Note that by putting the minus sign *over* the characteristic we indicate that it alone is negative, and that the mantissa, as always, is positive.

USE OF LOGARITHM TABLES

Logarithm tables give mantissas calculated to four-place, five-place accuracy, and upwards, depending on the table and its purpose. A four-place table insures an accuracy within 0.5% when we work with three-figure numbers.

The Table (pp. 256–257) has typical features. It contains (1) a column to the left and a row at the top to guide us in locating the mantissas of 3-figure numbers, (2) the 4-place mantissas of all 3-figure numbers, and (3) columns of proportional parts providing us with a quick means of calculating more accurate mantissas when given numbers of 4-figure accuracy—a process called *interpolation*.

To find the logarithm of a number:

First, determine the characteristic, then find the mantissa in the log table.

Examples:

Find the log of 262.

$262 = 2.62 \times 10^2$

By inspection of the ten factor, the characteristic $= 2$.
To find the mantissa, focus attention on the digits *262*.
In the left-hand column in the log table find *26;* opposite it and in the column numbered *2* is the desired mantissa 0.4183. (The table omits the 0.)

Therefore, $\log 262 = 2.4183$, *answer*.

Find the log of 2627.

$2627 = 2.627 \times 10^3$

By inspection of the ten factor, the characteristic = 3.
In the left-hand column in the table find *26;* opposite it and in the column numbered *2* find the mantissa 0.4183; opposite *26* and in column *7* under proportional parts find 11 (meaning 0.0011 but written without zeros) and add it to 0.4183 to obtain the desired mantissa 0.4194.

Therefore, log 2627 = 3.4194, *answer.*

Find the log of 0.002627.

$0.002627 = 2.627 \times 10^{-3}$

By inspection of the ten factor, the characteristic = $\bar{3}$.
The mantissa is determined as in the preceding example.
Therefore, log 0.002627 = $\bar{3}$.4194, *answer.*

To find the antilogarithm of a logarithm:

When a problem is solved by logarithms, the result is expressed as the *logarithm* of the answer. This necessitates the finding of the *antilogarithm* or *the number corresponding to the logarithm.* If the mantissa of a logarithm is known, its antilogarithm can be found by a *reverse reading* of the log table.

Examples:

Find the antilogarithm of the logarithm 1.7604.

The mantissa 0.7604 is found in the column numbered *6* opposite *57,* and the resulting figure is 576.
The characteristic is 1 and, the required number is 5.76×10^1 or 57.6, *answer.*

Find the antilogarithm of the logarithm 3.7607.

Since the mantissa 0.7607 is not found in the log table, interpolation must be used. In the log table, 0.7607 falls *between 0.7604 and 0.7612;* therefore, the resulting figure must be between *576 and 577.*
The *given* mantissa is 0.0003 (or 3 units) more than the mantissa 0.7604. Therefore, opposite 0.7604 find 3 in the column *4* of proportional parts. Then the required figure is *5764.*
The characteristic is 3 and the required number is $5.764 \times 10^3 = 5764$, *answer.*

SOME LOGARITHMIC COMPUTATIONS

As shown in the first example below, when a negative number is "added" it is actually subtracted; and as shown in the third example, when a negative number is "subtracted" it is actually *added*.

The fourth example shows the curious but consistent fact that, in subtracting one logarithm from another, if you *borrow* from a negative characteristic (as *1* is borrowed from the -1 of the minuend) you *increase* the value of the negative characteristic (as the -1 becomes -2, which is canceled out when the *2* of the subtrahend is "subtracted" from it).

Examples:

Multiply (5.25×10^3) by (8.92×10^{-6}) by (7.56×10^5).

$$\log (5.25 \times 10^3) = 3.7202$$
$$\log (8.92 \times 10^{-6}) = \overline{6}.9504$$
$$\log (7.56 \times 10^5) = 5.8785$$

Total: 4.5491

Antilogarithm of $4.5491 = 3.541 \times 10^4 = 35410$, or, (retaining only 3 significant figures), 35400, *answer*.

Divide 29600 by 5.544.

$$29600 = 2.96 \times 10^4$$
$$5.544 = 5.544 \times 10^0$$
$$\log (2.96 \times 10^4) = 4.4713$$
$$\log (5.544 \times 10^0) = 0.7438$$

Difference: 3.7275

Antilogarithm of $3.7275 = 5.34 \times 10^3 = 5340$, *answer*.

Divide 7500 by 0.627.

$$7500 = 7.50 \times 10^3$$
$$0.627 = 6.27 \times 10^{-1}$$
$$\log (7.50 \times 10^3) = 3.8751$$
$$\log (6.27 \times 10^{-1}) = \overline{1}.7973$$

Difference: 4.0778

Antilogarithm of $4.0778 = 1.196 \times 10^4 = 11960$, or (retaining only 3 significant figures), 12000, *answer*.

Divide 0.191 by 0.0452.

$0.191 = 1.91 \times 10^{-1}$

$0.0452 = 4.52 \times 10^{-2}$

$\log (1.91 \times 10^{-1}) = \bar{1}.2810$

$\log (4.52 \times 10^{-2}) = \bar{2}.6551$

Difference: 0.6259

Antilogarithm of $0.6259 = 4.226 \times 10^0 = 4.226$ or (retaining only 3 significant figures) 4.23, *answer.*

Find the value of $\dfrac{(4.54 \times 10^6) \times (3.25 \times 10^3)}{(1.21 \times 10^8)}.$

$\log (4.54 \times 10^6) = 6.6571$

$\log (3.25 \times 10^3) = 3.5119$

Total: $10.1690 = \log$ of numerator

$\log (1.21 \times 10^8) = 8.0828 = \log$ of denominator

Difference: 2.0862

Antilogarithm of $2.0862 = 1.219$ or $1.22 \times 10^2 = 122,$
answer.

Practice Problems

1. Find the logarithm of each of the following numbers.

(a)	2245	(f)	0.7245
(b)	5.265	(g)	215000
(c)	7000	(h)	0.0001372
(d)	187.9	(i)	68.78
(e)	0.002934	(j)	6.2×10^6

2. Find the antilogarithm corresponding to each of the following logarithms.

(a)	4.4512	(f)	2.1668
(b)	1.1523	(g)	0.0261
(c)	0.3302	(h)	$\bar{3}.8902$
(d)	$\bar{1}.1105$	(i)	1.9234
(e)	2.7892	(j)	$\bar{2}.1234$

3. Compute each of the following by means of logarithms.

    (a) 23.87×954.6

    (b) 8542×0.8562

    (c) 655.7×0.02253

    (d) $(8.235 \times 10^2) \times (4.296 \times 10^{-4}) \times (2.325 \times 10^3)$

    (e) $26.74 \times 5.987 \times 106.7$

4. Compute each of the following by means of logarithms.

    (a) $9525 \div 1.267$

    (b) $2500 \div 12.65$

    (c) $0.2925 \div 56.85$

    (d) $(1.658 \times 10^4) \div (4.689 \times 10^2)$

    (e) $0.491 \div 0.0357$

5. Find the value of each of the following by means of logarithms.

    (a) $\dfrac{(6.29 \times 10^2) \times (1.23 \times 10^4)}{(9.75 \times 10^4)}$

    (b) $\dfrac{1{,}667{,}000 \times 0.4101}{(6.31 \times 10^3)}$

    (c) $\dfrac{(7.32 \times 10^2)}{(4.315 \times 10^{-4}) \times (5.795 \times 10^3)}$

Table of Logarithms

Three-figure numbers	0	1	2	3	4	5	6	7	8	9	Proportional parts (for interpolation)								
											1	2	3	4	5	6	7	8	9
10	0000	0043	0086	0128	0170	0212	0253	0294	0334	0374	4	8	12	17	21	25	29	33	37
11	0414	0453	0492	0531	0569	0607	0645	0682	0719	0755	4	8	11	15	19	23	26	30	34
12	0792	0828	0864	0899	0934	0969	1004	1038	1072	1106	3	7	10	14	17	21	24	28	31
13	1139	1173	1206	1239	1271	1303	1335	1367	1399	1430	3	6	10	13	16	19	23	26	29
14	1461	1492	1523	1553	1584	1614	1644	1673	1703	1732	3	6	9	12	15	18	21	24	27
15	1761	1790	1818	1847	1875	1903	1931	1959	1987	2014	3	6	8	11	14	17	20	22	25
16	2041	2068	2095	2122	2148	2175	2201	2227	2253	2279	3	5	8	11	13	16	18	21	24
17	2304	2330	2355	2380	2405	2430	2455	2480	2504	2529	2	5	7	10	12	15	17	20	22
18	2553	2577	2601	2625	2648	2672	2695	2718	2742	2765	2	5	7	9	12	14	16	19	21
19	2788	2810	2833	2856	2878	2900	2923	2945	2967	2989	2	4	7	9	11	13	16	18	20
20	3010	3032	3054	3075	3096	3118	3139	3160	3181	3201	2	4	6	8	11	13	15	17	19
21	3222	3243	3263	3284	3304	3324	3345	3365	3385	3404	2	4	6	8	10	12	14	16	18
22	3424	3444	3464	3483	3502	3522	3541	3560	3579	3598	2	4	6	8	10	12	14	15	17
23	3617	3636	3655	3674	3692	3711	3729	3747	3766	3784	2	4	6	7	9	11	13	15	17
24	3802	3820	3838	3856	3874	3892	3909	3927	3945	3962	2	4	5	7	9	11	12	14	16
25	3979	3997	4014	4031	4048	4065	4082	4099	4116	4133	2	3	5	7	9	10	12	14	15
26	4150	4166	4183	4200	4216	4232	4249	4265	4281	4298	2	3	5	7	8	10	11	13	15
27	4314	4330	4346	4362	4378	4393	4409	4425	4440	4456	2	3	5	6	8	9	11	13	14
28	4472	4487	4502	4518	4533	4548	4564	4579	4594	4609	2	3	5	6	8	9	11	12	14
29	4624	4639	4654	4669	4683	4698	4713	4728	4742	4757	1	3	4	6	7	9	10	12	13
30	4771	4786	4800	4814	4829	4843	4857	4871	4886	4900	1	3	4	6	7	9	10	11	13
31	4914	4928	4942	4955	4969	4983	4997	5011	5024	5038	1	3	4	6	7	8	10	11	12
32	5051	5065	5079	5092	5105	5119	5132	5145	5159	5172	1	3	4	5	7	8	9	11	12
33	5185	5198	5211	5224	5237	5250	5263	5276	5289	5302	1	3	4	5	6	8	9	10	12
34	5315	5328	5340	5353	5366	5378	5391	5403	5416	5428	1	3	4	5	6	8	9	10	11
35	5441	5453	5465	5478	5490	5502	5514	5527	5539	5551	1	2	4	5	6	7	9	10	11
36	5563	5575	5587	5599	5611	5623	5635	5647	5658	5670	1	2	4	5	6	7	8	10	11
37	5682	5694	5705	5717	5729	5740	5752	5763	5775	5786	1	2	3	5	6	7	8	9	10
38	5798	5809	5821	5832	5843	5855	5866	5877	5888	5899	1	2	3	5	6	7	8	9	10
39	5911	5922	5933	5944	5955	5966	5977	5988	5999	6010	1	2	3	4	5	7	8	9	10
40	6021	6031	6042	6053	6064	6075	6085	6096	6107	6117	1	2	3	4	5	6	8	9	10
41	6128	6138	6149	6160	6170	6180	6191	6201	6212	6222	1	2	3	4	5	6	7	8	9
42	6232	6243	6253	6263	6274	6284	6294	6304	6314	6325	1	2	3	4	5	6	7	8	9
43	6335	6345	6355	6365	6375	6385	6395	6405	6415	6425	1	2	3	4	5	6	7	8	9
44	6435	6444	6454	6464	6474	6484	6493	6503	6513	6522	1	2	3	4	5	6	7	8	9
45	6532	6542	6551	6561	6571	6580	6590	6599	6609	6618	1	2	3	4	5	6	7	8	
46	6628	6637	6646	6656	6665	6675	6684	6693	6702	6712	1	2	3	4	5	6	7	7	8
47	6721	6730	6739	6749	6758	6767	6776	6785	6794	6803	1	2	3	4	5	5	6	7	8
48	6812	6821	6830	6839	6848	6857	6866	6875	6884	6893	1	2	3	4	4	5	6	7	8
49	6902	6911	6920	6928	6937	6946	6955	6964	6972	6981	1	2	3	4	4	5	6	7	8
50	6990	6998	7007	7016	7024	7033	7042	7050	7059	7067	1	2	3	3	4	5	6	7	8
51	7076	7084	7093	7101	7110	7118	7126	7135	7143	7152	1	2	3	3	4	5	6	7	8
52	7160	7168	7177	7185	7193	7202	7210	7218	7226	7235	1	2	2	3	4	5	6	7	7
53	7243	7251	7259	7267	7275	7284	7292	7300	7308	7316	1	2	2	3	4	5	6	6	7
54	7324	7332	7340	7348	7356	7364	7372	7380	7388	7396	1	2	2	3	4	5	6	6	7

Table of Logarithms—(Continued)

hree-igure mbers	0	1	2	3	4	5	6	7	8	9	1	2	3	4	5	6	7	8	9
														Proportional parts (for interpolation)					
55	7404	7412	7419	7427	7435	7443	7451	7459	7466	7474	1	2	2	3	4	5	5	6	7
56	7482	7490	7497	7505	7513	7520	7528	7536	7543	7551	1	2	2	3	4	5	5	6	7
57	7559	7566	7574	7582	7589	7597	7604	7612	7619	7627	1	2	2	3	4	5	5	6	7
58	7634	7642	7649	7657	7664	7672	7679	7686	7694	7701	1	1	2	3	4	4	5	6	7
59	7709	7716	7723	7731	7738	7745	7752	7760	7767	7774	1	1	2	3	4	4	5	6	7
60	7782	7789	7796	7803	7810	7818	7825	7832	7839	7846	1	1	2	3	4	4	5	6	6
61	7853	7860	7868	7875	7882	7889	7896	7903	7910	7917	1	1	2	3	4	4	5	6	6
62	7924	7931	7938	7945	7952	7959	7966	7973	7980	7987	1	1	2	3	3	4	5	6	6
63	7993	8000	8007	8014	8021	8028	8035	8041	8048	8055	1	1	2	3	3	4	5	5	6
64	8062	8069	8075	8082	8089	8096	8102	8109	8116	8122	1	1	2	3	3	4	5	5	6
65	8129	8136	8142	8149	8156	8162	8169	8176	8182	8189	1	1	2	3	3	4	5	5	6
66	8195	8202	8209	8215	8222	8228	8235	8241	8248	8254	1	1	2	3	3	4	5	5	6
67	8261	8267	8274	8280	8287	8293	8299	8306	8312	8319	1	1	2	3	3	4	5	5	6
68	8325	8331	8338	8344	8351	8357	8363	8370	8376	8382	1	1	2	3	3	4	4	5	6
69	8388	8395	8401	8407	8414	8420	8426	8432	8439	8445	1	1	2	2	3	4	4	5	6
70	8451	8457	8463	8470	8476	8482	8488	8494	8500	8506	1	1	2	2	3	4	4	5	6
71	8513	8519	8525	8531	8537	8543	8549	8555	8561	8567	1	1	2	2	3	4	4	5	5
72	8573	8579	8585	8591	8597	8603	8609	8615	8621	8627	1	1	2	2	3	4	4	5	5
73	8633	8639	8645	8651	8657	8663	8669	8675	8681	8686	1	1	2	2	3	4	4	5	5
74	8692	8698	8704	8710	8716	8722	8727	8733	8739	8745	1	1	2	2	3	4	4	5	5
75	8751	8756	8762	8768	8774	8779	8785	8791	8797	8802	1	1	2	2	3	3	4	5	5
76	8808	8814	8820	8825	8831	8837	8842	8848	8854	8859	1	1	2	2	3	3	4	5	5
77	8865	8871	8876	8882	8887	8893	8899	8904	8910	8915	1	1	2	2	3	3	4	4	5
78	8921	8927	8932	8938	8943	8949	8954	8960	8965	8971	1	1	2	2	3	3	4	4	5
79	8976	8982	8987	8993	8998	9004	9009	9015	9020	9026	1	1	2	2	3	3	4	4	5
80	9031	9036	9042	9047	9053	9058	9063	9069	9074	9079	1	1	2	2	3	3	4	4	5
81	9085	9090	9096	9101	9106	9112	9117	9122	9128	9133	1	1	2	2	3	3	4	4	5
82	9138	9143	9149	9154	9159	9165	9170	9175	9180	9186	1	1	2	2	3	3	4	4	5
83	9191	9196	9201	9206	9212	9217	9222	9227	9232	9238	1	1	2	2	3	3	4	4	5
84	9243	9248	9253	9258	9263	9269	9274	9279	9284	9289	1	1	2	2	3	3	4	4	5
85	9294	9299	9304	9309	9315	9320	9325	9330	9335	9340	1	1	2	2	3	3	4	4	5
86	9345	9350	9355	9360	9365	9370	9375	9380	9385	9390	1	1	2	2	3	3	4	4	5
87	9395	9400	9405	9410	9415	9420	9425	9430	9435	9440	0	1	1	2	2	3	3	4	4
88	9445	9450	9455	9460	9465	9469	9474	9479	9484	9489	0	1	1	2	2	3	3	4	4
89	9494	9499	9504	9509	9513	9518	9523	9528	9533	9538	0	1	1	2	2	3	3	4	4
90	9542	9547	9552	9557	9562	9566	9571	9576	9581	9586	0	1	1	2	2	3	3	4	4
91	9590	9595	9600	9605	9609	9614	9619	9624	9628	9633	0	1	1	2	2	3	3	4	4
92	9638	9643	9647	9652	9657	9661	9666	9671	9675	9680	0	1	1	2	2	3	3	4	4
93	9685	9689	9694	9699	9703	9708	9713	9717	9722	9727	0	1	1	2	2	3	3	4	4
94	9731	9736	9741	9745	9750	9754	9759	9763	9768	9773	0	1	1	2	2	3	3	4	4
95	9777	9782	9786	9791	9795	9800	9805	9809	9814	9818	0	1	1	2	2	3	3	4	4
96	9823	9827	9832	9836	9841	9845	9850	9854	9859	9863	0	1	1	2	2	3	3	4	4
97	9868	9872	9877	9881	9886	9890	9894	9899	9903	9908	0	1	1	2	2	3	3	4	4
98	9912	9917	9921	9926	9930	9934	9939	9943	9948	9952	0	1	1	2	2	3	3	4	4
99	9956	9961	9965	9969	9974	9978	9983	9987	9991	9996	0	1	1	2	2	3	3	3	4

17

APPENDIX G

PROBLEMS IN H–ion CONCENTRATION AND pH

WHEN the hydrogen-ion concentration of solutions is expressed quantitatively, it varies from a value of nearly 1 for a normal solution of a strong acid to about 1×10^{-14} for a normal solution of a strong alkali. Consequently, there is a variation of about 100,000,000,000,000 in the numerical values within these two limits. The use of ordinary notation for handling numbers of such magnitude in computations that involve hydrogen-ion concentration is impracticable.

In order to simplify the statement of hydrogen-ion concentration, it is convenient to use logarithmic notation, with the mantissa usually rounded off to one or two places of decimals. It has become customary, therefore, to speak of the hydrogen-ion concentration of a given solution in terms of its pH value which is defined as the *logarithm of the reciprocal of the hydrogen-ion value.* Mathematically, this statement may be expressed as

$$pH = \log \frac{1}{[H^+]}$$

and since the logarithm of a reciprocal equals the negative logarithm of a number, this equation may also be written

$$pH = -\log [H^+]$$

Therefore pH value may also be defined as the *negative logarithm of the hydrogen-ion value.*

Now, the reciprocal, or negative, of a logarithm always contains a *negative mantissa.* *Log* (7×10^{-8}), for example, equals $\overline{8}.8451$ or approximately $\overline{8}.8$, which is interpreted as $-8 + 0.8$. Its reciprocal is $-(-8 + 0.8)$, or $8 - 0.8$. In expressing pH value we eliminate the negative by borrowing *1* from the characteristic and adding it to the mantissa:

$$8 - 0.8 = (8 - 1) + (1 - 0.8) = 7 + 0.2, \text{ or } 7.2$$

If you say this is merely an elaborate way of subtracting *0.8* from *8.0*, you are quite right; but the importance of doing it this way becomes clear when you reverse the process.

Given $pH = 7.2$, to convert it to $-\log$ [H⁺] as the first step in ascertaining the H-ion concentration, you must add *1* to the characteristic and subtract it from the mantissa:

$$7.2 \text{ or } 7 + 0.2 = (7 + 1) + (0.2 - 1) = 8 - 0.8$$

Now you can proceed: if $8 - 0.8 = -\log$ [H⁺], then $\log$ [H⁺] $= -(8 - 0.8) = -8 + 0.8$ or $\bar{8}.8$.

To calculate the pH value of a solution, given its H-ion concentration:

Examples:

The H-ion concentration of a certain solution is 5×10^{-6}. Calculate the pH value of the solution.

$$\text{pH} = -\log \text{[H}^+\text{]} = -\log (5 \times 10^{-6})$$
$$\log (5 \times 10^{-6}) = \bar{6}.6990 \text{ or } \bar{6}.7, \text{ or } -6 + 0.7$$
$$-\log (5 \times 10^{-6}) = -(-6 + 0.7) = 6 - 0.7$$
$$\text{pH} = (6 - 1) + (1 - 0.7) = 5.3, \text{ answer.}$$

The H-ion concentration of a certain solution is 0.00012 gram-ion per liter. Calculate the pH value of the solution.

$$0.00012 = 1.2 \times 10^{-4}$$
$$\text{pH} = -\log \text{[H}^+\text{]} = -\log (1.2 \times 10^{-4})$$
$$\log (1.2 \times 10^{-4}) = \bar{4}.08, \text{ or } -4 + 0.08$$
$$-\log (1.2 \times 10^{-4}) = -(-4 + 0.08) = 4 - 0.08$$
$$\text{pH} = (4 - 1) + (1 - 0.08) = 3.92, \text{ answer.}$$

To calculate the H-ion concentration of a solution, given its pH value:

Examples:

The pH value of a certain solution is 11.1. Calculate the H-ion concentration of the solution.

$$\text{pH} = 11.1 = -\log \text{[H}^+\text{]}$$
$$-\log \text{[H}^+\text{]} = (11 + 1) + (0.1 - 1) = 12 - 0.9$$
$$\log \text{[H}^+\text{]} = -(12 - 0.9) = -12 + 0.9, \text{ or } \bar{12}.9$$
$$\text{H-ion concentration} = \text{antilog } \bar{12}.9 = 7.94 \times 10^{-12},$$

answer.

The pH value of a certain solution is 5.7. Express the H-ion concentration of the solution as gram-ion per liter.

pH $= 5.7 = -\log [H^+]$
$-\log [H^+] = (5 + 1) + (0.7 - 1) = 6 - 0.3$
$\log [H^+] = -(6 - 0.3) = -6 + 0.3 = \bar{6}.3$
H-ion concentration $=$ antilog $\bar{6}.3 = 2.0 \times 10^{-6}$, or
0.000002 gram-ion per liter, *answer.*

Practice Problems

1. The H-ion concentration of a certain solution is 2.5×10^{-11}. Calculate the pH value of the solution.

2. The H-ion concentration of a certain buffer solution is 2.85×10^{-10}. Calculate the pH value of the solution.

3. The H-ion concentration of a certain buffer solution is 0.000000603 gram-ion per liter. Calculate the pH of the solution.

4. The H-ion concentration of a certain solution is 0.0000036 gram-ion per liter. Calculate the pH of the solution.

5. The H-ion concentration of a buffer solution is 4.4×10^{-8}. Calculate the pH value of the solution.

6. The pH value of a certain solution is 6.5. Calculate the H-ion concentration of the solution.

7. A certain elixir has a pH of 2.2. Calculate the H-ion concentration of the elixir.

8. A prescription for a collyrium calls for a buffer solution having a pH value of 7.2. Calculate the H-ion concentration of the buffer solution.

9. A solution of a certain alkaloidal salt has a pH of 4.3. Express the H-ion concentration of the solution as gram-ion per liter.

10. A 1-100 solution of atropine sulfate has a pH value of 5.4. Calculate the H-ion concentration of the solution.

APPENDIX H

MISCELLANEOUS PROBLEMS IN DISPENSING PHARMACY

PROBLEMS INVOLVING THE RELATIONSHIP BETWEEN PREPARATIONS OF VEGETABLE DRUGS

THE unavailability of a preparation of a vegetable drug may necessitate a replacement by an equivalent amount of some other preparation of the drug. If, for example, a prescription calls for an extract which is not available, an equivalent amount of the corresponding fluidextract or tincture may be used providing that the physician's intent is fulfilled and that the replacement will present no compounding difficulties.

To calculate the amount of a tincture equivalent to its corresponding extract:

Example:

℞	Stramonium Extract	0.015 Gm.
	Cocoa Butter	q.s.
	Ft. suppos. tales no. x	
	Sig. One at night.	

Stramonium tincture (10%) is the only preparation of stramonium available. If 1 Gm. of the extract represents 4 Gm. of the drug, how many ml. of the tincture should be used?

0.015 Gm. × 10 = 0.150 Gm. of extract needed

Stramonium extract		*Stramonium*		*Stramonium tincture*
1 Gm.	represents	4 Gm.	represented by	40 ml.

Therefore, the extract is 40 times as strong as the tincture.

By the proportion:

1 (Gm.):0.15 (Gm.) = 40 (ml.):x
x = 6 ml., *answer.*

Dispensing note: The volume of the tincture must be reduced by evaporation at a controlled temperature before incorporation with the cocoa butter.

> ℞ Belladonna Extract   gr. $\frac{1}{8}$
>   Milk Sugar   q.s.
>   Ft. cap. tales no. 40
>   Sig. One capsule as directed.

Only belladonna tincture (10%) is available. If 1 Gm. of belladonna extract represents 4 Gm. of the drug, how much belladonna tincture should be used?

If the problem is in the apothecaries' system, it is generally best to convert the required quantity of the extract to the metric system.

$\frac{1}{8}$ gr. $\times$ 40 = 5 gr. = 0.325 Gm. of extract needed

Belladonna extract		Belladonna		Belladonna tincture
1 Gm.	represents	4 Gm.	represented by	40 ml.

Therefore, the extract is 40 times as strong as the tincture.

By the proportion:

1 (Gm.):0.325 (Gm.) = 40 (ml.):x
x = 13 ml., *answer.*

Dispensing note: The tincture must be evaporated to dryness at a controlled temperature before incorporation with the milk sugar.

To calculate the amount of an extract equivalent to its corresponding tincture:

> ℞ Belladonna Tincture   0.6 ml.
>   Calcium Lactate   0.3 Gm.
>   Ft. cap. tales no. 20
>   Sig. One capsule as directed.

One (1) Gm. of belladonna extract represents 4 Gm. of the drug. How much belladonna extract should be used to replace the tincture (10%) in this prescription?

0.6 ml. $\times$ 20 = 12 ml. of tincture needed
Belladonna tincture is $\frac{1}{40}$ as strong as the extract.

By the proportion:
40 (ml.):12 (ml.) = 1 (Gm.):x
x = 0.3 Gm., *answer.*

PROBLEMS INVOLVING THE USE OF TABLETS TO OBTAIN DESIRED QUANTITIES OF MEDICINAL SUBSTANCES

There can be little justification for the use of tablets or dispensing tablets as a standard procedure for obtaining small quantities of medicinal substances, since greater accuracy may be achieved by the use of the aliquot method (see Chapter I). The availability of materials, however, may restrict the choice of the method that can be employed for this purpose to the use of tablets.

To obtain a desired quantity of a medicinal substance by the use of tablets:

Example:

> ℞ Atropine Sulfate   gr. $\frac{1}{1000}$
> Ft. T.T. no. 50
> Sig. One tablet in each feeding.

The only source of atropine sulfate is in the form of dispensing tablets each containing $\frac{1}{4}$ gr. Explain how you would obtain the amount of atropine sulfate needed for the prescription.

$\frac{1}{1000}$ gr. $\times$ 50 = $\frac{1}{20}$ gr. of atropine sulfate needed
One dispensing tablet = $\frac{1}{4}$ gr. = $\frac{5}{20}$ gr. of atropine sulfate

Since one dispensing tablet contains $\frac{5}{20}$ gr. of atropine sulfate or *5 times* the amount needed, $\frac{1}{5}$ of the tablet will contain the required quantity or $\frac{1}{20}$ gr.
Assuming a desired accuracy of 5% and a balance sensitivity of $\frac{1}{30}$ gr., the required amount of atropine sulfate may be obtained as follows:

Step 1. Weigh *one* dispensing tablet (the tablet contains active ingredient and diluent).

Step 2. Powder the tablet in a mortar and dilute it with enough lactose to make 5 grains of dilution.

Step 3. Take 1 gr. of the dilution, *answer.*

Dispensing note: The amount of diluent (Step 2) should be large enough to insure that the aliquot (Step 3) can be weighed with the desired accuracy.

> ℞ Atropine Sulfate   gr. $\frac{1}{10}$
> Aromatic Elixir ad   ℥ iv
> Sig. ℥i before meals.

The only source of atropine sulfate is in the form of dispensing tablets each containing $\frac{1}{4}$ gr. Explain how you would obtain the amount of atropine sulfate needed for the prescription.

Amount of atropine sulfate needed $= \frac{1}{10}$ gr. $= \frac{2}{20}$ gr.

One dispensing tablet $= \frac{1}{4}$ gr. $= \frac{5}{20}$ gr. of atropine sulfate

Since one dispensing tablet contains $\frac{5}{20}$ gr. of atropine sulfate or $2\frac{1}{2}$ *times* the amount needed, $\frac{2}{5}$ of the tablet will contain the required quantity or $\frac{1}{10}$ *gr.*
The required quantity of atropine sulfate may be obtained as follows:

Step 1. Dissolve *one* dispensing tablet in enough distilled water to make 5 ml. of dilution.

Step 2. Take 2 ml. of the dilution, *answer.*

℞	Scopolamine Hydrobromide	0.0065	Gm.
	Morphine Hydrochloride	0.5	Gm.
	Ethylmorphine Hydrochloride	1.0	Gm.
	Distilled Water ad	25.0	ml.
	Sig. Use as directed.		

Only tablets, each containing $\frac{1}{150}$ gr. of scopolamine hydrobromide, are available. How many tablets should be used to obtain the amount of scopolamine hydrobromide needed in the prescription?

0.0065 Gm. $= \frac{1}{10}$ gr. of scopolamine hydrobromide needed

Changing $\frac{1}{10}$ gr. to a fraction having 150 as the denominator, $\frac{1}{10}$ gr. $= \frac{15}{150}$ gr. of scopolamine hydrobromide needed

Since the available tablets contain $\frac{1}{150}$ gr. of scopolamine hydrobromide, $\frac{15}{150} \div \frac{1}{150} = 15$ tablets, *answer.*

Practice Problems

1. ℞   Belladonna Extract   gr. $\frac{1}{10}$
         Phenobarbital   gr. ss
         Milk Sugar   gr. iii
         Ft. cap. tal. no. xxiv
         Sig. One capsule as directed.

Only belladonna tincture (10%) is available. If 1 Gm. of belladonna extract represents 4 Gm. of the drug, how much belladonna tincture should be used in the prescription?

2. ℞ Belladonna Extract   0.12
     Ichthammol   2.00
     Theobroma Oil   12.00
     Div. in suppos. no. vi.
     Sig. One at night.

Belladonna tincture (10%) is the only preparation of belladonna available. If 1 Gm. of belladonna extract represents 4 Gm. of the drug, how much of the tincture should be used in compounding the prescription?

3. ℞ Belladonna Tincture   0.3 ml.
     Aspirin   0.3 Gm.
     Ft. cap. tales no. 24
     Sig. One capsule b.i.d.

One (1) Gm. of belladonna extract represents 4 Gm. of the drug. How much belladonna extract could be used to replace the tincture (10%) in this prescription?

4. ℞ Belladonna Extract   0.005
     Ascorbic Acid   0.050
     Barbital   0.250
     Ft. cap. tales no. xxxvi
     Sig. One capsule b.i.d.

The only preparation of belladonna available is the tincture (10%). If 1 Gm. of the extract represents 4 Gm. of the drug, how many milliliters of the tincture should be used?

5. ℞ Tr. Belladonna   ♏ x
     Ft. T.T. no. 50
     Sig. One tablet as directed.

One (1) Gm. of belladonna extract represents 4 Gm. of the drug. How many milligrams of the extract should be used to replace the tincture (10%) in this prescription?

6. ℞ Hydrastis Extract
     Tannic Acid aa   0.2
     Carbowax Base   q.s.
     Ft. suppos. tal. no. xii
     Sig. Insert one at night.

Only hydrastis tincture (20%) is available. If 1 Gm. of the extract represents 4 Gm. of the drug, how many milliliters of the tincture should be used in compounding the prescription?

7. ℞   Belladonna Extract   0.015
       Aluminum Hydroxide   0.15
       Magnesium Trisilicate 0.25
       Ft. cap. tal. no. 60
       Sig. One capsule t.i.d.

Only belladonna tincture (10%) is available. If 1 Gm. of the extract represents 4 Gm. of the drug, how many milliliters of the tincture should be used in compounding the prescription?

8. ℞   Atropine Sulfate   gr. $\frac{1}{100}$
       Aspirin   gr. v
       Ft. pulv. tales no. xii
       Sig. One powder as directed.

The only source of atropine sulfate is in the form of dispensing tablets each containing $\frac{1}{4}$ gr. Explain how you would obtain the amount of atropine sulfate needed for the prescription.

9. ℞   Quinine Sulfate   gr. ii
       Arsenic Trioxide   gr. $\frac{1}{50}$
       Strychnine Sulfate gr. $\frac{1}{40}$
       Lactose   q.s.
       Ft. cap. tales no. xvi
       Sig. One capsule b.i.d.

Only $\frac{1}{30}$-gr. tablets of strychnine sulfate are available. How many tablets should be used to obtain the required quantity of strychnine sulfate?

10. ℞   Atropine Sulfate   gr. $\frac{1}{2000}$
       Lactose   q.s.
       Ft. T.T. tales no. 60
       Sig. One in each feeding.

The only source of atropine sulfate is in the form of dispensing tablets each containing $\frac{1}{4}$ gr. Explain how you would obtain the amount of atropine sulfate needed for the prescription.

11. ℞   Strychnine Sulfate   0.02
       Ferrous Sulfate Elixir 120.0
       Sig. 4 ml. t.i.d.

The only source of strychnine sulfate is in the form of dispensing tablets each containing $\frac{1}{2}$ gr. Explain how you would obtain the amount of strychnine sulfate needed for the prescription.

12. ℞ Dihydromorphinone Hydrochloride gr. $\frac{3}{4}$
      Tolu Balsam Syrup ad ℥vi
      Sig. ℥i for cough.

The only source of dihydromorphinone hydrochloride is in the form of tablets each containing $\frac{1}{32}$ gr. How many tablets should be used to obtain the required amount of dihydromorphinone hydrochloride?

13. ℞ Strychnine Sulfate gr. $\frac{1}{120}$
      Iron and Ammonium Citrate gr. v
      Ft. cap. tal. no. xxiv
      Sig. One capsule b.i.d.

The only source of strychnine sulfate is in the form of dispensing tablets each containing $\frac{1}{4}$ gr. Explain how you would obtain the amount of strychnine sulfate needed for the prescription.

14. How many $\frac{1}{150}$-gr. tablets of atropine sulfate should be used in compounding an eight-ounce prescription which is to contain $\frac{1}{500}$ gr. of atropine sulfate in each dessertspoonful?

15. ℞ Atropine Sulfate gr. $\frac{1}{250}$
      Acetylsalicylic Acid gr. iii
      Phenacetin gr. ii
      Citrated Caffeine gr. i
      Ft. pulv. tales no. xx
      Sig. One powder every 4 hours.

Only tablet triturates, each containing $\frac{1}{150}$ gr. of atropine sulfate, are available. How many should be used in compounding the prescription?

16. ℞ Suppos.
      Morphine Sulfate gr. $\frac{1}{4}$
      Atropine Sulfate gr. $\frac{1}{150}$
      Disp. tales no. vi
      Sig. Use as directed.

The atropine sulfate is available only in the form of dispensing tablets each containing $\frac{1}{4}$ gr. Explain how you would obtain the atropine sulfate needed for the prescription.

17. ℞ Colchicine gr. $\frac{1}{100}$
      Lactose q.s.
      Ft. chart. tales no. xv
      Sig. One powder every 3 hours.

Only colchicine granules, each containing $\frac{1}{120}$ gr., are available. Explain how you would obtain the colchicine needed for the prescription.

18. ℞   Atropine Sulfate   gr. $\frac{1}{1000}$
         Purified Water ad   ℥i
         Dispense ℥i
         Sig. ℥i in each feeding.

Only tablet triturates, each containing $\frac{1}{100}$ gr. of atropine sulfate, are available. How many tablet triturates should be used in compounding the prescription?

APPENDIX I

SOME COMMERCIAL PROBLEMS

DISCOUNTS

ONE of the more important discounts that the retail pharmacist encounters in everyday practice is the so-called *trade discount* which is a deduction from list prices of merchandise. Pharmaceutical manufacturers and wholesalers issue catalogues to retail practitioners and allow certain discounts from the list prices that are quoted on the items appearing in their catalogues.

To compute the net cost of merchandise, given the list price and the discount:

Example:

The list price of an elixir is $12.75 per gallon, less 40%. What is the net cost of the elixir per gallon?

List price Discount Net cost
$$100\% - 40\% = 60\%$$
$$\$12.75 \times 0.60 = \$7.65, \textit{answer.}$$

To compute the net cost of merchandise, given the list price and the series discount:

Frequently, several discounts are allowed. For example, the list price on some merchandise may be subject to deductions of *40%, 10%, and 5%.* This chain of deductions is usually referred to as a *series discount.* In such cases, the discounts in the series cannot be figured by adding them; rather, the first discount is deducted from the list price and each successive discount is taken upon the balance remaining after the preceding discount has been deducted. The order in which the discounts in a series discount are taken is immaterial.

Example:

A certain ointment lists at $5.00 per lb., less discounts of 40%, 10%, and 5%. What is the net cost of the ointment per lb.?

$100\% - 40\% = 60\%$ $100\% - 10\% = 90\%$ $100\% - 5\% = 95\%$
$\quad$ \$5.00 $\times$ 0.60 = \$3.00, cost after 40% is deducted
$\quad$ \$3.00 $\times$ 0.90 = \$2.70, cost after 10% is deducted
$\quad$ \$2.70 $\times$ 0.95 = \$2.57, net cost, *answer.*

To compute a single discount equivalent to a series discount:

This is done by subtracting each discount in the series from 100% and multiplying together the net percentages. The product thus obtained is subtracted from 100% to give the single discount equivalent to the series discount.

Example:

$\quad$ *Calculate the single discount equivalent to a series discount of 40%, 10%, and 5%.*

$100\% - 40\% = 60\%$ $100\% - 10\% = 90\%$ $100\% - 5\% = 95\%$
$\quad$ 0.60 $\times$ 0.90 $\times$ 0.95 = 0.513 or 51.3% = % to be paid
$\quad$ Discount = 100% − 51.3% = 48.7%, *answer.*

MARKUP

The term *markup*, sometimes used interchangeably with the term *margin* or *margin of profit (gross profit)*, refers to the difference between the cost of merchandise and its selling price. For example, if a pharmacist buys an article for \$1.50 and sells it for \$2.50, the markup (or gross profit) as a dollars-and-cents item is \$1.00.

Markup percentage (percentage of gross profit) refers to the markup (gross profit) divided by the selling price. The expression of the per cent of markup may be somewhat ambiguous since it may be based on either the cost or the selling price of merchandise. In modern retail practice, this percentage is invariably based on selling price, and when reference is made to markup percentage (or % of gross profit), it means the % that the markup is of the selling price. However, if a pharmacist chooses, for the sake of convenience, to base percentage markup on the cost of merchandise, he may do so providing he does not overlook the fact that the markup on cost must yield the desired percentage of gross profit on the selling price.

To calculate the selling price of merchandise to yield a given % of gross profit on the cost:

Example:

$\quad$ *The cost of 100 tablets is \$1.50. What should be the selling price per hundred tablets to yield a $66\frac{2}{3}\%$ gross profit on the cost?*

Cost $\times$ % of gross profit = Gross profit
$1.50 $\times$ 66$\frac{2}{3}$% = $1.00

Cost + Gross profit = Selling price
$1.50 + $1.00 = $2.50, *answer.*

To calculate the selling price of merchandise to yield a given % of gross profit on the selling price:

Example:

The cost of 100 tablets is $1.50. What should be the selling price per hundred tablets to yield a 40% gross profit on the selling price?

Selling price = 100%

Selling price — Gross profit = Cost
100%   —   40%   = 60%

By the proportion:

60 (%):100 (%) = $1.50:x
x = $2.50, *answer.*

To calculate the percentage markup on the cost that will yield a desired % of gross profit on the selling price:

Example:

What should the percentage markup on the cost of an item be to yield a 40% gross profit on the selling price?

Selling price = 100%

Selling price — Gross profit = Cost
100%   —   40%   = 60%

By the proportion:

$\begin{pmatrix} \text{Cost} \\ \text{as \% of selling} \\ \text{price} \end{pmatrix}$: $\begin{pmatrix} \text{Selling} \\ \text{price} \\ \text{as \%} \end{pmatrix}$ = $\begin{pmatrix} \text{Gross profit} \\ \text{as \% of} \\ \text{selling price} \end{pmatrix}$: x

x = % gross profit on the cost

60 (%):100 (%) = 40 (%):x
x = 66$\frac{2}{3}$%, *answer.*

Practice Problems

1. Calculate the single discount equivalent to each of the series discounts listed below.

(a) 40%, 5%, and 5%

(b) 20%, 10%, 5%, and 5%

(c) 20%, 10%, and 5%

(d) 40%, 5%, and 2%

(e) 25%, 10%, 10%, and 2%

(f) 10%, 10%, and 2%

2. If an ointment is listed at $4.50 per pound, less 40%, what is the net cost of 10 pounds?

3. If a certain preparation is listed at $24.00 per dozen, less $33\frac{1}{3}\%$, what is the net cost per item?

4. A fluidextract is listed at $10.25 per gallon, less 40%. What is the net cost of f℥ xii?

5. A pharmacist received a bill of goods amounting to $150, less discounts of 10% and 5%. What is the net amount of the bill?

6. If a gross of bottles of cough syrup costs $80.00, less 40% and 2%, what is the net cost per bottle?

7. A certain preparation is listed at $25.75 per dozen, less 40% and 15%. What is the net cost per unit?

8. A certain ointment is listed at $8.00 per dozen tubes, less 40%, 10%, and 5%. What is the net cost of a single tube?

9. A certain proprietary lists at $12.00 per dozen, less 40% and 15%. What is the net cost per unit?

10. The list price on a certain tablet is $18.00 per 5 M, less 40%. What is the net cost of 100 tablets?

11. Calculate the difference in the net cost of a bill of goods amounting to $500 if the bill is discounted at 40% and if it is discounted at 30% and 10%.

12. ℞ Glycerin   ℥ ii
      Boric Acid Solution
      Witch Hazel aa ad   ℥ viii
      Sig. Apply to affected areas.

Witch hazel is listed at $3.00 per gallon, less 40%. What is the net cost of the amount needed in compounding the prescription?

13. ℞ Codeine Phosphate   0.3
        Hydriodic Acid Syrup
        Cobenzil aa   120.0
        Sig. 4 ml. for cough.

Cobenzil is listed at $24.67 per gallon, less 40%. What is the net cost of the amount needed in compounding the prescription?

14. ℞ Hydriodic Acid Syrup
        Compound Cocillana Syrup aa ad Oi
        Sig. 4 ml. every two or three hours.

Compound cocillana syrup is listed at $16.50 per gallon, less 40%. What is the net cost of the amount needed in compounding the prescription?

15. ℞ Belladonna Tincture   15.0
        Phenobarbital Elixir ad   120.0
        Sig. 4 ml. in water a.c.

Belladonna tincture is listed at $3.75 per pint, less 40%, and phenobarbital elixir is listed at $10.00 per gallon, less 40%. Calculate the net cost of the ingredients in the prescription.

16. ℞ Aluminum Acetate Solution   10.0
        Lanolin   20.0
        Zinc Oxide Paste   30.0
        Sig. Apply to hands.

Zinc oxide paste is listed at $8.75 per 5 lb., less 40% and 5%. What is the net cost of the amount needed in the prescription?

17. An article costs $0.75. At what price must a pharmacist sell it to realize a gross profit of $66\frac{2}{3}\%$ on the cost?

18. A certain article is listed at $4.00 per dozen, less 40%. At what price must the article be sold to yield a gross profit of $66\frac{2}{3}\%$ on the cost?

19. A bottle of tablets is listed at $3.00 with discounts of 40% and 5%. At what price must it be sold to yield a gross profit of 40% on the selling price?

20. A bottle of mouth wash costs 75 cents. At what price must it be sold to yield a gross profit of 40% on the selling price?

21. A jar of cleansing cream is sold for 75 cents, thereby yielding a gross profit of 60% on the cost. What did it cost?

18

22. A certain proprietary is sold for 85 cents, thereby yielding a gross profit of 35% on the selling price. What did it cost?

23. A certain preparation is listed at $5.00 per dozen, less 40%. At what price must it be sold to yield a gross profit of 50% on the selling price?

24. If chloroform (specific gravity 1.475) costs $0.50 per pound, at what price per pint must it be sold to yield a gross profit of 50% on the selling price?

25. A certain fluidextract is listed at $7.50 per gallon, less 40%. At what price should f℥ iv be sold in order that a gross profit of 50% on the selling price might be realized?

26. A pharmacist buys glycerin (specific gravity 1.25) for 50 cents per pound. At what price must he sell f℥ viii in order to realize a gross profit of 50% on the selling price?

27. A pharmacist buys 20,000 tablets for $100.00 with discounts of 40% and 10%. At what price per hundred must he sell the tablets in order to realize a gross profit of 40% on the selling price?

28. A pharmacist buys a bottle of multiple vitamin capsules for $5.00 less discounts of 40% and 10%. At what price must the capsules be sold to yield a profit of 50% on the selling price?

29. Calculate the difference between a single discount of 40% and a series discount of 25% and 15%.

30. A pharmacist purchases an oil for 90 cents per liter. If he sold 1 pt. of it for $1.00, what percentage of gross profit on the selling price did he realize?

31. A pharmacist sells a bottle of tablets for $3.75, thereby realizing a gross profit of 60% on the cost. Calculate the cost of the tablets.

32. A pharmacist finds that he can realize a gross profit of 40% on the selling price if he sells a medicine for $1.50 per bottle. What percentage of gross profit does this represent if based on the cost of the medicine?

33. A pharmacist sells a jar of a cosmetic cream for $2.50, thereby realizing a profit of 60% on the selling price. Calculate the cost of the cosmetic cream.

34. A certain cough syrup lists at $20.00 per gallon with discounts of 40% and 15%. What is the net cost of f℥ vi of the cough syrup?

35. A pharmacist finds that he can realize a gross profit of 60% on the selling price if he sells an item for $5.00. What percentage of gross profit does this represent if based on the cost of the item?

36. A pharmacist bought 5 gallons of an elixir for $20.00 ,which was 20% off the list price. He sold 4 gallons of the elixir at 10% off the list and the balance at 10% above list. What was the percentage of gross profit, the basis of the calculation to be the selling price?

37. A pharmacist buys one dozen bottles of an ophthalmic solution listed at $24.00 per dozen. He receives a discount of 40% off the list price plus a 2% discount for paying the bill before the 10th of the month. At what price per unit must he sell the solution in order to realize a gross profit of 50% on the selling price?

38. At what price must a pharmacist mark an item that costs $1.30 so that he can reduce the selling price 25% for a special sale and still make 35% on the cost price?

39. A pharmacist bought a bill of goods at a discount of 30%, 10%, and 10%. The total discount amounted to $129.90. Calculate the original amount of the bill.

APPENDIX J
DILUTION TABLE

Each column indicates the total number of parts by volume of weak solution of the ratio strength specified at the top that can be made by diluting ONE part by volume of any of the stronger solutions of the percentage strengths given in the left-hand column.

For example, a 1:4000 solution can be made by diluting 1 ml. of 1% solution to 40 ml., or by diluting 1 ml. of 2% solution to 80 ml., or 1 ml. of 3% solution to 120 ml.; and so on.

Again, when 1 ml. of 5% solution is diluted to 10 ml., you get a 1:200 solution; when 1 ml. of 5% solution is diluted to 50 ml., you get a 1:1000 solution; and so on.

%	$\frac{1}{100}$	$\frac{1}{200}$	$\frac{1}{300}$	$\frac{1}{400}$	$\frac{1}{500}$	$\frac{1}{600}$	$\frac{1}{700}$	$\frac{1}{800}$	$\frac{1}{900}$	$\frac{1}{1000}$	$\frac{1}{2000}$	$\frac{1}{3000}$
0.1	...	...	...	...	...	...	...	...	...	(1)	2	3
0.2	...	...	...	...	(1)	1.2	1.4	1.6	1.8	2	4	6
0.3	...	...	...	1.2	1.5	1.8	2.1	2.4	2.7	3	6	9
0.4	...	...	1.2	1.6	2.0	2.4	2.8	3.2	3.6	4	8	12
0.5	...	(1)	1.5	2.0	2.5	3.0	3.5	4.0	4.5	5	10	15
0.6	...	1.2	1.8	2.4	3.0	3.6	4.2	4.8	5.4	6	12	18
0.7	...	1.4	2.1	2.8	3.5	4.2	4.9	5.6	6.3	7	14	21
0.8	...	1.6	2.4	3.2	4.0	4.8	5.6	6.4	7.2	8	16	24
0.9	...	1.8	2.7	3.6	4.5	5.4	6.3	7.2	8.1	9	18	27
1	(1)	2	3	4	5	6	7	8	9	10	20	30
2	2	4	6	8	10	12	14	16	18	20	40	60
3	3	6	9	12	15	18	21	24	27	30	60	90
4	4	8	12	16	20	24	28	32	36	40	80	120
5	5	10	15	20	25	30	35	40	45	50	100	150
6	6	12	18	24	30	36	42	48	54	60	120	180
7	7	14	21	28	35	42	49	56	63	70	140	210
8	8	16	24	32	40	48	56	64	72	80	160	240
9	9	18	27	36	45	54	63	72	81	90	180	270
10	10	20	30	40	50	60	70	80	90	100	200	300
11	11	22	33	44	55	66	77	88	99	110	220	330
12	12	24	36	48	60	72	84	96	108	120	240	360
13	13	26	39	52	65	78	91	104	117	130	260	390
14	14	28	42	56	70	84	98	112	126	140	280	420
15	15	30	45	60	75	90	105	120	135	150	300	450
16	16	32	48	64	80	96	112	128	144	160	320	480
17	17	34	51	68	85	102	119	136	153	170	340	510
18	18	36	54	72	90	108	126	144	162	180	360	540
19	19	38	57	76	95	114	133	152	171	190	380	570
20	20	40	60	80	100	120	140	160	180	200	400	600
21	21	42	63	84	105	126	147	168	189	210	420	630
22	22	44	66	88	110	132	154	176	198	220	440	660
23	23	46	69	92	115	138	161	184	207	230	460	690
24	24	48	72	96	120	144	168	192	216	240	480	720
25	25	50	75	100	125	150	175	200	225	250	500	750
30	30	60	90	125	150	180	210	240	270	300	600	900
35	35	70	105	140	175	210	245	280	315	350	700	1050
40	40	80	120	160	200	240	280	320	360	400	800	1200
45	45	90	135	180	225	270	315	360	405	450	900	1350
50	50	100	150	200	250	300	350	400	450	500	1000	1500

To make up a desired quantity of dilute solution, select a quantity of the strong that when multiplied by the total number of parts will give the desired quantity or any insignificant excess. One liter of 1:10000 solution may be made by diluting 5 ml. of 2% solution to 200 × 5 ml. or 1000 ml.

To make very dilute solutions, proceed by steps. Dilute 1 ml. of 30% solution to 300 ml., making a 1:1000 or 0.1% solution; then dilute 1 ml. of this to 1000 ml. to get a 1:1000000 solution.

This table is valid for all solutions except if expansion or contraction occurs when active ingredient is mixed with diluent.

%	$\frac{1}{4000}$	$\frac{1}{5000}$	$\frac{1}{10000}$	$\frac{1}{25000}$	$\frac{1}{50000}$	$\frac{1}{100000}$	$\frac{1}{200000}$	$\frac{1}{500000}$	$\frac{1}{1000000}$
0.1	4	5	10	25	50	100	200	500	1000
0.2	8	10	20	50	100	200	400	1000	2000
0.3	12	15	30	75	150	300	600	1500	3000
0 4	16	20	40	100	200	400	800	2000	4000
0 5	20	25	50	125	250	500	1000	2500	5000
0 6	24	30	60	150	300	600	1200	3000	6000
0.7	28	35	70	175	350	700	1400	3500	7000
0 8	32	40	80	200	400	800	1600	4000	8000
0 9	36	45	90	225	450	900	1800	4500	9000
1	40	50	100	250	500	1000	2000	5000	10000
2	80	100	200	500	1000	2000	4000	10000	20000
3	120	150	300	750	1500	3000	6000	15000	30000
4	160	200	400	1000	2000	4000	8000	20000	40000
5	200	250	500	1250	2500	5000	10000	25000	50000
6	240	300	600	1500	3000	6000	12000	30000	60000
7	280	350	700	1750	3500	7000	14000	35000	70000
8	320	400	800	2000	4000	8000	16000	40000	80000
9	360	450	900	2250	4500	9000	18000	45000	90000
10	400	500	1000	2500	5000	10000	20000	50000	100000
11	440	550	1100	2750	5500	11000	22000	55000	110000
12	480	600	1200	3000	6000	12000	24000	60000	120000
13	520	650	1300	3250	6500	13000	26000	65000	130000
14	560	700	1400	3500	7000	14000	28000	70000	140000
15	600	750	1500	3750	7500	15000	30000	75000	150000
16	640	800	1600	4000	8000	16000	32000	80000	160000
17	680	850	1700	4250	8500	17000	34000	85000	170000
18	720	900	1800	4500	9000	18000	36000	90000	180000
19	760	950	1900	4750	9500	19000	38000	95000	190000
20	800	1000	2000	5000	10000	20000	40000	100000	200000
21	840	1050	2100	5250	10500	21000	42000	105000	210000
22	880	1100	2200	5500	11000	22000	44000	110000	220000
23	920	1150	2300	5750	11500	23000	46000	115000	230000
24	960	1200	2400	6000	12000	24000	48000	120000	240000
25	1000	1250	2500	6250	12500	25000	50000	125000	250000
30	1200	1500	3000	7500	15000	30000	60000	150000	300000
35	1400	1750	3500	8750	17500	35000	70000	175000	350000
40	1600	2000	4000	10000	20000	40000	80000	200000	400000
45	1800	2250	4500	11250	22500	45000	90000	225000	450000
50	2000	2500	5000	12500	25000	50000	100000	250000	500000

REVIEW PROBLEMS

1. A liquid contains 500 mcg. of a medicament per ml. Estimate the number of mg. of the medicament that 1 gallon of the liquid will contain.

2. Estimate the number of $\frac{1}{120}$-gr. tablets that can be made from 62.5 mg. of atropine sulfate.

3. A pharmacist weighed 0.015 Gm. of a substance on a balance sensitive to 0.004 Gm. Estimate the percentage of error that he may have incurred.

4. A pharmacist weighed 1 grain of atropine sulfate on a balance sensitive to 5 mg. Estimate the percentage of error that he may have incurred.

5. A pharmacist weighed 24 mg. of amphetamine sulfate on a balance sensitive to 0.005 Gm. Estimate the percentage of error that he may have incurred.

6. A sample of alcohol measured 10.3 ml. and weighed 8.05 Gm. Estimate the specific gravity of the sample.

7. A glass stopper loses 20.560 Gm. when suspended in water and 30.232 Gm. when suspended in a certain liquid. Estimate, to one decimal place, the specific gravity of the liquid.

8. A glass stopper loses 10.560 Gm. when suspended in water and 14.362 Gm. when suspended in a certain liquid. Estimate the specific gravity of the liquid.

9. Sulfuric acid has a specific gravity of 1.84. Estimate its specific volume.

10. A chemical costs $4.00 per lb. Estimate the approximate cost of ℥vi.

11. A prescription for 240 ml. of a liquid contains 15 mg. of atropine sulfate and has a dose of 8 ml. (a) Calculate the fraction of a grain of atropine sulfate that is contained in each dose. (b) **Assuming** a balance sensitivity of 10 mg., explain how you would **obtain** the 15 mg. of atropine sulfate with an error not greater than 5%. Use distilled water as the diluent.

12. How many 300-mg. tablets can be made from $\frac{1}{4}$ lb. of chloral hydrate?

13. A prescription calls for 18 gr. of phenacaine hydrochloride. If the phenacaine hydrochloride costs \$2.50 per 10 Gm., what is the cost of the amount needed for the prescription?

14. The estimated minimum daily requirement of riboflavin is 2 mg. How many micrograms of riboflavin are there in a capsule containing 3 times the minimum daily requirement?

15. A pharmacist weighed 20 mg. of strychnine alkaloid on a balance having a sensitivity of 5 mg. Calculate the maximum potential error in terms of percentage.

16. If a 90-ml. mixture contains 0.01 Gm. of morphine sulfate in each 5 ml., how many grains does the entire preparation contain?

17. If homatropine hydrobromide costs \$1.47 a gram, what is the cost of 2 grains?

18. A formula for capsules calls for $\frac{1}{100}$ gr. of nitroglycerin, $\frac{1}{16}$ gr. of phenobarbital, and $\frac{3}{4}$ ℳ of hyoscyamus tincture. What quantity (metric) of each ingredient is required to prepare 1000 capsules?

19. A certain injectable solution contains 30 micrograms of vitamin B_{12} per ml. How many milligrams of vitamin B_{12} are there in a 10-ml. vial of the solution?

20. ℞ Acetylsalicylic Acid   0.200
        Phenacetin   0.130
        Citrated Caffeine   0.06
        Codeine Phosphate   0.016
        M. et Ft. caps. tales no. 100
        Sig. One for pain.

How many grains of codeine phosphate are left in an original $\frac{1}{8}$-oz. bottle after the amount required for the prescription is used?

21. How many grains of strychnine sulfate are required to make f℥ ss of a solution containing $\frac{1}{84}$ gr. of the salt in each five minims of the solution?

22.   Thymol Iodide   8 Gm.
        Castor Oil   15 ml.
        Zinc Oxide Ointment, a sufficient quantity,
                    To make   100 Gm.

How much of each ingredient is required to prepare 5 lb. of the ointment?

23. The dose of a drug is 500 micrograms. How much should be given to a child 10 years old?

24. A formula for powders calls for $\frac{1}{4}$ gr. of belladonna extract, $\frac{1}{30}$ gr. of strychnine sulfate, and enough lactose to make 3 grains. How much of each ingredient should be used in preparing 25 powders?

25. A f℥ vi mixture contains, in each teaspoonful, $\frac{1}{6}$ gr. of codeine phosphate. How many grains of the salt are contained in the entire mixture?

26. Assuming a balance sensitivity of 0.008 Gm., what is the smallest amount, expressed in milligrams, that can be weighed with an error not greater than 5%?

27. A certain vehicle contains 0.05 ml. of amaranth solution per 100 ml. of finished product. Using a 10-ml. graduate, calibrated in units of 1 ml., explain how you would measure the amaranth solution required for 500 ml. of the vehicle. Use water as the diluent.

28. ℞   Iodine   gr. ss
        Mineral Oil   ℥ i
        Sig. Nasal spray.

In compounding, the pharmacist weighed the iodine on a torsion balance insensitive to quantities less than $\frac{1}{30}$ gr. Calculate the percentage of error that he might have incurred.

29. A volume of gas was collected at a barometric pressure of 762 mm. and a temperature of 25° C. Calculate (a) the equivalent pressure in inches and (b) the corresponding temperature on the F. scale.

30. How many grains of a chemical are left in a $\frac{1}{2}$-oz. bottle after enough of it is used to make 10,000 tablets, each containing $\frac{1}{250}$ gr.?

31. A manufacturer recommends that his product be stored at a temperature not exceeding 40° F. Express this temperature on the centigrade scale.

32. A pharmacist bought 4 oz. of phenobarbital. How many capsules, each containing $1\frac{1}{2}$ grains, can he prepare from this amount?

33. If sulfanilamide costs $2.50 per lb., what will be the cost of the sulfanilamide in 50 three-grain powders?

34. ℞ Menthol   gr. v
       Rose Oil   ♏ ss
       Liquid Petrolatum ad   ℥ i
       Sig. Nasal spray.

Change the quantities in this prescription to the metric system.

35. ℞ Menthol   0.05
       Tartar Emetic   0.015
       Potassium Citrate   4.0
       Orange Syrup ad   120.0
       Sig. 4 ml. t.i.d.

In compounding this prescription, the pharmacist weighed the 15 mg. of tartar emetic on a torsion balance having a sensitivity of 2 mg. Calculate the percentage of error that he may have incurred.

36.   Coal Tar   50 Gm.
      Bentonite   80 Gm.
      Water   300 ml.
      Hydrophilic Ointment   80 Gm.
      Zinc Oxide Paste, to make   1000 Gm.

How much of each ingredient should be used in preparing ℥ iv of the ointment?

37. If iodine costs $3.61 a pound, and iodine tincture contains 20 Gm. of iodine in a liter, what will be the cost of the iodine in one pint of the tincture?

38.   Aminophyllin   0.25 Gm.
      Phenobarbital Sodium   50 mg.
      Benzocaine   30 mg.
      Theobroma Oil ad   2.0 Gm.

Calculate the quantity of each ingredient to be used in preparing 250 suppositories.

39. ℞ Atropine Sulfate   gr. $\frac{1}{500}$
       Lactose ad   gr. iii
       Ft. chart. no. xxx
       Sig. One powder as directed.

Assuming a balance sensitivity of $\frac{1}{8}$ gr., explain how you would weigh the atropine sulfate with an error not greater than 5%.

40. Witch Hazel   12 ml.
     Glycerin   5 ml.
     Boric Acid Solution ad   100 ml.

How much of each ingredient should be used in preparing 5 gallons of the lotion?

41. ℞ Sol. Sodium Thiocyanate   ℥vi
        ℥i = gr. iii
        Sig. ℥i t.i.d.

How many grains of sodium thiocyanate are required in compounding the prescription?

42. How many tablets, each containing 10 micrograms, can be made from 0.250 Gm. of vitamin B_{12}?

43. ℞ Aspirin   0.2 Gm.
        Phenacetin   0.15 Gm.
        Caffeine   30 mg.
        Ft. caps. no. 100
        Sig. One capsule for pain.

Change the quantities in this prescription to the apothecaries' system.

44. Tannic Acid   gr. ii
     Belladonna Extract   gr. ¼
     Cocoa Butter ad   ℨss

Calculate the quantity of each ingredient in the formula that will be required to prepare 200 suppositories.

45. ℞ Strychnine Sulfate   0.0325
        Iron and Ammonium Citrate 6.0
        Aromatic Elixir ad   120.0
        Sig. 4 ml. a.c.

Change the quantities in this prescription to the apothecaries' system.

46. In compounding a prescription for ℥ss of a 20% sulfathiazole ointment, a pharmacist used 45 grains of sulfathiazole instead of the 48 grains that he should have used. Calculate the percentage of error that he may have incurred.

47. If an average No. 1 capsule weighs 90 mg., and no capsule in the lot varies in weight by more than plus or minus 10% of this average, what is the maximum percentage of error that could be incurred by using a capsule of this lot as a tare in filling other capsules of this lot with five grains of a medicinal substance?

48. In compounding a prescription for a saturated solution of potassium iodide, a pharmacist used ℥ vii of potassium iodide instead of the 455 grains called for. Calculate the percentage of error on the basis of what he should have used.

49. A pharmacist bought 1 oz. of a chemical from a wholesaler. He dispensed at different times, ℥ ii, 20 gr., ℈ iss, and ℥ ss. How many grains of the chemical were left?

50. If 1 f℥ of a solution contains 15 gr. of a chemical, how many grams would be contained in 180 ml.?

51. A vitamin liquid contains, in each 0.5 ml., the following:

Thiamine Hydrochloride	1 mg.
Riboflavin	400 mcg.
Ascorbic Acid	50 mg.
Nicotinamide	2 mg.

Calculate the quantity, expressed in grams, of each ingredient in 30 ml. of the liquid.

52. The dose of a certain antibiotic is 5 mg. per kilo of body weight. How many milligrams should be used for a person weighing 145 lb.?

53. How many 0.000065-Gm. doses can be prepared from 15 gr. of atropine sulfate?

54. If ammonium bromide costs 75 cents per pound, what is the cost of the salt in f℥ iv of a solution containing 5 gr. per teaspoonful?

55. Set up a formula for 5 lb. of a glycerogelatin containing 10 parts, by weight, of zinc oxide, 15 parts, by weight, of gelatin, 40 parts, by weight, of glycerin, and 35 parts, by weight, of water.

56. The average adult dose of a solution is 0.2 ml. What is the dose, expressed in minims, for a child 8 years old?

57. ℞
Atropine Sulfate	gr. $\frac{1}{100}$
Bismuth Subgallate	gr. iii
Alum	gr. i
Cocoa Butter q.s.	℥ ss

Ft. suppos. tales no. x
Sig. One at night.

Assuming a balance sensitivity of $\frac{1}{16}$ gr., explain how you would obtain the correct amount of atropine sulfate with an error not greater than 5%. Use bismuth subgallate as the diluent.

58. How many milligrams of thiamine are required to prepare 5 liters of an elixir, each 4 ml. to contain 100 mcg. of thiamine?

59. A balance has a sensitivity of 6 mg. Explain how you would weigh 60 mg. of a medicinal substance with an error not greater than 5%. Use lactose as the diluent.

60. ℞ Scopolamine Hydrobromide 0.005
Codeine Phosphate 0.150
Papaverine Hydrochloride 0.150
Div. in caps. no. 10
Sig. One capsule every three hours.

Only apothecaries' weights are available, the smallest being $\frac{1}{2}$ grain. Assuming a balance sensitivity of $\frac{1}{12}$ gr., explain how you would weigh the scopolamine hydrobromide with an error not greater than 5%.

61. ℞ Codeine Sulfate gr. iv
Ammonium Chloride ℨi
Squill Syrup ℥iss
Tolu Syrup ad ℥iv
Sig. ℨi for cough.

Convert the quantities in this prescription to the metric system.

62. ℞ Hydrochloric Acid 0.24
Merbromin 1.20
Glycerin 6.00
Distilled Water ad 60.00
Sig. External use.

Convert the quantities in this prescription to the apothecaries' system.

63. The contents of a vial of penicillin G potassium weigh 120 mg. This quantity represents the equivalent of 200,000 units of penicillin. How many grains are needed to prepare one ounce of an ointment containing 500 units per Gm.?

64. ℞ Procaine Penicillin G 300,000 units
Buffered Crystalline Penicillin G 100,000 units
Crystalline Dihydrostreptomycin 1 Gm.
Water for Injection ad 3 ml.
Make a multiple-dose vial containing 5 doses.
Sig. For intramuscular use only. Sterile.

To permit withdrawal of the five doses prescribed, an excess volume of 0.80 ml. must be present in the 15 ml. vial. How much of each of the three antibiotics should be used in compounding the prescription?

65. Dover's Powder contains 10% of powdered opium. A pharmacist prepared 15 Gm. of the powder. He removed the required quantity of powdered opium from a new one-ounce bottle of it and for inventory purposes marked the bottle with the quantity of powdered opium remaining in it. How many grains of powdered opium remained in the bottle?

66. In checking the inventory of narcotics in a hospital pharmacy, the checker found it to be kept in the metric system. The inventory showed 124.4 Gm. (4 one-ounce original bottles) of codeine sulfate on hand at the beginning of the inventory period. The prescriptions on file showed that 96 Gm. of codeine sulfate had been dispensed. On weighing the contents of the one-ounce bottle that remained, the checker found that only 17.4 Gm. was left, instead of 28.4 Gm. that apparently should have remained. What error, if any, had been made in the inventory?

67. If the adult dose of a drug is 0.03 mg., what is the dose for a child 10 years old?

68.   Salicylic Acid   0.5 Gm.
        Precipitated Sulfur   4.5 Gm.
        Hydrophilic Ointment   35.0 Gm.

Calculate the quantity of each ingredient to be used in making 5 lb. of the ointment.

69. The initial dose of a drug is 0.25 mg. per kilogram of body weight. How many milligrams should be prescribed for a person weighing 154 lb.?

70. The adult dose of belladonna extract is 15 mg. Calculate the dose, in grains, for a child 8 years old.

71. The average adult dose of a certain solution is 0.3 ml. (a) What is the dose for a child 6 years old? (b) If the solution is to be dispensed in a dropper bottle, the dropper of which calibrates 30 drops per ml., how many drops should be given to obtain the correct dose for the child?

72. An elixir is to contain 0.25 mg. of an alkaloid in each ml. How many grains of the alkaloid will be required to prepare 5 liters of the elixir?

73. A patient shows a temperature of 103.5° F. on a clinical thermometer. What would this temperature be on the centigrade scale?

74. A pharmacist purchased 5 gallons of alcohol. He used at different times Oii, 2 gallons, 8f℥, and ½ gallon. What volume, expressed as a compound quantity, remained?

75. One liter of Sodium Bromide Elixir contains 175 Gm. of sodium bromide. The official average dose of the elixir is 4 ml. What quantity, expressed in grains, of sodium bromide is contained in each dose?

76. ℞   Atropine Sulfate   gr. $\frac{1}{10}$
     Distilled Water ad   ℥i
     Sig. Five minims in each feeding.

Calculate the amount of atropine sulfate in each dose.

77. ℞   Lugol's Solution   ℥i
     Sig. Ten drops in water once a day.

Lugol's solution contains 5% of iodine. If the dispensing dropper calibrates 25 drops per ml., calculate the amount, in milligrams, of iodine in each dose of the solution.

78. ℞   Cyanocobalamin   10 mcg. per ml.
     Disp. 10-ml. sterile vial.
     Sig. 1.5 ml. every other week.

(a) How many micrograms of cyanocobalamin will be administered in a period of twelve weeks?
(b) How many milligrams of cyanocobalamin will there be in 10 ml. of this preparation?

79. ℞   Sol. Atropine Sulfate   10 ml.
      1:1000
     Sig. Five drops t.i.d. as directed.

Assuming that a standard U.S.P. dropper (20 drops per ml.) is used to measure the prescribed dose, calculate the amount, in grains, of atropine sulfate in each dose.

80. If 232 Gm. of a liquid measure 263 ml., what is its specific gravity?

81. If 4 f℥ of a liquid weigh 1932 gr., what is its specific gravity?

82. If the specific gravity of a liquid is 1.32, what is its specific volume?

83. If 5000 ml. of a syrup weigh 6565 Gm., calculate (a) its specific gravity and (b) its specific volume.

84. The specific gravity of strong ammonia solution is 0.897 at 25° C. Calculate the weight, in grams, of 10 pt. of the solution.

85. A pharmacist measures 4 ml. of sulfuric acid. The weight of the acid, sp. gr. 1.84, is found to be 7.85 Gm. What is the percentage of error in the measurement?

86. A prescription has a volume of six fluidounces and a dose of one dessertspoonful. It contains ℥ss of nitroglycerin spirit, 1% w/w, sp. gr. 0.82. What quantity, in grains, of nitroglycerin is contained in the prescribed dose?

87. Find the specific gravity of a sample of alcohol whose percentage strength is 44.35% (v/v) at 15.56° C. (Use the alcoholometric table.)

88. An alcohol sample has a specific gravity of 0.9477 at 15.56° C. Find the percentage strength (v/v). (Use the alcoholometric table.)

89. A pycnometer weighs 23.57 Gm. Filled with distilled water, it weighs 47.35 Gm. Filled with another liquid, it weighs 44.75 Gm. Calculate the specific gravity of the liquid.

90. The weight of a plummet in air is 10.97 Gm. Submerged in distilled water, it weighs 8.62 Gm. Submerged in another liquid it weighs 8.12 Gm. Calculate the specific gravity of the liquid.

91. The specific gravity of a sample is 1.478. Calculate its specific volume.

92. A glass plummet weighs 39.63 Gm. in air, 24.63 Gm. in water, and 28.83 Gm. in ether. Calculate (a) the specific gravity and (b) the volume, in ml., of 5 lb. of ether.

93. In making a syrup with a specific gravity of 1.313, 6800 Gm. of sucrose are dissolved in sufficient water to make 8000 ml. How many milliliters of water are used?

94. A piece of glass weighs 250 grains in air, 135 grains when submerged in water, and 145 grains when submerged in a certain acid. Calculate (a) the specific gravity of the acid, (b) the specific gravity of the glass, and (c) the specific volume of the acid.

95. A prescription contains 0.48 Gm. of hydrochloric acid. Calculate the volume, in milliliters, of hydrochloric acid with a specific gravity of 1.18 to be used in compounding the prescription.

96. A saturated solution contains, in each 100 ml., 100 Gm. of a substance. If the solubility of the substance is 1 Gm. in 0.7 ml. of water, what is the specific gravity of the saturated solution?

97. A formula for 200 Gm. of an ointment contains 10 Gm. of glycerin. How many milliliters of glycerin having a specific gravity of 1.25 should be used in preparing 1 lb. of the ointment?

98. A bottle holds 50.3 Gm. of water. When 8.6 Gm. of an insoluble powder are introduced and the bottle is filled with water, the contents weigh 55.4 Gm. What is the specific gravity of the powder?

99. A piece of wax weighs 12.5 Gm. in air, and a sinker weighs 24.6 Gm. when submerged in water. When submerged together in water, the wax and sinker weigh 22.4 Gm. What is the specific gravity of the wax?

100. A crystal of a chemical weighs 8.34 Gm. in air and 5.86 Gm. when submerged in an oil with a specific gravity of 0.825. What is the specific gravity of the crystal?

101. What is the volume, in milliliters, of 2 kilograms of a liquid with a specific volume of 1.125?

102. What is the weight, in kilograms, of 5000 ml. of a liquid with a specific gravity of 1.09?

103. If a substance weighs 10.6 Gm. and displaces 12.5 Gm. of water, what is its specific gravity?

104. A pharmacist has in stock 2½ wine gallons of 90 proof brandy. How many proof gallons of alcohol does this amount contain?

105. A manufacturing pharmacist bought 50 proof gallons of spirits. How many wine gallons does this represent if the purchase was 70% (v/v) alcohol?

106. If a liquid is 1.475 times as heavy as water and it is bought for $2.75 a pound, what is the cost of 240 ml.?

107. If the specific volume of a liquid is 1.264, what is its specific gravity?

108. A prescription calls for 2.5 Gm. of nitroglycerin spirit having a specific gravity of 0.82. How many milliliters should be used in compounding the prescription?

109. Find the specific gravity of a sample of alcohol whose percentage strength is 25.75% (v/v). (Use the alcoholometric table.)

110. A sample of alcohol has a specific gravity of 0.8038 at 15.56° C. By reference to the alcoholometric table find its percentage strength (v/v).

111. How many proof gallons of alcohol are there in 55 wine gallons of diluted alcohol that contains 48.5% (v/v) of pure alcohol?

112. If alcohol is taxed at $10.50 per proof gallon, what is the tax on 30 wine gallons of 70% (v/v) alcohol?

113. If 7.5 ml. of a substance weigh 325 grains, what is its specific gravity?

114. What is the volume, in fluidounces, of 250 grams of a liquid having a specific gravity of 1.11?

115. How many gallons of "proof spirit" are equivalent to 80 wine gallons of 75% (v/v) alcohol?

116. Ferric Sulfate solution contains ferric sulfate corresponding to 10% (w/w) of iron. How many grams of iron are there in 250 ml. of the solution having a specific gravity of 1.43?

117. ℞ Sat. Sol. Magnesium Sulfate   500 ml.
Sig. For compresses.

The solubility of magnesium sulfate is 1 Gm. in 1 ml. of water at 25° C. The volume of the resulting solution is 1.5 ml. How many grams of magnesium sulfate and how many milliliters of water should be used in compounding the prescription?

118. ℞ Sol. Homatropine Hydrobromide   30.0
1%
Buffer to pH 6.75
Sig. Homatropine eye drops.

At $1.68 per $\frac{1}{8}$ oz., what is the cost of the homatropine hydrobromide needed in the prescription?

119. ℞ Mercury Bichloride   0.1%
Distilled Water ad   ℥xvi
Sig. Dilute and use as directed.

How many tablets, each containing 0.125 Gm. of mercury bichloride, should be used in compounding the prescription?

120. ℞ Arsenic Trioxide
Strychnine Sulfate aa   0.5 mg.
Cofron Elixir ad   8.0 ml.
Disp. 480 ml.
Sig. 8 ml. t.i.d.

19

Arsenious acid solution contains the equivalent of 1% of arsenic trioxide. How many milliliters of the solution should be used to obtain the arsenic trioxide needed in the prescription?

121. Given a solution of potassium permanganate prepared by dissolving sixteen 0.325-Gm. tablets in enough distilled water to make 2600 ml.,

    (a) What is the percentage strength of the solution?

    (b) What is the ratio strength of the solution?

    (c) How many milliliters should be used in preparing 2 liters of a 1:8000 solution?

122. ℞   Potassium Permanganate   6.0
         Distilled Water ad   250.0
         Sig. Dilute two tablespoonfuls to one quart.
What is the percentage strength of the dilution?

123. Given a salt solution of 1:1500 concentration, what is:

    (a) the percentage strength?

    (b) the weight, in grains, of the salt per pint?

    (c) the weight, in micrograms, of the salt per ml.?

    (d) the number of milliliters required to prepare 2 liters of a 1:2500 solution?

124. ℞   Zinc Sulfate   0.1
         Adrenalin Chloride Sol.
            1:3000
         Benzalkonium Chloride Sol.
            1:10000   aa   30.0
         Sig. Eye drops.

How many milliliters of a 1:1000 adrenalin chloride solution and how many milliliters of a 0.5% benzalkonium chloride solution should be used in compounding the prescription?

125. ℞   Mercury Bichloride   480.0
           (15 ml. diluted to 500 ml. = 1:4000 sol.)
         Make sol. and color blue.
         Sig. Use as directed.

How many tablets, each containing 0.125 Gm. of mercury bichloride, should be used in compounding the prescription?

126. ℞   Potassium Permanganate Sol.   Oii
           1:8000
         Sig. For irrigation.

The potassium permanganate is to be obtained by using a 3% (w/v) stock solution. How much of the stock solution should be used?

127. How many grams of 40.5% (MgO equivalent) magnesium carbonate are required to prepare 24 bottles of magnesium citrate solution so that each bottle will contain the equivalent of 6.0 Gm. of MgO?

128. The formula for Albright's Solution "G" calls for 4.37 Gm. of anhydrous sodium carbonate (Na_2CO_3 - 106) in 1000 ml. of finished product. In preparing 5 gallons of the solution, how many grams of monohydrated sodium carbonate ($Na_2CO_3.H_2O$-124) should be used?

129. ℞ Sol. Potassium Permanganate   240.0 ml.
            0.01%
        Sig. For irrigation.

How many milliliters of a 1:200 stock solution of potassium permanganate should be used in compounding the prescription?

130. How many grams of 99% (w/w) acetic acid should be used in preparing 475 Gm. of 36% (w/w) acid?

131. A syrup containing 62% (w/w) of sucrose has a specific gravity of 1.295. How much sucrose should be used in preparing 1000 ml. of the syrup?

132. Calculate the number of milliliters of 28% (w/w) ammonia solution having a specific gravity of 0.90 required to prepare 1 gallon of 5% (w/v) ammonia solution?

133. What is the solubility of a chemical if 500 Gm. of an aqueous saturated solution yield a 70 Gm. residue upon evaporation?

134. ℞   Sol. Phosphoric Acid   180 ml.
            1:2000
        Sig. For bladder irrigation.

How many milliliters of 85% (w/w) phosphoric acid having a specific gravity of 1.71 should be used in compounding the prescription?

135. You are directed to prepare 10 liters of Hydriodic Acid Syrup. Only one pint of diluted hydriodic acid (10% w/v) is available. If the syrup contains 1.4% (w/v) of hydriodic acid, how many milliliters of a 19% (w/w) solution of hydriodic acid, sp. gr. 1.20, should be used in addition to the available material in preparing the syrup?

136. Eight hundred and seventy Gm. of sucrose are dissolved in 470 ml. of water, and the resulting volume is 1010 ml. Calculate

(a) the percentage strength (w/v) of the solution, (b) the percentage strength (w/w) of the solution and (c) the specific gravity of the solution.

137. In preparing 750 ml. of a syrup, 550 Gm. of sucrose were used. If the specific gravity of the syrup was 1.25, how many milliliters of water were used in preparing it?

138. A sample of opium contains 9.75% of morphine and 28.5% of moisture. What percentage of morphine will it contain after drying?

139. ℞   Nux Vomica Tincture   100.0
          Compound Gentian Tincture   200.0
          Compound Cinchona Tincture   60.0
          Aromatic Elixir   100.0
          Syrup ad   500.0
          Sig. 8 ml. before meals.

Nux vomica tincture contains 70% (v/v) of alcohol; compound gentian tincture, 45% (v/v) of alcohol; compound cinchona tincture, 50% (v/v) of alcohol; and aromatic elixir, 22% (v/v) of alcohol. Calculate the percentage of alcohol (v/v) in the prescription.

140. ℞   Calomel   0.6
          Alcohol 70% ad   15.0
          Sig. Use in right ear.

(a) How many milliliters of 95% (v/v) alcohol should be used in preparing 15 ml. of 70% (v/v) alcohol? (b) What is the percentage (w/v) of calomel in the prescription?

141. How many grams of a greaseless ointment base should be added to 4500 Gm. of an ointment containing 675 Gm. of sulfathiazole to prepare an ointment containing 5% of sulfathiazole?

142. ℞   Phenol $\frac{1}{4}$ %
          Alcohol   10%
          Tragacanth $\frac{1}{2}$ %
          Aluminum Sulfate $\frac{1}{10}$%
          Water ad   200.0 ml.
          Sig. Astringent lotion.

How much of each ingredient should be used in compounding the prescription?

143. ℞   Potassium Arsenite Solution   20.0
          Nux Vomica Tincture   30.0
          Essence of Pepsin ad   240.0
          Sig. Teaspoonful t.i.d.

Potassium arsenite solution contains the equivalent of 1% of arsenic trioxide. How many milligrams of arsenic trioxide will the patient receive per day?

144. In compounding a prescription for f℥i of a $\frac{1}{2}$% solution of copper sulfate, a pharmacist filtered the solution, losing f℥i. If he adjusted the volume to f℥i after the filtration, (a) what was the concentration of copper sulfate in the resulting product, and (b) what percentage of error did he incur?

145. ℞ Hydriodic Acid Syrup   30.0
       Terpin Hydrate Elixir   30.0 (42% of alcohol)
       Tolu Balsam Syrup   30.0
       Anise Water ad   120.0
       Sig. 4 ml. for cough.

If a concentration of 28% of alcohol is desired in the final product, how many milliliters of anise water should be replaced with alcohol?

146. ℞ Pine Tar   5 parts
       Zinc Oxide Paste   50 parts
       Disp. 240 Gm.
       Sig. Apply.

How many grams of pine tar should be used in compounding the prescription?

147. Ferric chloride tincture is prepared by diluting 350 ml. of ferric chloride solution, sp. gr. 1.35, with enough alcohol to make 1000 ml. If the solution contains the equivalent of 10% by weight of iron, how many milligrams of iron are represented in the usual dose of 0.6 ml. of the tincture?

148. A formula for a cosmetic cream calls for 0.04% of a mixture of 65 parts of methylparaben and 35 parts of propylparaben. How many grams of each should be used in formulating 10 lb. of the cream?

149. ℞ Phenol   50.0
       Glycerin   50.0
       Witch Hazel ad   500.0
       Sig. Dilute and use as directed.

In compounding the prescription, a pharmacist used 50 ml. of liquefied phenol (88% of phenol). Calculate the percentage of error that he may have incurred.

150. On June first you purchased 1 oz. of cocaine hydrochloride. During the month you dispensed the following:

| Cocaine ointment 3% | 1 ounce |
| Cocaine Solution 1% | 2 ounces |

Nausea powders each containing $\frac{1}{12}$ gr. of cocaine—no. 60

How many grains of cocaine hydrochloride were left in stock for the July first narcotic inventory?

151. On June first you had in stock $\frac{1}{2}$ oz. of cocaine hydrochloride. During the month you dispensed the following:

    (a) ℞   Cocaine Hydrochloride   1.25%
               Hydrophilic Ointment ad   ℥ ii
               Sig. Apply.

    (b) ℞   Cocaine Hydrochloride   4%
               Distilled Water ad   ℥ iv
               Sig. Use as directed.

    (c) ℞   Cocaine Hydrochloride   gr. $\frac{1}{10}$
               Cerium Oxalate   gr. iii
               D.T.D. cap. no. 100
               Sig. One capsule for nausea.

How many grains of cocaine hydrochloride were left for your July first narcotic inventory?

152. A preparation is to be made from opium tincture and must contain 0.06% of morphine. If opium tincture contains 10% of opium and if the opium contains 10% of morphine, how many milliliters of the tincture should be used to prepare 120 ml. of the product?

153. A manufacturing pharmacist has on hand four lots of belladonna tincture, containing 25 mg., 27 mg., 33 mg., and 35 mg. of alkaloids per 100 ml. How many gallons of each lot should he use to prepare 16 gallons of belladonna tincture containing 30 mg. of alkaloids per 100 ml.?

154. How much low alcoholic elixir (8%) and how much high alcoholic elixir (78%) should be used in preparing 1 gallon of iso-elixir containing 56% (v/v) alcohol?

155. U-80 insulin contains 80 units per ml. How many minims should be used to obtain 45 units of insulin?

156. A prescription calls for f℥ iv of a 15% solution of colloidal silver iodide. (a) How many grains of colloidal silver iodide should be used in compounding the prescription? (b) If colloidal silver iodide costs $1.35 per oz., what is the cost of the amount needed in the prescription?

157. ℞   Atropine Sulfate Tablets   gr. $\frac{1}{2000}$
     Make 80 such tablets.
     Sig. One tablet as directed.

How many grains of a 1:20 trituration should be used to obtain the atropine sulfate needed for the prescription?

158. A prescription calls for 48 capsules each containing $\frac{1}{40}$ gr. of strychnine sulfate. How many grains of a 10% trituration of strychnine sulfate should be used in compounding the prescription?

159. How many grams of mercury bichloride should be used in preparing 5 gallons of an 0.025% (w/v) solution?

160. How would you prepare f℥iv of a 4% (w/v) solution of cocaine hydrochloride?

161. If 30 grains of strong silver protein are dissolved in enough water to make f℥ii, what is the percentage strength (w/v) of the solution?

162. How many grams of zinc sulfate must be dissolved in 450 Gm. of water to make a 15% (w/w) solution?

163. How many grains of aniline violet should be used in preparing f℥vi of a 0.25% solution?

164. How much 4% (w/v) solution can be made from $\frac{1}{8}$ oz. of cocaine hydrochloride?

165. The specific gravity of a 64.7% (w/w) solution of sucrose in water is approximately 1.313. How many grams of sucrose and how many milliliters of water will be required to make 8000 ml. of a 64.7% (w/w) aqueous solution? What will be the percentage strength (w/v) of the solution?

166. How many grains of mercury bichloride are required to prepare 8 Gm. of an ophthalmic ointment containing 0.02% of mercury bichloride?

167. How much 0.1% (w/v) solution can be made from 5 Gm. of atropine sulfate?

168.   Stearic Acid   25%
        Potassium Hydroxide   q.s.
        Glycerin   8%
        Water ad   500 Gm.

How many grams of 88% potassium hydroxide should be used to saponify 35% of the stearic acid in the formula? The saponification value of stearic acid is 208.

169. A cold cream formula calls for 350 Gm. of white wax. The white wax to be used has an acid value of 23. How many grams of sodium borate which has an equivalent weight of 191 should be used in formulating the cream?

170. ℞   Nux Vomica Tincture   60.0
       Iso-Alcoholic Elixir ad   250.0
       Sig. 4 ml. t.i.d.

Nux vomica tincture contains 70% (v/v) of alcohol. How many milliliters of low alcoholic elixir (8%) and how many milliliters of high alcoholic elixir (78%) should be used in compounding the prescription?

171. How much of a 1:200 stock solution of atropine sulfate should be used in preparing f℥iv of a solution to contain $\frac{1}{200}$ gr. of atropine sulfate in each fluidrachm?

172. What volume of 0.1% solution can be made from 20 grains of methylrosaniline chloride?

173. How many grains of potassium iodide should be used in preparing ℥ss of the official solution of potassium iodide? The official solution is prepared by dissolving 100 Gm. of potassium iodide in sufficient distilled water to make 100 ml.

174. ℞   Sol. Mercury Oxycyanide   1:4000   10.0 ml.
       Sig. Use in the eyes.

If the mercury oxycyanide is to be obtained from a 0.04% solution, how many milliliters should be used?

175. How many grains of mercury bichloride should be used in preparing f℥iv of a solution such that f℥ii diluted to a quart will yield a 1:5000 solution?

176. ℞   Sol. Silver Nitrate   250.0
       (8 ml. diluted to a liter = 1:2500 sol.)
       Sig. Use as directed.

How much silver nitrate should be used in compounding the prescription?

177. How much sodium fluoride should be used in making one quart of a solution such that 10 ml. diluted to two quarts will give a 1:1,000,000 solution of fluorine?

178. How many milliliters of 95% (v/v) alcohol and of 30% (v/v) alcohol should be mixed to make 4000 ml. of 50% (v/v) alcohol?

179. How many pints of 95% (v/v) alcohol should be mixed with 12 pints of 22% (v/v) alcohol to make 60% (v/v) alcohol?

180. What is the percentage (v/v) of alcohol in a mixture of 600 ml. of 78% (v/v) alcohol, 1500 ml. of 42% (v/v) alcohol, and 800 ml. of 35% (v/v) alcohol?

181. How much mercury bichloride and how much 95% (v/v) alcohol should be used in preparing 1 gallon of a 1:1000 solution of mercury bichloride in 70% (v/v) alcohol?

182. How many grams of 95% (w/w) sodium hydroxide must be added to 1200 Gm. of a 5% (w/w) sodium hydroxide solution to raise the concentration to 9% (w/w)?

183. Calculate the number of milliliters of a 25% (w/v) stock solution of mild silver protein that should be used in preparing 60 ml. of a 10% (w/v) solution?

184. How much water should be added to 5 lb. of 28% (w/w) ammonia solution having a specific gravity of 0.90 to make 10% (w/v) ammonia solution?

185. In what proportion should two lots of a drug containing 2.35% and 4.25% of alkaloids be mixed to obtain a mixture containing 3.55% of alkaloids?

186. How many milliliters of 36% (w/v) solution of aluminum citrate are required to prepare 120 ml. of a 6% (w/v) solution?

187. ℞ Silver Nucleinate Solution
      20%   f℥ ss
      Sig. For the nose.
(a) How many grains of silver nucleinate should be used in compounding the prescription? (b) If silver nucleinate costs $1.20 per oz., what is the cost of the amount used in compounding the prescription?

188. Camphor liniment contains 20% (w/w) of camphor in cottonseed oil. How many grams of camphor and how many milliliters of cottonseed oil having a specific gravity of 0.915 are required to make 5 kilograms of camphor liniment?

189. White's ophthalmic ointment contains 1:3000 of mercury bichloride and 5:3000 of sodium chloride. Express these concentrations in terms of percentage.

190. ℞ Sol. Atropine Sulfate   ℥ iv
       0.05%
       Sig. As directed.

A stock solution contains 1 grain of atropine sulfate per fluidrachm. How many minims of the stock solution should be used in compounding the prescription?

191. If 1096 Gm. of ferrous iodide syrup having a specific gravity of 1.37 contain 58 Gm. of ferrous iodide, what is the percentage strength (w/v)?

192. How many minims of a stock solution containing 2 gr. of hyoscine to the fluidounce should be used in preparing a f℥ iv prescription, each teaspoonful dose of which is to contain 0.5 mg. of hyoscine?

193. ℞ Phenol Solution   240 ml.
            1:10
        Sig. As directed.

Phenol glycerite contains, in each 100 ml., 18 Gm. of phenol. How many milliliters of phenol glycerite should be used in compounding the prescription?

194. ℞ Resorcinol Monoacetate   10.0 ml.
        Castor Oil   5.0 ml.
        Ethyl Alcohol 85% ad   200.0 ml.
        Sig. Apply to scalp.

How many milliliters of 95% (v/v) ethyl alcohol and how much water should be used in compounding the prescription?

195. ℞ Neocalamine   20.0
        Liquefied Phenol   2.5
        Bentonite   2.5
        Lime Water ad   125.0
        Sig. For external use.

How many milliliters of 5% (w/v) bentonite magma should be used to obtain the bentonite needed for the prescription?

196. ℞ Precipitated Sulfur   12.5%
        Zinc Oxide Ointment ad   ℥ii
        Sig. Apply.

How many grains of precipitated sulfur should be used in compounding the prescription?

197. How many milliliters of water should be added to 10 lb. of phenol crystals (98% of phenol) to prepare liquefied phenol (88% of phenol)?

198. A hospital pharmacist has on hand 14 liters of iodine tincture (2%). How many milliliters of strong iodine tincture (7%) should he mix with it in order to get a product that will contain 3.5% of iodine?

199. ℞ Potassium Iodide Solution 10%
Ephedrine Sulfate Solution 3% aa ad ℥ ii
Sig. Use as directed.

How many minims of a saturated solution of potassium iodide (100%) should be used in compounding the prescription?

200. Saponated benzyl benzoate contains, in each 100 ml., 100 Gm. of benzyl benzoate. How many milliliters of saponated benzyl benzoate should be used in preparing 20 liters of benzyl benzoate lotion containing 25% (v/v) of benzyl benzoate? The specific gravity of benzyl benzoate is 1.120.

201. You have on hand 5 liters of a sodium hypochlorite solution, properly buffered and assaying 0.405%. How many milliliters of Hyclorite (4.05%) should be added to it to make Dakin's Solution (0.5%)?

202. Belladonna leaf contains 0.35% of alkaloids. Sixty ml. of a tincture prepared from this drug contain 22.05 mg. of alkaloids. Calculate the percentage strength of the tincture.

203. ℞ Sodium p-Aminobenzoate
Potassium p-Aminobenzoate
Equal parts of each to make a 10% solution
Dispense 250 ml.
Sig. Use as directed.

How many grams of p-aminobenzoic acid, of sodium bicarbonate, and of potassium bicarbonate should be used in compounding the prescription?

$$NH_2C_6H_4COOH + NaHCO_3 = NH_2C_6H_4COONa + H_2O + CO_2$$
$$NH_2C_6H_4COOH + KHCO_3 = NH_2C_6H_4COOK + H_2O + CO_2$$

204. ℞ Hydrochloric Acid 10% (w/w) 1000 ml.
Sig. Ten drops as directed.

In compounding the prescription, the pharmacist used 100 ml. of 37% (w/w) hydrochloric acid having a specific gravity of 1.18. If the specific gravity of the prescribed dilution is 1.05, what percentage of error was incurred in compounding the prescription?

205. ℞ Sol. Potassium Citrate 120.0
4 ml. = 0.3 Gm.
Sig. 4 ml. every 4 hours.

Assuming that no potassium citrate is available, how much potassium bicarbonate and how much citric acid are required to make the potassium citrate for this prescription?

$$3KHCO_3 + H_3C_6H_5O_7 = K_3C_6H_5O_7 + 3H_2O + 3CO_2$$

206. ℞ Sol. Histamine Phosphate 15.0 ml.
1:10000
Sig. As directed.

In compounding, the pharmacist used 5 ml. of a solution containing 0.275 mg. of histamine phosphate per ml. Calculate the percentage of error that he may have incurred.

207. How many milliliters of 36% (w/w) hydrochloric acid having a specific gravity of 1.17 are required to prepare 5 gallons of 10% (w/v) hydrochloric acid?

208. How many grams of mercury bichloride are required to prepare the ammoniated mercury needed to make 1000 Gm. of 5% ammoniated mercury ointment?

$$HgCl_2 + 2NH_4OH = HgNH_2Cl + NH_4Cl + 2H_2O$$

209. How many grams of 85% KOH are required to saponify completely 1350 ml. of a fixed oil having a specific gravity of 0.925 and a saponification value of 190?

210. How many grams of potassium chloride should be used in making a liter of a solution containing 5 mEq of potassium per ml.?

211. A proprietary product contains 3 gr. of $FeSO_4.2H_2O$ in each tablet. How much $FeSO_4.7H_2O$ does this represent?

212. In the monograph on Ferrous Sulfate Tablets, the U.S.P. states that an "equivalent amount of exsiccated ferrous sulfate may be used in place of $FeSO_4.7H_2O$ in preparing ferrous sulfate tablets." How many grams of exsiccated ferrous sulfate (179) could be used to replace the $FeSO_4.7H_2O$ (278) in preparing 10,000 tablets, each containing 0.3 Gm. of the hydrated salt?

213. The formula for Benedict's Solution calls for 100 Gm. of anhydrous sodium carbonate (Na_2CO_3—106) per liter of finished product. You are directed to prepare 5 liters of the solution. In checking the stock of the ingredients you find that only 250 Gm. of anhydrous sodium carbonate are available. How many grams of monohydrated sodium carbonate ($Na_2CO_3.H_2O$—124) should be used in addition to the anhydrous salt that is available?

214. A hospital requests you to prepare 5000 ml. of a solution of sodium p-aminosalicylate ($NH_2C_6H_3OHCOONa$—175), each 5 ml.

to contain 1 Gm. of p-aminosalicylic acid. How many grams of p-aminosalicylic acid ($NH_2C_6H_3OHCOOH - 153$) and how many grams of sodium bicarbonate ($NaHCO_3 - 84$) should be used in preparing the solution?

215. In making 500 ml. of potassium citrate solution, 40 Gm. of potassium bicarbonate ($KHCO_3 - 100$) and 30 Gm. of citric acid ($H_3C_6H_5O_7 - 210$) are used. How many grams of potassium citrate ($K_3C_6H_5O_7 - 324$) are there in the finished product?

216. The formula for sodium phosphate solution calls for 755 Gm. of sodium phosphate per liter of finished product. You are directed to prepare 4 liters of the solution. In checking the stock of the ingredients, you find that only 5 lb. of sodium phosphate are available. How many grams of exsiccated sodium phosphate (142) should be used in addition to the sodium phosphate (268) that is available?

217 How many grains of cocaine hydrochloride were left in a 1-oz. bottle after the following prescriptions have been dispensed?

℞ #1—Cocaine hydrochloride solution 4% f℥i

℞ #2—50 nausea powders each containing $\frac{1}{12}$ gr. of cocaine hydrochloride

218. ℞ Potassium Arsenite Solution   15.0
   Nux Vomica Tincture   30.0
   Essence of Pepsin ad   240.0
   Sig. ℥i t.i.d.

Potassium arsenite solution contains 1% of arsenic. What fraction of a grain of arsenic is contained in each dose of the prescription?

219. The adult dose of aureomycin is 250 mg. What would be the dose for a child 2 years old?

220. Calculate the quantity of ephedrine sulfate and of chlorobutanol required to make 500 ml. of a solution such that 30 ml. diluted to 100 ml. will represent 1:500 of ephedrine sulfate and 1:3000 of chlorobutanol.

221. ℞ Atropine Sulfate   0.5
   Benzalkonium Chloride Solution 100.0
     1:5000
   Sig. For the eye.

How many milliliters of a 12.8% solution of benzalkonium chloride should be used in compounding the prescription?

222. The solubility of salicylic acid in water is 1 Gm. in 460 ml. Calculate the percentage strength (w/w) of a saturated solution.

223. ℞ Salol   15.0   (Treat as a volatile oil)
        Expressed Almond Oil   40.0   (Fixed oil)
        Orange Syrup   100.0
        Water ad   240.0
        Sig. 4 ml. ex aq.

How many grams of acacia and how many milliliters of water should be used in preparing the primary of this emulsion?

224. ℞ Nitroglycerin   0.00075
        Phenobarbital   0.03
        Theobromine   0.5
        Ft. cap. tal. no. 20
        Sig. One capsule p.c.

How many milliliters of 1% (w/w) nitroglycerin spirit having a specific gravity of 0.82 should be used in compounding the prescription?

225.   White Wax   7.0 Gm.
        Sodium Borate   0.5 Gm.
        Precipitated Sulfur   5.0 Gm.
        Rose Water   17.5 ml.
        Mineral Oil   40.0 Gm.

How many milliliters of mineral oil having a specific gravity of 0.900 should be used in preparing 15 lb. of the medicated cream?

226. ℞ Sodium Fluoride   q.s.
        Distilled Water ad   500 ml.
        Sig. Sodium Fluoride Solution. 12 drops contain sodium fluoride = to 0.01 mg. of fluorine.

Assuming that a standard U.S.P. dropper (20 drops = 1 ml.) is to be used to measure the 12 drops, how much sodium fluoride should be used in compounding the prescription?

227. ℞ Solution Calcium Chloride   480 ml.
            10%
        Sig. Use as directed.

How many grams of calcium carbonate and how many milliliters of 35% (w/w) hydrochloric acid having a specific gravity of 1.18 should be used to prepare the calcium chloride ($CaCl_2.2H_2O$) for this prescription?

$$CaCO_3 + 2HCl + H_2O = CaCl_2.2H_2O + CO_2$$

228. ℞   Calcium Gluconate   0.5
         Phenobarbital   0.03
         Belladonna Extract   0.01
         Ft. caps. tales no. 40
         Sig. One capsule b.i.d.

Only belladonna tincture (10%) is available. If 1 Gm. of belladonna extract represents 4 Gm. of the drug, how many milliliters of belladonna tincture should be used in compounding the prescription?

229. ℞   Atropine Sulfate   gr. $\frac{1}{250}$
         Sodium Bicarbonate   gr. v
         Aspirin   gr. v
         Ft. pulv. no. xx
         Sig. One p.r.n.

Assuming that the atropine sulfate is available only in the form of dispensing tablets, each containing $\frac{1}{4}$ gr., explain how you would obtain the correct amount of atropine sulfate.

230. ℞   Belladonna Extract   gr. $\frac{1}{8}$
         Opium   gr. i
         Cocoa Butter q.s.
         Ft. suppos. no. xxiv
         Sig. One at night.

The only preparation of belladonna available is the tincture (10%). If 1 Gm. of the extract represents 4 Gm. of the drug, how much of the tincture should be used in compounding the prescription?

231. ℞   Pyribenzamine   gr. $\frac{3}{8}$
         Lactose   q.s.
         Ft. chart. no. x
         Sig. One, and repeat as directed.

Only tablets, each containing 50 mg. of Pyribenzamine, are available. How many tablets should be used in compounding the prescription?

232. If some hot water bottles are listed at $40 a dozen, with discounts of 50%, 15%, and 2%, what is the cost of one bottle?

233. Find the net amount of a bill of goods for $1240, with discounts of 20%, 12%, and 5%.

234. A certain preparation is listed at $5.00 per dozen, less 40% and 10%. At what price per unit must the preparation be sold to yield a gross profit of $66\frac{2}{3}$% on the cost?

235. Five gross of bottles cost $25.00, less discounts of 8%, 3%, and 1%. Calculate the net cost per bottle.

236. ℞   Potassium Permanganate   q.s.
         Distilled Water ad   250.0
         Ft. sol. 1:5000
         Sig. Irrigation.

How much of a stock solution containing 10 gr. of potassium permanganate per f℥i should be used in compounding the prescription?

237. ℞   Belladonna Tincture (65% alcohol)   30.0
         High Alcoholic Elixir (75% alcohol)   140.0
         Distilled Water ad   240.0
         Sig. 4 ml. ex aq.

Calculate the percentage of alcohol in the finished product.

238. ℞   Nitroglycerin   gr. $\frac{1}{400}$
         Lactose   q.s.
         Ft. tabs. tales no. 100
         Sig. One p.r.n.

How many milliliters of 1% (w/w) nitroglycerin spirit having a specific gravity of 0.82 should be used in compounding the prescription?

239. A pharmacist buys a bottle of vitamin capsules at $7.50 less discounts of 40% and 5%. At what price must the capsules be sold to yield a gross profit of 40% on the selling price?

240. What is the weight, in kilograms, of 5 gallons of a mixture of equal parts of simple syrup having a specific gravity of 1.313 and distilled water?

241. How many milliliters of a syrup having a specific gravity of 1.350 should be added to 5 liters of a syrup having a specific gravity of 1.250 to make a product having a specific gravity of 1.313?

242. Terpin hydrate elixir contains 40% (v/v) of glycerin. If glycerin (specific gravity 1.25) is bought for $28.62 for 50 lb., what is the cost of the amount needed to prepare 5 gallons of the elixir?

243. ℞   Potassium Arsenite Solution (5% alcohol)   40.0
         Compound Gentian Tincture (45% alcohol)   100.0
         Iso-Alcoholic Elixir q.s. ad   480.0
         Sig. 4 ml. as directed.

How many milliliters of low (10%) and how many milliliters of high (75%) alcoholic elixir should be used to give an alcoholic concentration of 45% in the finished product?

244. ℞ Nitroglycerin Spirit   3.0
       Lobelia Tincture   15.0
       Hydriodic Acid Syrup ad   120.0
       Sig. 4 ml. p.r.n.

Assuming that nitroglycerin is available only in the form of tablets, each containing $\frac{1}{100}$ gr., how many tablets should be used in compounding the prescription? Nitroglycerin Spirit (sp. gr. 0.82) contains 1% (w/w) of nitroglycerin.

245. ℞ Magnesium Oxide   gr. ii
       Papaverine Hydrochloride   gr. i
       Pyribenzamine   gr. $\frac{1}{3}$
       Ft. cap. D.T.D. no. xxiv
       Sig. One capsule as directed.

How many tablets, each containing 50 mg. of Pyribenzamine, should be used in compounding the prescription?

246. How many milliliters of purified water must be added to 1 lb. of wool fat to convert it to lanolin containing 25% of water?

247. In a solubility determination, 100 Gm. of a chemical dissolved in 300 ml. of distilled water at 25° C., and the volume of the resulting solution was 340 ml. Calculate the percentage strength (w/v) of the solution.

248. How many grams of ichthammol should be added to 5 lb. of 10% ichthammol ointment to make an ointment containing 50% of ichthammol?

249. How many grains of petrolatum should be mixed with the official 1% yellow mercuric oxide ointment to make ʒi of 0.25% ointment?

250. ℞ Atropine Sulfate   gr. $\frac{1}{250}$
       Ft. cap. tal. no. 60
       Sig. One as directed.

How many grains of a 1:12 trituration of atropine sulfate should be used in compounding the prescription?

251. ℞ Sat. Sol. Potassium Iodide   ʒi
       Sig. Ten drops in water.

Potassium Iodide Solution, N.F., contains 100 Gm. of potassium iodide in 100 ml. of solution. In compounding the pre-

20

scription, a pharmacist used ℥vii of potassium iodide and enough water to make one fluidounce. Calculate the percentage of error on the basis of the correct quantity of potassium iodide that he should have used.

252. ℞   Stearic Acid   40.0
           Liquid Petrolatum   10.0
           Triethanolamine   10.0
           Coconut Oil Soap   80.0
           Distilled Water   50.0
           Glycerin   10.0
           Sig. Apply at night.

How many grams of 85% KOH should be used in preparing the coconut oil soap required for making 2 lb. of this cream? Coconut oil soap contains 40% (w/w) of coconut oil, and the saponification value of coconut oil is 260.

253. ℞   Copaiba   10.0   (Treat as a volatile oil)
           Expressed Almond Oil   10.0   (Fixed oil)
           Syrup   20.0
           Distilled Water ad   120.0
           Sig. 4 ml. p.c.

How many grams of acacia and how many milliliters of water should be used in preparing the primary of this emulsion?

254. ℞   Epinephrine Bitartrate   0.60
           Sodium Bisulfite   0.01
           Sodium Chloride   0.20
           Distilled Water ad   30.0
           Sig. Use in the eyes.

How many milliliters of a 0.9% sodium chloride solution should be used to obtain the sodium chloride for the prescription?

255. A formula for a cosmetic cream calls for 5 lb. of stearic acid. How many grams of 88% potassium hydroxide are required to neutralize 30% of the stearic acid? The saponification value of stearic acid is 208.

256. In preparing 1000 Gm. of coconut oil soap, you are directed to use 400 Gm. of coconut oil having a saponification value of 260. How many milliliters of dekanormal solution of potassium hydroxide should be used to saponify the oil?

257. The formula for medicinal soft soap calls for 380 Gm. of a vegetable oil and 91.7 Gm. of potassium hydroxide (85%). On the basis of these figures, what must be the saponification value of a

vegetable oil in order that it may be used in the manufacture of the soap?

258. ℞ Atropine Sulfate   0.00013
        Aspirin   0.3
        Phenacetin   0.03
        Ft. caps. tales no. xx
        Sig. One capsule every three hours.

If the atropine sulfate is available only in the form of tablets, each containing $\frac{1}{150}$ gr., how many tablets should be used in compounding the prescription?

259. ℞ Quinine Sulfate   gr. ii
        Arsenic Trioxide   gr. $\frac{1}{50}$
        Strychnine Sulfate   gr. $\frac{1}{40}$
        Lactose   q.s.
        Ft. caps. tales no. xv
        Sig. One capsule a.c.

(a) How many grains of a 1 : 10 trituration of arsenic trioxide should be used in compounding the prescription? (b) If the strychnine sulfate is available only in the form of tablets, each containing $\frac{1}{30}$ gr., how many tablets should be used?

260. What is the solubility of a chemical if 1200 Gm. of a saturated alcoholic solution yield a 75-Gm. residue upon evaporation? The specific gravity of alcohol is 0.8.

261. ℞ Scopolamine Hydrobromide   0.25%
        Phenacaine Hydrochloride   0.5%
        Sodium Chloride   q.s.
        Distilled Water ad   50.0
        Ft. isoton. sol.
        Sig. For the eyes.

How many milliliters of 0.9% sodium chloride solution should be used in compounding the prescription?

262. ℞ Procaine Hydrochloride   2%
        Ephedrine Hydrochloride   0.1%
        Sodium Chloride   q.s.
        Distilled Water ad   1000 ml.
        Ft. isoton. sol.
        Sig. For injection.

How many grams of sodium chloride should be used in compounding the prescription?

263. ℞   Ephedrine Sulfate
    Phenacaine Hydrochloride aa   0.5%
    Dextrose   q.s.
    Distilled Water ad   30.0
    Ft. isoton. sol.
    Sig. Use in the nostrils.

How many grams of dextrose should be used in compounding the prescription?

264. ℞   Tubocurarine Chloride   0.6
    Chlorobutanol   0.5%
    Sodium Chloride   q.s.
    Distilled Water ad   20.0
    Ft. isoton. sol.
    Sig. To be administered by the nurse.

Tubocurarine chloride (786) is a 3-ion electrolyte, dissociating 85%. How many grams of sodium chloride should be used in compounding the prescription?

265. ℞   Phenobarbital Sodium   15 mg. per ml.
    Sodium Chloride   q.s.
    Distilled Water ad   20 ml.
    Ft. isoton. sol. and sterilize.
    Sig. To be administered by the M.D.

How many grams of sodium chloride should be used in compounding the prescription?

266. A prescription has a volume of f℥iv and a dose of a half teaspoonful. It contains one and a half fluidrachms of nitroglycerin spirit (1% w/w) having a specific gravity of 0.82. Calculate the amount of *nitroglycerin* in each dose.

267. ℞   Quinine Sulfate   gr. iii
    Arsenic Trioxide   gr. $\frac{1}{80}$
    Nux Vomica Extract   gr. $\frac{1}{12}$
    Ft. cap. tales no. xx
    Sig. One capsule t.i.d. a.c.

The tincture (10%) is the only preparation of nux vomica available. If 1 Gm. of the extract represents 6 Gm. of the drug, how much of the tincture should be used in compounding the prescription?

268. ℞   Ephedrine Hydrochloride   2%
         Chlorobutanol   0.2%
         Dextrose   q.s.
         Distilled Water ad   120.0
         Ft. isoton. sol.
         Sig. Nasal spray.

How many grams of anhydrous dextrose should be used in compounding the prescription?

269.   Papaverine Hydrochloride   50 mg. per ml.
         Sodium Chloride   q.s.
         Distilled Water ad   30.0 ml.
         Label: Papaverine Injection—1 ml. = 50 mg.

Papaverine hydrochloride has a molecular weight of 376. Its dissociation factor is 1.8. How many grams of sodium chloride should be used to make this solution isotonic with the blood?

270. ℞   Turpentine Oil   20%
         Licorice Syrup
         Water aa ad   ℥ vi
         Sig. Teaspoonful.

How many grams of acacia and how many milliliters of water should be used in preparing the primary of this emulsion?

271. ℞   Holocaine Hydrochloride   0.5%
         Zinc Sulfate   0.5%
         Boric Acid   q.s.
         Distilled Water ad   ℥ ii
         Ft. isoton. sol.
         Sig. One drop in right eye.

How many milliliters of a 3% boric acid solution should be used in compounding the prescription?

272. ℞   Belladonna Tincture   60.0
         Sodium Phenobarbital   1.0
         Peppermint Water ad   240.0
         Sig. 4 ml. once a day.

Belladonna tincture contains 0.03% (w/v) of alkaloids. Express the amount, in milligrams, of alkaloids represented in each dose of the prescription.

273. ℞   Digitoxin Solution (Oral)   ℥ ii
         M. et Ft. sol.—0.01 mg. per ♏ ii
         Sig. ♏ iv in a.m. with meals.

If the dispensing dropper calibrates 600 drops per f℥i, how many milligrams of digitoxin should be used in compounding the prescription?

274. If some toothbrushes are bought at $4.50 a dozen, less 40% and 2%, what is the net cost of one toothbrush, and at what price must it be sold so that a gross profit of 50% on the selling price will be realized?

275. Calculate the pH of a solution in which the H-ion concentration is 5.9×10^{-6}.

276. A certain elixir has a pH of 4.1. Calculate its H-ion concentration.

277. ℞ Potassium Acetate   50.0
      Wintergreen Water ad   500.0
      Sig. 4 ml. ex aq.

Assuming that no potassium acetate is available, how much potassium bicarbonate and how much 36% (w/w) acetic acid, specific gravity 1.050, will be required to make the potassium acetate for this prescription?

$$KHCO_3 + HC_2H_3O_2 = KC_2H_3O_2 + CO_2 + H_2O$$

278. ℞ Tyrothricin   500 micrograms per Gm.
      Hydrophilic Ointment q.s. ad 100 Gm.
      Sig. Apply as directed.

How many milliliters of a 2.5% tyrothricin solution should be used to obtain the tyrothricin needed for this prescription?

279. A pharmacist buys 5000 capsules for $45.00 with discounts of 40% and 5%. At what price per hundred must he sell the capsules in order to realize a gross profit of 50% on the selling price?

280. ℞ Ichthammol   250 Gm.
      Hydrophilic Petrolatum ad 1000 Gm.
      Sig. Use as directed.

In compounding, you discover that through an error 1000 Gm. of hydrophilic petrolatum were used. How many grams of ichthammol should be added to the resulting product in order to make one containing the intended concentration of ichthammol?

281.   Sorbitan Sesquioleate   5%
         Petrolatum   45%
         Water   50%

A mixture (1 and 9) of the first two ingredients absorbs 18 times its weight of water. How much additional water can be added to 2000 Gm. of the above product to obtain one containing the maximum amount of water that can be absorbed?

282. ℞ Sol. Atropine Sulfate   120.0
          (4 ml. = gr. $\frac{1}{1000}$)
          Sig. 4 ml. as directed.

Assuming that the atropine sulfate is available only in the form of tablets, each containing $\frac{1}{4}$ gr., explain how you would obtain the amount of atropine sulfate needed for this prescription.

283. The pH value of a certain buffer solution is 9.2. Calculate the H-ion concentration of the solution.

284. A prescription specialty lists at $14.50 per pint, less discounts of 40% and 2%. At what price must f℥i of the specialty be sold to yield a gross profit of 50% on the selling price?

285. Calculate the pH of a solution in which the H-ion concentration is 0.000000092 gram-ion per liter.

286. A gas occupies a volume of 1140 ml. at 27° C. and 775 mm. pressure. Calculate the volume of the gas at standard temperature and pressure.

287. ℞ Atropine Sulfate   2%
          Boric Acid   q.s.
          Distilled Water ad   100 ml.
          Ft. isoton. sol.
          Sig. For the eyes.

(a) How many grams of boric acid should be used? (b) Boric Acid Solution, N. F., contains 5% of boric acid. How many milliliters of the solution should be used to obtain the amount of boric acid needed in the prescription? (c) You are directed to sterilize this prescription at a temperature not exceeding 105° C. Calculate the corresponding F. temperature.

ANSWERS TO PRACTICE PROBLEMS

NOTE: *Answers are given to all problems in Chapter I (Some Fundamental of Measurement and Calculation) and Appendix F (Exponential and Logarithmic Notation); elsewhere, only the answers to odd-numbered problems are given.*

Chapter I

ROMAN NUMERALS

(Page 12)

1. (a) xviii
   (b) lxiv
   (c) lxxii
   (d) cxxvi
   (e) xcix
   (f) xxxvii
2. (a) 45
   (b) 1000
   (c) 48
   (d) 64
   (e) 16
   (f) 84
3. (a) 5, 15, 80, 4
   (b) $1\frac{1}{2}$, 40, 6, $\frac{1}{2}$

SIGNIFICANT FIGURES

(Page 19)

1. (a) Six
   (b) Four
   (c) Three
   (d) Three
   (e) Seven
   (f) One
2. (a) Two
   (b) Three
   (c) Two
   (d) Four
   (e) Five
   (f) Two
   (g) Four
   (h) Three

SIGNIFICANT FIGURES *(continued)*

   (i) Two
   (j) Two
3. (a) 32.8
   (b) 200
   (c) 0.0363
   (d) 21.6
   (e) 0.00944
   (f) 1.08
   (g) 27.1
   (h) 0.862
   (i) 3.14
4. (a) 0.001
   (b) 34.795
   (c) 0.005
   (d) 6.130
   (e) 14.900
5. 330.8 grains
6. 420.5 grams
7. 38 grains
8. 40 grains
9. (a) 6.38
   (b) 1.0
   (c) 90.2
   (d) 240 grains
   (e) 6.0 grams
   (f) 210.55 grams
   (g) 0.068 grain
   (h) 0.054 gram
   (i) 630
   (j) 230
   (k) 2.6
   (l) 0.0267
   (m) 140
   (n) 23.808

ESTIMATION

(*Page 25*)

NOTE: *Estimated answers will vary with methods used. Some calculated answers are here given in parentheses for comparison.*

1. Six zeros
2. Four zeros
3. Three zeros
4. Two zeros
5. 20,500
   (*19,881*)
6. 22,000
   (*21,405*)
7. 14,500
   (*14,320*)
8. 36,000
   (*35,314*)
9. 3500
   (*3580*)
10. 28,000
    (*28,985*)
11. $20 \times 20 = 400$
    (*374*)
12. $30 \times 30 = 900$
    (*868*)
13. $8 \times 50 = 400$
    (*384*)
14. $20 \times 38 = 760$
    (*722*)
15. $30 \times 60 = 1800$
    (*1736*)
16. $40 \times 77 = 3080$
    (*3003*)
17. $40 \times 40 = 1600$
    (*1638*)
18. $120 \times 90 = 10,800$ or $11,000$
    (*11,500*)
19. $360 \times 100 = 36,000$
    (*35,770*)

ESTIMATION (*continued*)

20. $473 \times 100 = 47,300$
    (*48,246*)
21. $600 \times 200 = 120,000$
    (*121,584*)
22. $600 \times 120 = 72,000$
    (*73,688*)
23. $650 \times 20 = 13,000$
    (*12,825*)
24. $1000 \times 13 = 13,000$
    (*12,974*)
25. $7000 \times 800 = 5,600,000$
    (*5,435,670*)
26. $1000 \times 1000 = 1,000,000$
    (*1,042,956*)
27. $8000 \times 10,000 = 80,000,000$
    (*82,286,560*)
28. $7000 \times 20 = 140,000$
    (*136,477*)
29. $5000 \times 1000 = 5,000,000$
    (*4,917,078*)
30. $2300 \times 6000 = 13,800,000$
    (*13,875,543*)
31. $2\frac{1}{2} \times 14 = 35$
    (*$36\frac{1}{4}$*)
32. $800 \div 3 = 266$
    (*$266\frac{2}{3}$*)
33. $21 \times 7 = 147$
    (*$142\frac{2}{6}$*)
34. $\frac{3}{4} \times 800 = 600$
    (*612*)
35. $840 \div 3 = 280$
    (*283.76*)
36. $6 \times 7000 = 42,000$
    (*41,557*)
37. $2 \times 700 = 1400$
    (*1438.812*)
38. $0.02 \times 500 = 10$
    (*9.4304*)
39. $(7 \times 7000) \div 100 = 490$
    (*504.6426*)
40. $100 \times 0.0031 = 0.31$
    (*0.3038*)

Estimation (continued)

41. $6 \times 70 = 420$
(*411.079*)
42. $7500 \div 10 = 750$
(*728.8947*)
43. $170 \div 20 = 8.5$
(*9.0*)
44. $(\frac{2}{3} \times 165)$ or $110 \div 10 = 11$
(*11*)
45. $180 \div 100 \div 20 = 0.09$
(*0.08*)
46. $300 \div 15 = 20$
(*21.39*)
47. $16 \div 320 = \frac{1}{20}$ or 0.05
(*0.05*)
48. $3600 \div 4 = 900$
(*900*)
49. $8400 \div 7 = 1200$
(*1200.7*)
50. $1100 \div 100 = 11$
(*11*)
51. $9800 \div 5 = 1960$
(*2000*)
52. $1700 \div 6 = 283$
(*298.5*)
53. $0.01 \div 5 = 0.002$
(*0.002149*)
54. $200 \div 4 = 50$
(*48.6*)
55. $19 \div 0.25 = 19 \times 4 = 76$
(*73.9*)
56. $19 \div 50 = 38 \div 100 = 0.38$
(*0.409*)
57. $460 \div 8 = 57.5$
(*57.3*)
58. $4500 \div 0.50 = 4500 \times 2 = 9000$
(*9340*)
59. 90,000
60. 300
61. 3
62. 0.01 or $\frac{1}{100}$
63. 3.5

Estimation (continued)

64. 100
65. 100
66. 20
67. 160
68. $1,250
69. $400
70. $225
71. $400
72. 0.9 Gm.
73. 750 doses
74. $15
75. $10

Percentage of Error

(*Page 29*)

1. $6\frac{2}{3}$ or 6.7%
2. 8%
3. 5%
4. 2.4%
5. 6.3%
6. 1.4%
7. 0.1%
8. 5.2%
9. 6.7%
10. 0.24 gram
11. $1\frac{2}{3}$ grains
12. 0.2 gram
13. 8.33%
14. 2.4 grains

Aliquot Method of Measuring

(*Page 34*)

1. (a) 100 ml.
(b) 3 mg.
2. Weigh 120 mg.
Dilute to 1500 mg.
Weigh 150 mg.

ALIQUOT METHOD OF MEASURING
(continued)

3. Weigh   80 mg.
   Dilute to   1600 mg.
   Weigh   100 mg.
4. Weigh   1 gr.
   Dilute to   10 gr.
   Weigh   1 gr.
5. Weigh   300 mg.
   Dilute to   6000 mg.
   Weigh   400 mg.
6. Weigh   4 gr.
   Dilute to   20 gr.
   Weigh   5 gr.
7. Weigh   160 mg.
   Dilute to   4000 mg.
   Weigh   200 mg.
8. Weigh   3 gr.
   Dilute to   16 gr.
   Weigh   4 gr.
9. Measure   1 ml.
   Dilute to   10 ml.
   Measure   6 ml.
10. Measure   1 ml.
    Dilute to   8 ml.
    Measure   6 ml.
11. Measure   1 ml.
    Dilute to   10 ml.
    Measure   2 ml.
12. Measure   1 ml.
    Dilute to   8 ml.
    Measure   1 ml.
13. Measure   5 ℳ
    Dilute to   50 ℳ
    Measure   20 ℳ
14. Weigh   2 gr.
    Dissolve in enough
    alcohol to make   25 ml.
    Measure   2 ml.
15. Weigh   0.090 Gm.
    Dissolve in enough
    water to make   6 ml.
    Measure   1 ml.

COMMON AND DECIMAL FRACTIONS

(Page 41)

1. (a) $\frac{37}{32}$ gr. or $1\frac{5}{32}$ gr.
   (b) $\frac{13}{600}$ gr.
   (c) $\frac{77}{480}$ gr.
2. (a) $\frac{209}{64}$ or $3\frac{17}{64}$ gr.
   (b) $\frac{1}{120}$ gr.
   (c) $\frac{5}{6}$ gr.
3. (a) $\frac{225}{48}$ or $4\frac{11}{16}$
   (b) $\frac{105}{4}$ or $26\frac{1}{4}$
   (c) $\frac{9}{2500}$
4. (a) $\frac{48}{3}$ or 16
   (b) $\frac{1}{60000}$
   (c) $\frac{25}{2}$ or $12\frac{1}{2}$
5. $\frac{189}{200}$ grain
6. 75 doses
7. $\frac{59}{160}$ grain
8. $\frac{223}{60}$ or $3\frac{43}{60}$ grains
9. $\frac{1}{90}$ grain
10. $\frac{1}{300}$ grain
11. 80 doses
12. 2.048
13. 1.565
14. 2000 doses
15. $\frac{1}{40}$ grain
16. $\frac{1}{96}$ grain
17. $\frac{8}{75}$ grain
18. 2 grains

Chapter II

RATIO AND PROPORTION

(Page 48)

1. $32.40
3. 0.91 gram
5. $7.59
7. 40 pounds
9. 25.6 grams
11. 80 grains
13. 14 grains
15. $72\frac{1}{2}$ pounds

Chapter III

THE METRIC SYSTEM

(Page 58)

1. 502.550 Gm.
3. 0.000025 Gm.
5. 0.0005 Gm.
7. 500 doses
9. 0.1125 mg.
11. 1006.650 Gm.
13. 250 ml.
15. 0.0985 Gm., or 98.5 mg.
17. 83.33 ml.
    5.4 mg.
19. 1,256,000 mcg.
    1256 mg.
    0.001256 Kg.
21. 2.69375 or 2.694 Gm.
23. 114 Gm.
25. 30 mg.
27. 3999.5 mg.—which rounds off to what you started with: 4000 mg., or 4 Gm.
29. 152.625 or 152.6 Gm.
31. 4.60 Gm.
33. 23.88 mg.
35. 20,410 Gm. per 25.4 mm.
37. 0.125 mg.
39. 134.759 Gm.
41. 0.625 mg.
43. 35.09 Gm.
45. 9 Gm.
    13 Gm.
    0.26 Gm.
47. 363.025 or 363.0 mg.
49. 368.25 or 368 mg.
51. 4 tablets
53. 0.0125 Gm.
    12.5 Gm.
    0.125 Gm.
55. 13 mcg.
57. 300 mg.

Chapter IV

THE COMMON SYSTEMS

(Page 68)

1. (a) 150 gr.
   (b) 1050 gr.
   (c) 530 gr.
   (d) 90 gr.
3. (a) ℨ ½℈ 8 gr., or
       ℨ 1℈ 18 gr.
   (b) ℨ 2℈ ½℈ 5 gr., or
       ℨ ½℈ 1℈ 5 gr.
   (c) ℨ 1℈ 1℈ ½℈, or
       ℥ 1½℈
   (d) ℈ ½℈ 5 gr.
   (e) ℈ ½℈ 6 gr., or
       ℈ 1℈ 16 gr.
5. 1 qt. 10 f℥
7. 16 doses
9. 320 bottles
11. 350 capsules
13. 218.75 or 218 tablets
15. 8 f℥
17. ½ gr.
    1½ gr.
    6 gr.
19. 72 cents
21. 6562 doses
23. 1750 tablets
25. 84.4 gr.
27. 370 gr.

Chapter V

CONVERSION

(Page 75)

1. $3\frac{3}{20}$ in.
   $4\frac{7}{10}$ in.
3. $31\frac{1}{2}$ in.
5. 4.93 ml.
7. 8.161 L.
9. 0.0000394 in., or
   $\frac{1}{25400}$ in.

Conversion (*continued*)

1. 3.94 or 4 in.
3. 12,123.7 or 12,120 ml.
5. 30.9 or 31 gr.
   2.76 or $2\frac{3}{4}$ in.
7. 308 tablets
9. (a) $\frac{1}{926}$ Gm., or
      1.08 or 1.1 mg.
   (b) 7.39 or 7.4 ml.
   (c) 24.375 or 24 mg.
   (d) 1.84 or 1.8 ml.
   (e) 0.325 mg.
21. 89.8 lb. per 3.0 in.
23. 0.00077 or $\frac{1}{1300}$ gr.
25. 12 cents
27. 2392 or 2400 tablets
29. 65 mcg.
31. 0.65 mg.
33. 50 doses
35. 1.04 Gm.

Chapter VI
Calculation of Doses
(*Page 84*)

Note: *In calculating the number of* *ses contained in a specified quantity* *medicine, disregard any fractional* *mainder.*

1. 800 doses
3. 30 doses
5. 48 doses
7. 2 teaspoonfuls
9. 4 teaspoonfuls
11. 6 f℥
13. $\frac{1}{130}$ gr.
15. $\frac{1}{240}$ gr.
17. $\frac{1}{4}$ gr.
19. $\frac{1}{13}$ gr.
21. $1\frac{1}{2}$ gr.
23. 33 mg.
    0.33 ml.
25. $\frac{4}{65}$ gr.

Calculation of Doses (*continued*)

27. 5.6 or 6 ℳ
    $\frac{1}{8}$ gr.
29. $\frac{4}{5}$ gr.
31. 180 gr. or ℥ iii
    240 ℳ or f℥ vi
33. $\frac{1}{4}$ gr.
35. 60 ℳ
37. 96 gr.
39. 12 gr.
41. $\frac{19}{65}$ gr.
43. 1.84 Gm.
45. 0.025 Gm.
47. 2 gr.
49. $\frac{1}{360}$ gr.
51. $\frac{1}{13}$ gr.
53. $\frac{1}{550}$ gr.
55. $\frac{1}{3000}$ gr.
57. (a) 0.125 ml.
    (b) 3 drops

Chapter VII
Reducing and Enlarging Formulas
(*Page 94*)

1.   45   ml.
       0.9 Gm.
       3.6 Gm.
   ad 180   ml.
3.   0.57 Gm.
       0.34 Gm.
       568   Gm.
       568   Gm.
       272   Gm.
       114   Gm.
   ad 2270   Gm., or 5 lb.
5.   1725   Gm.
       90.8 Gm.
       416   Gm.
       227   ml.
   ad 4540   Gm., or 10 lb.

REDUCING AND ENLARGING FORMULAS

(continued)

7.		4.73 Gm.
		2.36 Gm.
		2.36 Gm.
	9.46 or	9.5 ml.
		2.36 Gm.
		14.2 Gm.
	0.47 or	0.5 ml.
	ad 473	ml., or 1 pt.
9.		113.5 Gm.
		113.5 Gm.
		227 Gm.
	Total:	454 Gm., or 1 lb.
11.		200 ml.
		50 ml
		750 ml.
	Total:	1000 ml., or 1 L.
13.		430 ml.
		860 ml.
		1075 ml.
	Total:	2365 ml., or 5 pt.
15.	118.3 or	118 ml.
	59.13 or	59 ml.
	177.4 or	177 Gm.
	ad 2365	ml., or 5 pt.
17.	353.1 or	353 Gm.
		25 Gm.
	100.9 or	101 Gm.
	201.8 or	202 Gm.
		1589 Gm.
	Total:	2270 Gm., or 5 lb.
19.		640 gr., or ʒi ʒii ℈ii
		1280 gr., or ʒii ʒv ℈i
	Total:	1920 gr., or ʒiv

REDUCING AND ENLARGING FORMUL

(continued)

21.		0.180 Gm.	
		2.340 Gm.	
		0.036 Gm.	
		0.288 Gm.	
	ad 3.60	Gm.	
23.	2649.5 or	2650 ml.	
	8516.25 or	8516 Gm.	
		ad 18925 ml., or 5 gal.	
25.	2499 or	2500	Gm.
	454.4 or	454	Gm.
	170.4 or	170	Gm.
		852	Gm.
		ad 11.36 Kg., or 25 lb.	
27.		0.062 Gm.	
		0.034 Gm.	
	ad 240	ml.	
29.		1.60 Gm.	
	0.667 or	0.68 Gm.	
		1.20 Gm.	
		13.3 Gm.	
31.		0.744 Gm.	
		0.444 Gm.	
	ad 60	ml.	
33.		37.85 Gm.	
		56.78 Gm.	
		113.6 Gm.	
		2650. ml.	
	ad 3785.	ml., or 1 gal.	
35.		9.46 Gm.	
		166. ml.	
		47. ml.	
	ad 473.	ml., or 1 pt.	

Chapter VIII

DENSITY, SPECIFIC GRAVITY, AND SPECIFIC VOLUME

(Page 106)

1. 0.812 Gm. per ml.
3. 1.83 Gm. per ml.

DENSITY, SPECIFIC GRAVITY, AND
SPECIFIC VOLUME (*continued*)

5. 0.9375
7. 1.313
9. 1.18
11. 1.235, or 1.24
13. 1.134, or 1.13
15. 0.893
17. 1.19, or 1.2
19. 1.169, or 1.17
21. 0.8633
23. 1.831
25. 0.788
27. 0.836
29. 3.237
31. 10.6
33. 2.498, or 2.50
35. 1.531, or 1.53
37. 2.137
39. 0.237
41. 2.00
43. 7.00
45. 1.110
47. 1.096, or 1.10
49. 0.5476
51. 1.212, or 1.21

Chapter IX

WEIGHTS AND VOLUMES OF LIQUIDS

(*Page 114*)

1. 116 Gm.
3. 190.4 or 190 Gm.
5. 9.2 Kg.
7. 8.12 Kg.
9. 1108 or 1110 gr.
11. 7.37 or 7.4 lb.
13. 205.8 or 206 Gm.
15. 4.97 Kg.

WEIGHTS AND VOLUMES OF LIQUIDS
(*continued*)

17. Using *1 gr. = 0.065 Gm.:*
2157 gr.
Using *1 Gm. = 15.432 gr.:*
2164 gr.
Both results should be rounded
off to 2160 gr.
19. 13.17 or $13\frac{1}{5}$ lb.
21. 58.47 or 58.5 ml.
23. 546.4 or 546 ml.
25. 367.9 or 368 ml.
27. 4348 or 4350 ml.
29. 1101 or 1100 ml.
31. $58\frac{7}{10}$ ℳ
33. 4.73 or $4\frac{7}{10}$ pt.
35. 29.2 or $29\frac{1}{5}$ pt.
37. $23.23
39. $0.19
41. $46.76
43. $0.65
45. 1938 ml.
47. 181.05 or 181.1 Gm.
49. 15.5 ml.
120.77 or 120.8 ml.

Chapter X

PERCENTAGE PREPARATIONS

(*Page 134*)

1. 12.5 Gm.
3. 0.48 Gm.
5. 0.3 Gm.
7. 45 Gm.
9. 7.5 mg.
11. 4.5 or 4.55 gr.
13. 45 or 45.5 gr.
15. 1.14 or $1\frac{1}{7}$ gr., or
1.125 or $1\frac{1}{8}$ gr.
17. 1.46 gr., or 1.44 gr.
19. 27 gr.
$67\frac{1}{2}$ gr.

PERCENTAGE PREPARATIONS
(*continued*)

21. 25 Gm.
23. 0.35%
25. 0.4%
    2%
27. 0.44%
    4.4%
29. 3.3%
31. 177 ml.
33. 6.15 L.
35. 50,444 or 50,400 ml.
37. 50 f℥
39. 378.5 or 379 ml.
41. 2838 or 2840 ml.
43. 709.5 or 710 ml.
45. 0.250 Gm.
    7.50 ml.
47. 96 ℳ
49. 24 ℳ and $11\frac{1}{4}$ gr.
51. 2.2%
53. 5%
55. 20.8%
57. 30 mg.
59. 37.5%
61. 800 ml.
63. 1.875 or 1.88 Gm.
65. 882.1 or 882 Gm.
67. 363 Gm.
69. 10 Gm. in 240 Gm. or 264 ml.
71. 241 gr. in 1365 gr. or 3 f℥
73. 20 Gm.
75. 25%
77. 16.5%
79. 25 Gm.
81. 227 Gm.
83. 12 gr.
85. 1.2 Gm.
    150 mg.
87. 30.6%
89. 0.24 Gm.
91. 24 gr.
93. 5.9%

PERCENTAGE PREPARATIONS
(*continued*)

95. 9.5%
97. 5%
99. (a) 1:800
    (b) 1:40
    (c) 1:125
    (d) 1:$166\frac{2}{3}$ or 6:1000
    (e) 1:300
    (f) 1:2000
101. 1:2000
103. 1:588
105. 1:1182 or 1:1200
107. 1:1,000,000
109. 0.25 Gm.
111. 30 mg.
113. 0.015 Gm.
115. 6 mg.
117. 0.1 Gm.
     0.0033 Gm.
119. 0.3 gr.

Chapter XI

DILUTION AND CONCENTRATION

(*Page 172*)

1. 1:3200
3. 4%
5. 15%
7. 32%
9. 20,000 ml.
11. 425 ml.
13. 544 Gm.
15. 84.6 or $84\frac{3}{5}$ lb.
17. 6944 or 6940 ml.
19. 1600 ml.
21. 12 f℥
23. 40 ml.
25. 40 ml.
27. 10.9 or 11 ml.
29. 108ℳ and 36 ℳ

DILUTION AND CONCENTRATION
(*continued*)

31. 461 ℔ or 7 f℥ 40 ℔
33. 3 ml.
35. 0.75 ml.
37. 10 ml.
39. 5.45 or 5.5 ml.
41. 80 ml.
    120 ml.
43. 36 ml.
45. 7.5 ml.
47. 48 ℔
49. (a) 12.5 Gm.
    (b) 500 ml.
51. 92.1 or 92 gr.
53. 5.208 or 5.21 Gm.
55. 17.06 or 17.1 gr.
57. 500 ml.
59. 900 ml.
61. 1667 ml.
63. 2125 Gm., or 2125 ml.
65. Enough to make 4150 ml.
67. 557 ml.
69. 50.5 or 51 ml.
    Enough to make 120 ml.
71. 115.7 or 116 ml.
73. 245.6 or 246 ml.
75. 770.4 or 770 ml.
77. 99.5 or 100 ml.
79. 14.5%
81. 351.9 or 352 ml.
83. 4.95% (w/w)
    4.125 or 4.13% (w/v)
85. 5.36 Gm.
87. 0.25 Gm.
    9.75 Gm.
89. 1000 Gm.
91. 4.76%
93. 0.050 Gm.
95. 8 gr.
97. 5 mg.
99. $\frac{3}{5}$ gr.
101. 2 gr.

DILUTION AND CONCENTRATION
(*continued*)

103. 4 gr.
105. 8.8%
107. 7.25%
109. 2.575 or 2.58%
111. 21.95 or 22%
113. 39.4%
115. 55.3%
117. 70:12
119. 5:2
121. 27:1.5, or 54:3, or 18:1
123. 25:25:30, or 5:5:6
125. 5:5:12.
127. 5:5:5:15, or 1:1:1:3.
129. 2175 ml.
131. 34.4 or 34 ml. or 35 ml.
     145.6 or 146 ml. or 145 ml.
     ——————   ——————
     Total: 180 ml.   180 ml.
133. 2200 Gm.
     300 Gm.
135. 400 Gm.
     2400 Gm.
     1200 Gm.
      800 Gm.
137. 66.66 or 66.7 Gm.
139. 431 Gm.
      431 Gm.
      431 Gm.
     1207 Gm.
141. 300 ml.
143. 44.1 or 44 Gm.
145. 750 Gm.
147. 37.5 Gm.
149. 22,500 ml.
151. (a) 8%
     (b) 164.7 or 165 Gm.
153. 0.855
155. 44.2 or 44 ml.
     55.8 or 56 ml.

Chapter XII

Isotonic Solutions

(Page 197)

1. 1.73%
3. −0.036° C.
5. 3.3 gr.
7. 0.720 Gm.
9. 0.396 Gm.
11. 0.500 Gm.
13. 2.35 or 2.4 gr.
15. 0.1095 or 0.110 Gm.
17. 0.410 Gm.
19. 0.467 Gm.
21. 0.690 Gm.
23. 0.372 Gm.
25. 17.8, or 18 ml.
27. 0.7 gr.
29. 0.103 Gm.
31. 0.290 Gm.

Chapter XIII

Chemical Problems

(Page 217)

1. 74.096, or 74.10
3. 46.068, or 46.07
5. 60.052, or 60.05
7. C: 64.81%
   H: 13.60%
   O: 21.59%
9. Na: 16.66%
   H: 2.92%
   P: 22.45%
   O: 57.97%
11. 1024 Gm.
13. 25.45%
15. 73.88%
17. 73.23 or 73 Gm.
19. 55.2 or 55 mg.
21. 0.165 Gm.

Chemical Problems *(continued)*

23. 79.5 or 80 mg.
25. 294.4 or 294 Gm.
27. 23.1 or 23 Gm.
    16.2 or 16 Gm.
29. 92.6 or 93 Gm.
    64.8 or 65 Gm.
31. 678.6 or 679 Gm.
    232.3 or 232 Gm.
33. 640.6 or 641 Gm.
35. 47.6 Gm.
    145 ml.
37. 585 Gm.
39. 2.1 Gm.
41. 3.639 Gm.
43. 14.73 or 14.7 Gm.
45. 64.4 or 64 mg.
47. 14.28 or 14.3 Gm.
49. 3570.8 or 3570 Gm. (rounding off
    to three significant figures)
51. 372.8 mg.
53. 4 mEq
55. 4 mEq
57. 0.298%
59. 200 mEq
61. 225 Gm.
63. 11.8 or 12 Gm.
65. 200
67. (a) 8.59 or 8.6 Gm.
    (b) 19.3 Gm.
69. 11.36 or 11.4 Gm.
71. 7.5 Gm.
73. 1.452 or 1.45 Gm.
75. 19.9 L.
77. 140 L.
79. 218.7 or 219 Gm.
81. 365.7 or 366 Gm.
83. 112 L.
    113.5 L.
85. 7 L.
    7.69 or 7.7 L.
87. 110 ml.

Appendix A

THERMOMETRY

(Page 231)

1. 50° F.
3. 39.2° F.
5. 25° C.
7. 37° C.
9. 23° F. to 572° F.
11. 159.8° F.
13. −40° C.
15. 86° F. to 95° F.
17. 68° F.
19. 35.6° F. to 50° F.

Appendix B

PROOF STRENGTH

(Page 235)

1. 102.6 proof gallons
3. 490 proof gallons
5. $83\frac{1}{3}$ wine gallons
7. $3\frac{57}{100}$ wine gallons
9. $99.65
11. $324.90
13. $27.80

Appendix C

ALCOHOLOMETRIC TABLES

(Page 239)

1. 53.10% (v/v)
3. 26.50% (v/v)
5. 87.226 or 87.23% (v/v)
7. 0.82575 or 0.8258
9. 0.96998 or 0.9700

Appendix D

SOLUBILITY RATIOS

(Page 243)

1. 1:5.25, or 1 Gm. in
   5.25 ml. of water

SOLUBILITY RATIOS *(Continued)*

3. 1:2.67, or 1 Gm. in
   2.67 ml. of water
5. 5.5714 or 5.57% (w/w)
7. 59.5 Gm.
   178.57 or 178.6 ml.

Appendix E

EMULSION NUCLEUS

(Page 245)

1. 7.5 Gm.
   15 ml.
3. ℥ii
   f℥ss
5. 7.5 Gm.
   15 ml.
7. 8.75 Gm.
   17.5 ml.
9. 2 Gm.
   4 ml.

Appendix F

EXPONENTIAL NOTATION

(Page 249)

1. (a) 1.265×10^4
   (b) 5.5×10^{-9}
   (c) 4.51×10^2
   (d) 6.5×10^{-2}
   (e) 6.25×10^8
2. (a) 4,100,000
   (b) 0.0365
   (c) 0.00000513
   (d) 250,000
   (e) 8695.6
3. (a) $17.5 \times 10^7 = 1.75 \times 10^8$
   (b) $16.4 \times 10^{-4} = 1.64 \times 10^{-3}$
   (c) 6.0×10^0
   (d) $12 \times 10^7 = 1.2 \times 10^8$
   (e) $36 \times 10^2 = 3.6 \times 10^3$

EXPONENTIAL NOTATION (*continued*)

4. (a) 3.0×10^3
   (b) 3.0×10^{-10}
   (c) 3.0×10^9
5. (a) 8.52×10^4, or 8.5×10^4
   (b) 3.58×10^{-5}, or 3.6×10^{-5}
   (c) 2.99×10^3, or 3.0×10^3
   (a) 6.441×10^6, or 6.4×10^6
   (b) 6.6×10^{-3}
6. (c) 6.94×10^3, or 6.9×10^3

LOGARITHMIC NOTATION

(*Page 254*)

1. (a) 3.3512
   (b) 0.7214
   (c) 3.8451
   (d) 2.2739
   (e) $\bar{3}.4675$
   (f) $\bar{1}.8600$
   (g) 5.3324
   (h) $\bar{4}.1373$
   (i) 1.8375
   (j) 6.7924
2. (a) $2.827 \times 10^4 = 28,270$
   (b) $1.42 \times 10^1 = 14.2$
   (c) $2.139 \times 10^0 = 2.139$
   (d) $1.29 \times 10^{-1} = 0.129$
   (e) $6.154 \times 10^2 = 615.4$
   (f) $1.468 \times 10^2 = 146.8$
   (g) $1.062 \times 10^0 = 1.062$
   (h) $7.766 \times 10^{-3} = 0.007766$
   (i) $8.383 \times 10^1 = 83.83$
   (j) $1.329 \times 10^{-2} = 0.01329$
3. (a) 22,790
   (b) 7315
   (c) 14.76
   (d) 822.6
   (e) 17,090
4. (a) 7517
   (b) 197.6
   (c) 0.00517

LOGARITHMIC NOTATION (*continued*)

   (d) 35.37
   (e) 13.75 or 13.8
5. (a) 79.36 or 79.4
   (b) 108.5 or 109
   (c) 292.8 or 293

Appendix G

PROBLEMS IN H-ion CONCENTRATION AND pH

(*Page 260*)

1. 10.6
3. 6.22 or 6.2
5. 7.36 or 7.4
7. 6.31×10^{-3}, or 6.3×10^{-3}
9. 5.01×10^{-5}, or 5.0×10^{-5}

Appendix H

MISCELLANEOUS PROBLEMS IN DISPENSING PHARMACY

(*Page 264*)

1. 6.2 ml.
3. 0.180 Gm., or 180 mg.
5. 770 mg.
7. 36 ml.
9. 12 tablets
11. Dissolve 1 tablet in enough of the elixir to make 6.5 ml., and use 4 ml. of the dilution
13. Powder 1 tablet, dilute it to 5 gr with iron and ammonium citrate and take 4 gr. of the dilution
15. 12 tablet triturates
17. 18 granules

Appendix I

SOME COMMERCIAL PROBLEMS

(*Page 272*)

1. (a) 45.85 or 45.9%

SOME COMMERCIAL PROBLEMS
(*continued*)

   (b) 35%
   (c) 31.6%
   (d) 44.14 or 44.1%
   (e) 40.465 or 40.5%
   (f) 20.62 or 20.6%
 3. $1.33
 5. $128.25
 7. $1.09
 9. 51 cents
11. $15
13. 46 cents
15. 25 cents

SOME COMMERCIAL PROBLEMS
(*continued*)

17. $1.25
19. $2.85
21. 47 cents
23. 50 cents
25. 28 cents
27. 45 cents
29. 3.75%
31. $2.34
33. $1.00
35. 150%
37. $2.35
39. $300

INTERNATIONAL ATOMIC WEIGHTS

1955

Oxygen: 16.0000

Names	*Symbols*	*Accurate atomic weights*	*Approximate atomic weights*
Actinium	Ac	227	227
Aluminum	Al	26.98	27
Americium	Am	[243]	243
Antimony	Sb	121.76	122
Argon	A	39.944	40
Arsenic	As	74.91	75
Astatine	At	[210]	210
Barium	Ba	137.36	137
Berkelium	Bk	[249]	249
Beryllium	Be	9.013	9
Bismuth	Bi	209.00	209
Boron	B	10.82	11
Bromine	Br	79.916	80
Cadmium	Cd	112.41	112
Calcium	Ca	40.08	40
Californium . . .	Cf	[249]	249
Carbon	C	12.011	12
Cerium	Ce	140.13	140
Cesium	Cs	132.91	133
Chlorine	Cl	35.457	35
Chromium	Cr	52.01	52
Cobalt	Co	58.94	59
Copper	Cu	63.54	64
Curium	Cm	[245]	245
Dysprosium . . .	Dy	162.51	163
Erbium	Er	167.27	167
Europium	Eu	152.0	152
Fluorine	F	19.00	19
Francium	Fr	[223]	223
Gadolinium . . .	Gd	157.26	157
Gallium	Ga	69.72	70
Germanium . . .	Ge	72.60	73
Gold	Au	197.0	197
Hafnium	Hf	178.50	179
Helium	He	4.003	4
Holmium	Ho	164.94	165
Hydrogen	H	1.0080	1
Indium	In	114.82	115
Iodine	I	126.91	127
Iridium	Ir	192.2	192
Iron	Fe	55.85	56
Krypton	Kr	83.80	84
Lanthanum . . .	La	138.92	139
Lead	Pb	207.21	207
Lithium	Li	6.940	7
Lutetium	Lu	174.99	175
Magnesium . . .	Mg	24.32	24
Manganese . . .	Mn	54.94	55
Mendelevium . . .	Mv	[256]	256